The Junior Medical Officer's Guide to the Hospital Universe

The Junior Medical Officer's Guide to the Hospital Universe

A Survival Manual

John Shi
Junior Doctor
New South Wales, Australia

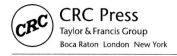

CRC Press
Taylor & Francis Group
Boca Raton London New York

CRC Press is an imprint of the
Taylor & Francis Group, an **informa** business

First edition published 2023
by CRC Press
4 Park Square, Milton Park, Abingdon, Oxon, OX14 4RN

and by CRC Press
6000 Broken Sound Parkway NW, Suite 300, Boca Raton, FL 33487-2742

CRC Press is an imprint of Informa UK Limited

The right of John Shi to be identified as author of this work has been asserted in accordance with sections 77 and 78 of the Copyright, Designs and Patents Act 1988.

This book contains information obtained from authentic and highly regarded sources. While all reasonable efforts have been made to publish reliable data and information, neither the author[s] nor the publisher can accept any legal responsibility or liability for any errors or omissions that may be made. The publishers wish to make clear that any views or opinions expressed in this book by individual editors, authors or contributors are personal to them and do not necessarily reflect the views/opinions of the publishers. The information or guidance contained in this book is intended for use by medical, scientific or health-care professionals and is provided strictly as a supplement to the medical or other professional's own judgement, their knowledge of the patient's medical history, relevant manufacturer's instructions and the appropriate best practice guidelines. Because of the rapid advances in medical science, any information or advice on dosages, procedures or diagnoses should be independently verified. The reader is strongly urged to consult the relevant national drug formulary and the drug companies' and device or material manufacturers' printed instructions, and their websites, before administering or utilizing any of the drugs, devices or materials mentioned in this book. This book does not indicate whether a particular treatment is appropriate or suitable for a particular individual. Ultimately it is the sole responsibility of the medical professional to make his or her own professional judgements, so as to advise and treat patients appropriately. This book is not intended to give legal or financial advice and is sold with the understanding that the author is not engaged in rendering legal, accounting or other professional services or advice. If legal or financial advice or other expert assistance is required, the services of a competent professional should be sought to ensure you fully understand your obligations and risks. This book may include information regarding the products and services by third parties. We do not assume responsibility for any third party materials or opinions. Any reliance on the third party material is at your own risk. The author and publisher make no representations, warranties or guarantees, express or implied, about the completeness, accuracy, or reliability of the information, products, services, or related graphics contained in this book for any purpose. The information is provided 'as is' to be used at your own risk. The authors and publishers have also attempted to trace the copyright holders of all material reproduced in this publication and apologize to copyright holders if permission to publish in this form has not been obtained. If any copyright material has not been acknowledged please write and let us know so we may rectify in any future reprint.

Trademark notice: Product or corporate names may be trademarks or registered trademarks and are used only for identification and explanation without intent to infringe.

British Library Cataloguing-in-Publication Data
A catalogue record for this book is available from the British Library

ISBN: 9781032403236 (hbk)
ISBN: 9781032397405 (pbk)
ISBN: 9781003352501 (ebk)

DOI: 10.1201/9781003352501

Typeset in Minion Pro, designed by Robert Slimbach, from Adobe Originals
by Evolution Design & Digital Ltd (Kent)

For my colleagues.

Contents

Author

John Shi is a Trainee Doctor who has both studied to be, and trained as, a Doctor in a range of medical settings in New South Wales, Australia, including in public hospitals ranging from primary to quaternary centres as well as private general practice clinics. Dr Shi has also held teaching positions with multiple universities and has been recognised with various teaching awards.

Glossary

ACAT: Aged Care Assessment Team. Assesses aged care patients for various services, e.g. RACF, respite.

ADLs: Activities of daily living.

Admin: Short for Administration. Bane of existence (across multiple industries).

Admission: The act of the patient coming into Hospital to stay (for a bit).

ADO: Allocated day off. A day, legitimately, you have off work.

After Hours: Outside of business hours, i.e. any time that is not about 8.30 a.m. to 5 p.m., Monday to Friday.

AHPRA: Australian Health Practitioner Regulation Agency. Regulates doctors (among other Healthcare Workers). Where you get Registration. Also where you get reported to if you've been bad.

AMH: Australian Medicines Handbook. Great simple medication reference.

AMO: Attending Medical Officer; see Boss.

AMS: Antimicrobial Stewardship. So your grandkids still have antibiotics to use.

AT: Advanced Trainee. Registrars on their final stretch to becoming a Boss.

ATOR: At time of reporting.

Ax: Assessment.

BAT call: Priority patient is arriving (likely someone who is dying. Now.). Make sure brown pants also arrive.

Blood(s): Can mean any of (1) bloods from patients to be taken/analysed; (2) blood to be transfused to a patient; (3) blood coming from a patient where it shouldn't physiologically be, e.g. drain, vomit, stools, sheets etc.; (4) blood's usual meaning.

Boss: aka AMO, Consultant, the Boss. The most upgraded version of you. Who you get to be in a million years. Meantime, your Boss.

BPT: Basic Physician Trainee. Often also the Med Reg. Generally highly stressed individual you consult for medical issues or is your Team Reg. On the way to becoming a Physician.

BSL: Blood sugar level; aka BGL (blood glucose level).

BTF: Between the flags. Zone of (relative) safety for both patients and swimmers; the latter in terms of surf, the former in terms of vital sign observations (chiefly NSW policy).

Cannula (IVC): Large needle that introduces plastic tubing that allows intravenous stuff to be given. At times, one of the banes of existence to put in.

Chase: Hounding after various things because they weren't there when you first looked for them.

CMO: Career Medical Officer. Often senior.

Code Black: Personal threat. Someone is doing/done something aggressive. You need more than medical knowledge.

Code Blue: Medical Emergency. If you're on, that means you.

Code [Insert colour]: Bad things of various colours happening. Know your local policy.

Community: Out of the Hospital.

Consent: Legal document stating patient agrees to something.

Consult: The act of requesting advice from another Team. Common bane of existence for JMOs and Regs.

Consultant: The peak tier of Doctor; see Boss.

COW: Computer on Wheels. Literally, a computer mounted on wheels, pushable through the Ward. Not to be confused with a common four-legged herbivore; see WOW.

Death Certificate: Certifies a patient (or anyone) has died.

Discharge (D/C): Can mean either (1) the act of a patient going home (exciting time for both patients and Healthcare Workers) or (2) the actual paperwork for Discharge (highly unexciting time for JMOs).

Document: Can mean any of (1) a written record of something; (2) the act of recording some medical occurrence; (3) see usual dictionary definition.

DPET: Directors of Prevocational Education and Training.

ED: Emergency Department, aka Accident and Emergency (A&E).

eMeds: Electronic Medications. What you use instead of Med Charts.

eMR: Electronic Medical Records. What you use instead of paper.

eTG: Therapeutic Guidelines. Great guidelines on many medical conditions, especially when you have no idea what to do.

Fluid Chart: See Med Chart. Similar document (less bulkiness), but for various fluids and infusions and much less baneful as it doesn't require recharting.

Geris: Geriatric Medicine or Aged Care.

Handover: The transfer of patient care to the next shift of Healthcare Workers assuming your responsibilities. So they know what they're working with and you can go home. The reverse is true when you receive handover.

HCW: Healthcare Workers.

HPC: History of Presenting Complaint. (Note that PC is presenting complaint.)

Hx: History.

ICU: Intensive Care Unit.

IDC: In-dwelling catheter.

IM: Intramuscular; into the muscle.

Inpatient: Patient staying inside the Hospital; see Outpatient.

Intern: Your first year as a Doctor.

ISBAR: Common handover format. Identify, Situation, Background, Assessment and Recommendation.

IV: Intravenous; into the vein.

Ix: Investigation.

JMO: Junior Medical Officer. Presumably you.

Jobs: The stuff Junior Medical Officers must do to make things happen. Can be one of the many banes of existence.

Letters: Consultant letters/notes about the patient, written in the community. One of many banes of existence to chase, especially when using fax machines.

List: Can mean any of (1) your list of patients; (2) list of procedures/operations to be done today; (3) classical dictionary definition of 'list' in noun and verb form.

LR: Life Round. The act of rounding for the purpose of optimising +/– saving your life.

MAR: Medication Administration Record. Electronic, more complicated and less flexible version of paper Medication Charts (you can't just cross things out with a pen).

MDO: Medical Defence Organisation. Your legal representation and indemnity insurance provider.

MDT: Multi-Disciplinary Team. Involves care by teams from multiple disciplines: Medical, Nursing and Allied Health. Often involves many meetings.

Med: Can be any of (1) Medical related (as opposed to other Specialties, e.g. Surgical); (2) Medication related; (3) related to Medicine in general; (4) consider classical dictionary definition.

Med Chart: Thick, multi-copy documents where all the patient's medications are charted. One of many banes of existences to rechart. Obviated with eMeds (though its own set of banes arise).

Med School: Medical School. Places that train doctors. You thought that it was hard. You will think differently.

MET call: Medical Emergency Team call. Sometimes known as Rapid Response. Highly suggestive of patient deterioration. Everyone is coming.

MIMS: Monthly Index of Medical Specialties. Great, but very complex and extensive, medication reference.

MMSE: Mini-mental state examination.

Mx: Management.

NBM: Nil by mouth. Literally.

NESB: Non-English-speaking background. Mainly to signify the patient cannot speak English, and not as relevant if they are of non-English-speaking background but can speak English.

NFR: Not for resuscitation.

NOK: Next of kin, not a misspelled act of aggression.

NUM: Nurse Unit Manager. Boss nurse of the Ward.

Obs: Observations or patient vital signs.

On Call/take: Patients are coming.

O/E: On examination.

O+G/O&G: Obstetrics and Gynaecology.

Ortho: Orthopaedics related.

Outpatient: Patient staying outside of (i.e. not 'in') the Hospital. See Inpatient.

PACS: Picture Archiving and Communication System. How to get images/videos onto eMR without crashing the system.

Paeds: Paediatric Medicine.

Pager: Indestructible, screaming piece of medieval equipment announcing someone wants you for something. One of many banes of existences to hear.

Pathology: Magical place that takes all your specimens, including blood, sweat, tears and all other excretions/bodily components, and generates meaningful results from them.

PEARL: Pupils equal and reactive to light.

PMHx: Past Medical History.

PO: *Per os. Per oral.* By the mouth.

Post take: Patients have come; keep calm and carry on.

PPI: Proton pump inhibitor.

PR: *Per rectum.* By the rectum. Also can mean performing a digital rectal examination.

Prescriber number: Allows you to prescribe medications. Need to know.

PRINT: Pre-Internship Student. One breath away from becoming a Doctor.

PRN: *Pro re nata*. As required.

Provider number: Allows you to participate in the Medicare programme. Especially used in ordering Investigations. Need to know.

RACF: Residential Aged Care Facility.

Radiology: Magical place that takes patients and looks inside them, generally without opening them. The difficulty is getting them there.

Red Zone: When a patient's vital signs fall very much out of certain criteria, suggestive of more severe deterioration (see Yellow Zone).

Reg: Registrar. The Underboss. You generally answer to them. Usually on the way to training in a Specialty.

Registration: Your recognition by AHPRA to practise (in your defined scope).

Resident (RMO): Resident Medical Officer. Second year or beyond as a Doctor, but not yet a Reg. May have 'Senior' appended onto name, e.g. SRMO if more than 2 years as a doctor.

RN: Registered Nurse.

ROM: Range of motion.

Rx: Treatment.

S8: Authority for Pharmacies to dispense restricted medications, especially opioids. Must be especially beautifully written or will certainly face rejection.

Script: Authority for Pharmacies to dispense medications. Must be beautifully written or beware rejection.

Scrubs: Hospital clothing that is generally more comfortable and practical.

SET: Surgical Education and Training. The trainee is often the Surg Reg. On the Surgical training programme.

SHx: Social History.

SRMO: Senior Resident Medical Officer.

Staff Specialist: Permanent Boss employed by the Hospital in question.

STAT: From Latin, *statum*, i.e. immediately. Usually as immediately as someone can get to it.

Stcth: Stethoscope. The thing that hangs around doctors' necks. Useful for listening to various things and doubles sub-optimally as a tendon hammer (this is not an endorsement).

Stickers: Patient labels that have all a patient's details printed on them and are sticky. Very useful and saves much writing.

Surg: Surgical related (as opposed to other Specialties, e.g. Medical).

Switch: The connector of all calls to the right places and knower of many things (contacts related).

Team: The group of Healthcare Workers that form one unit and habitually work together. Usually one Specialty.

Term: The rotation you're on. Where you'll be usually for a few months before your job almost completely changes (maybe).

Theatre: Place where Operations/procedures take place, not performances.

TOC: Take over care. When you do, someone else's patient is now yours. When others do, your patient is now someone else's.

Urinary retention: aka retention. The state of not emptying the bladder. Common in both patients and Healthcare Workers, especially Junior Medical Officers.

VMO: Visiting Medical Officer who is a Boss but generally not a Staff Specialist at the Hospital in question.

Ward: Where patients (and you) generally stay. Though in different places.

WOW: Workstation on Wheels. Not to be confused with a common emotional expression. Synonymous with COW.

WR: Ward Round. The act of seeing patients daily.

Yellow Zone (YZ): When a patient's vital signs fall out of certain criteria, suggestive of early deterioration; see also Red Zone.

CHAPTER 1

Introduction

Let me tell you the beginning. You tell me the end.

First of all, this isn't a book about Medicine. Go and find a good clinical textbook, paper or living.

We know – shock, horror – a book for JMOs (Junior Medical Officers) not about Medicine.

Doubtless a good many of you are, or will be, much better doctors than we are now. So, we won't presume to lecture you about Medicine. But that's irrelevant.

This book is about life in Medicine.

And *that* is vastly different from Medicine.

In fact, it's not Medicine at all, it's all those nitty, gritty, gross, irrelevant, frustrating, maddening, mundane, boring, stupid and ridiculous things that we have to plough through, before we even get a *glance* of that thing we call Medicine, a glimpse of the true reason we entered Medicine in the first place.

A place of luxury that isn't even always reserved for Bosses (Consultants), let alone JMOs.

It's called Admin.

And, of course, that's a most boring subject. We mean – who wants to talk about Admin? But there are two sorry facts of life. The first is that Admin must be done. The second is that if Admin is not done well in life, Admin *is* your life.

For only when it is sorted can there be any life left at all for Medicine, if, by then, you still want it there.

Hence, this book. For – though people become doctors for many reasons, like being good clinicians, helping people, fighting disease or whatever else it is you want to do – there's one thing we're sure of: you did *not* become a doctor for the sheer joy of doing colossal amounts of Admin. If that's what you wanted, you would've become a personal assistant or something.

Yet Admin must be done. It is only when you've cleared all *that* out, and maintained yourself in a reasonably functioning state, that you can possibly reach your reason for entering Medicine. Otherwise, you'll forever gaze at it from afar, or – perhaps worse – cease to gaze at it at all, your sight already burned everlastingly.

This book aims to prevent that. We want to save you time, energy and sanity. For it is only when you have those things that will you be *enabled* to access the world of Medicine itself.

And when you get there, go where you will.

We hope that you find this book useful and informative, one that answers questions which aren't asked – though they constantly knock loudly against the collective frontal bone – and, at the same time, mildly entertaining.

HOW TO USE THIS BOOK

PRN (pro re nata). Always PRN.

This is a super-practical guide.

Practical as in you can use it every day, almost every moment, of your working life, for at least the next 2 years and, for many, perhaps the next 10 years. And, for some, possibly even for all your working life (especially if you pursue a Hospital career).

This is a reference book. We know that you're busy and don't have time to eat, let alone read. So, it's fine if you read this only when you need to. It's not cheating to check references in an open-book exam. Life, in truth, *is* an open-book exam. And as open-book exams are usually the harder of the exams, then life would be the hardest of them all.

Yet, if you have the right tools, it isn't so bad. Make this one of your tools. There are only two things needed to make things work: have the right tools and remember to use them.

You are looking at this book. So, you have the right tool (we hope). Just remember to use it.

Use this book the way *you* like. Some may like to read it through, from end to end, in PRINT (Pre-Internship), but it works just as well if you're perusing it on the fly as an SRMO (Senior Resident Medical Officer).

Whatever helps you. Use it entirely on an ad hoc basis. Each section is virtually independent, so starting in the middle is as easy as the end – so jump about.

Only three tips we offer.

First, have this book with you. Somewhere easily accessible – your phone or tablet or USB – and *refer* to it. When there's a problem. When you want to improve. When you are bored. Whenever.

Second, know the *Contents* well. That'll help you find the solution to the problem. There's only six main sections (see below) and they follow in logical progression. Still, if you're too busy for that, just search for the keyword or check the index. That'll bring you to the section you need.

Third, if you're too busy to read a section, look for the *Key Points* box, usually at the end of a section or via Ctrl+F. This is the super-condensed version of the preceding section. This is the bite of info you need even when you don't have time for a bite to eat. You can always expand on the points you need in detail within the text.

This book aims to be comprehensive. Virtually every common scenario you could encounter will be here. And for the uncommon, you should be asking someone.

But as common things happen commonly (as doctors so often say), it's the common things that'll sap your time and energy most. So, if you sort them out well, you'll hopefully not only survive but thrive.

This book will go over the entire life cycle of the usual JMO.

Before the Term will cover what you need to prepare for the Term, including things to bring, things to do and people to know.

The Term will discuss all the common tasks of the JMO and how to maximise efficiency and efficacy without exhausting yourself while ensuring patient care within your role.

We'll tour the intricacies of the Hospital's eMR (electronic Medical Records) in *IT* and show you how to make this system your best personal assistant and administrative servant instead of the master of frustration. Think of Discharges, Ordering Bloods, Documenting and note trawling. Then think how their completion may be almost instantaneous, even automated. Read on.

We'll discuss *Organisation* and how to plan your working day, so as much as possible simply *happens* – reliably, safely and effortlessly. Think of a time when *all* the Jobs are done. And it's only 4.55 p.m. The day you might finally leave on time.

We'll explore the endless web of *Human Relations*, into the midst of which you'll be thrown on day 1, and how you may thread through it to your aid, without being strangled by it. Think of Radiology, Consults, your own Team and the endless other services the Hospital encompasses. Imagine if, when you asked for something (for patient care, that is), it just got done. With an understanding of the system, that's possible, even often.

Finally, we'll try to maximise your own chances of staying alive in *Life Rounds* with basic life tips to survive the ordeal called Internship and being a Doctor-in-Training. No, you have not graduated from eating, drinking, sleeping and seeking relief.

End of Term will close the circle by discussing the transition between Terms, how you'll tie up the loose ends and, most importantly, the Handover process, where you prepare to pass your Job to the next JMO and receive another Job as the next JMO.

A similar scheme will be followed in *After Hours*, where the JMO life cycle has been compressed from months into hours. And this vastly different work environment necessitates a new set of strategies for organising your tasks (whose very nature has changed), for looking after your patients (of whom you now know none) and for looking after yourself (in new ways to meet the new times) as you hold the fort through the night against the unknown legions of changing clinical conditions and await the relief of dawn's first light (and new JMOs).

Of course, no medical text would be complete without mentioning the greatest global pandemic in generations. While the clinical landscape of *COVID-19* continues to evolve, we delve into the administrative and practical aspects of the new Hospital terrain we work in.

Lastly, we'll discuss some serious life Admin, i.e. your actual working conditions and entitlements – financial and otherwise – in *Money Matters*,' where all those topics that people are so interested in, yet are so little discussed, will be clarified. From pay to working hours, from Overtime to Leave, all these interesting matters of common interest will be reviewed, with a focus on the Public Hospital Award, the chief document that governs your working life, the document that both you and the Hospital are mandated to abide by.

As commonly said, knowledge is power. We hope this book will give you knowledge. And, when armed with this knowledge, we hope you'll be empowered to better integrate this new thing 'work' with that old thing 'life'.

Disclaimer: We aim to offer helpful advice. However, it is general in nature. The advice in this book always defers to clinical judgement, Senior advice and official guidelines and protocols. This applies to the whole book.

EXHORTATION TO READ, AND *DO* THIS ASAP

Do it, now, for there is no time like now.

Many may well feel that the things we'll discuss here, especially the set-up of all your various systems, e.g. in eMR and organisation in general, are very helpful, even necessary perhaps. However, it's unfortunate many won't make use of them.

Many will say, 'I'll do it when I have more time.' But the problem is, you will never have *more* time. Besides, unless you make time, you'll never have time for anything, apart from compulsions and instant gratifications. And neither of those things, though required, will allow you to thrive, to be the *optimal* 'you'.

But you want to be the best 'you' possible. Yet that's only possible if you have time and energy. And you'll only have time and energy if you optimise your systems and harness every efficiency and synergy possible. The methods advocated here aim to enable that.

You'll thank yourself later for the immense savings that will accrue, even if you can't foresee them now. Savings in time, energy and sanity. The system you set up for yourself is like money in the bank. Let it work for you hard and early, and you'll benefit in ways you didn't even expect. Otherwise, even the easiest task will become just that much harder. And, like money, it is an excellent servant but a terrible master. Furthermore, money, though very useful, is yet limited, while the savings you'll amass here will help you in almost every way possible, for time, energy and sanity are universal currencies.

They'll help you reach your career goals faster.

They'll help you cope better on the Job.

They'll aid you in having a life outside the Wards.

They'll make Overtime that little bit more tolerable.

They'll make that final Blood Order that little bit easier.

So, set up your system at the very first opportunity. Do it in the first quiet moment you have. Do it during a lunch break. Do it in the Overtime that you must do. Do it during a quiet After Hours. Do it on the job itself.

For, although the first time you do this, things may seem like they're taking a hundred times longer than they should, once you're familiar with it, you'll bless yourself on how fast everything is.

It's just like walking. Remember how long it took to walk those first steps? Nearly a whole year.

But from then onwards? Do you regret the time you spent learning to walk?

Well, this is the same, for this *walking* through the eMR and the whole Hospital system is the one skill you must absolutely master if you're to do anything well or efficiently. And even when you've attained mastery, you should always seek ways to improve. Learn from your buddies, your Seniors, your colleagues. Then, on their foundations and inheriting their experience, you can establish and use the best system possible, and, perhaps, leave something even better to your juniors.

Remember with everything else – Overtime, late Boss Rounds, After Hours, Jobs, etc. – all these things you must do continuously. They will also keep changing. But this set-up, which will hardly change, you only need to do once.

So, *do* it once, and benefit always. You may not have time. But it will make time for you.

FOR ALL DOCTORS

There is no end.

Some may believe that, once they're out of the 2 years of Internship and Residency, they will be free. They'll have someone to do all that stuff they had to do. They'll at last only practise Medicine. They'll live in their utopia.

Sorry – truth.

Whether in the Hospital system or not, whether in public or private, you won't be free.

Why?

Unfortunately, the Admin that plagues us hasn't gone away. And unless you have very competent JMOs, all the time, every Term, you *will* be subject to the vicissitudes and storms of Admin. All the Jobs as a JMO, if not completed effectively, can hold up the operation of the whole Team. And even though they'll no longer be your duty per se as you move up the ranks, they can still swamp you and your Team if your JMO can't keep them at bay. And your JMOs *can't* always keep them at bay. Especially the day 1 JMO. Or the sick one. Or the one on ADO. Or the relieving one.

Remember the saying: Nothing one doesn't do oneself is ever done well. And the medical proverb that shares itself with intelligence agencies: Trust no one.

And the sorrier fact is that even Bosses (which many of you will become), sitting as they do at the absolute pinnacle of the medical spire, have their own distinct set of Admin duties to navigate, not the least of which is the Hospital system.

Hence, this book is not just a possession for JMOs, PRINT and Medical Students who wish to become good JMOs, but a possession for all doctors, from Regs (Registrars) to Bosses.

To liberate yourself from the mountains, or rather continents, of Admin that each of us has to do.

To effectively navigate and harness the IT system that was supposed to help us in the first place.

To empower you, through gaining adequate time, to engage in the clinical practice you love, or whatever else it is you love.

To free you from reliance upon others and to get things done, easily, effectively, precisely, completely.

And for the Seniors among you, this will help to ensure that you're not subject to the competency of inexperienced junior staff, which makes you tremble at the start of each Term as you wonder whether any of your instructions will be done at all. But, rather, be their true senior in every aspect, even in their Job, and be able to guide even the most inexperienced to an effective path. And in critical cases, when there's no one else, to act yourself in the most effective way possible.

Hence, there'll no longer be any bottleneck. You have opened them all yourself and the only rate-limiting step in your entire clinical chain will merely be the speed of the clinical decision and the actual practical logistics of all Investigations and Management, with no further administrative and technological roadblocks to hinder good patient care.

For JMOs, hopefully this becomes your lifesaver. Instead of the glorified secretary that we all know we are (at least most of the time), we can be that glorified secretary and so much more, perhaps even actual Doctors-in-Training, when we at last have the time to do something other than document your twentieth review of a day 3 cannula.

For Regs, this will help you best utilise and organise your Intern's time and energy (and perhaps even your own). For you have been there. And the Interns have not. So, this will help them out. And if they're helped out, then you'll be too because, after all, they are front line. And no resources are wasted if spent on the front line. For it's the front line that often makes all the difference to the whole campaign.

And for those sub-specialising, this book is an administrative foundation to build upon. It'll only get more complex, not simpler, so with these solid bases to work upon, your administrative future can only get easier and be more integrated into your practice. Use the principles here in your sub-specialty, and your administrative work as a Boss will be as streamlined as an SRMO on a busy Term.

Hence this guide, one that aims to help *all* doctors in the Hospital system to *be* doctors, instead of administrative machines, which sap time, energy and passion, and, at last, become the person that their first spark of inspiration had fired them to be.

CHAPTER 2

Before the Term

One does NOT simply, walk onto the job.

So, it's your first day and you're super-excited (and not a little scared) to be, at last, Doctor [insert name here].

And you're ready to start saving lives.

The problem is, if you only start being Doctor [insert name] at 8 a.m. (or a bit earlier) on day 1 of Term 1, you may be a little late already.

In truth, your job has often started before you've even quite left Med School and has certainly started a week before the contracted start date.

No, we don't mean Orientation (though that helps too).

We mean preparation.

The aim is not solely to impress (though you probably want to do that too); it's more to ease yourself into the job, rather than the job easing an avalanche over you.

But what should I prepare?

Quite simply, only three things: your stuff, your mind, your people. That is, be aware of *Things to Bring*, *Things to Do* and *People to Know*.

THINGS TO BRING

Day 1 – Intern: The Hospital is a battlefield. Go in well armed.

It's a common caricature to see how laden Interns are with useless tools, then failing to find the one thing they need. This is often because JMOs (Junior Medical Officers) are loaded with so many jobs, which they're expected to perform almost instantaneously, that, being in this permanent state of anxiety, they vary between carrying so many things that they can find nothing or carrying nothing at all and must find everything.

Now, there are a few props that you should definitely endow yourself with to make your work and life easier, while many others are so rarely used that they're best left in your locker and brought out PRN (*pro re nata*).

Props are essential to streamline your day, especially as you're the administrative centre of the Team. And as nobody really wants to do admin, but nothing can be done without it, you're expected to complete it in a way that's fast, accurate and effortless.

The main principle is *instantaneousness*. Avoid being the rate-limiting factor. The more of the Plan that you can make happen then and there, the more accurate it is, the quicker for you, the less you'll forget, the fewer jobs you'll be too busy to get to and the better it is for the patient.

That's the idea of props. It's *there*. And if you have it there, things will happen there, right now.

By doing this, you'll also have no jobs later but the hard ones, which naturally become much easier if they aren't bulwarked by a legion of easy ones.

So, consider carrying the things listed below to buoy rather than burden your day.

COMMON MEDICATIONS AND DOSES

Bring a Common Medications List (with doses)

> **NB:** MOST RELEVANT FOR STARTING INTERNS, LESS SO FOR THE SENIORS.

You know how they said in Med School not to remember doses?

That's a lie.

Well, not really for Med School. But they sort of wash their hands of you once you don that gown and cardboard hat, which we don't blame them for; else their hands would be way too full.

But, in the real world, you're the one charting most things. The Nurses are looking at you to write/type something, right now. So, while you may not need doses as a student, as a JMO, you sure do. It's then that you wished you remembered less about the Krebs cycle and more about how much ondansetron to give the patient who's teaching you what projectile really means.

People always say you'll pick it up. But that's time that you are struggling – all that time you're 'picking up'.

We know, it's hard to remember all doses. Even Regs don't remember everything. Hence, always look things up. In addition, many eMeds (electronic Medication systems) suggest common doses for you. But, for common things, every time you must look it up is time that could be spent wiser if you just knew. There is a search cost. But to stay safe and minimise the searching, there's a better way still.

Carry a Reference List

There are plenty of printouts around (see guidelines/hand-me-downs/preferences/drug availability). Hospital-specific ones are best as each has its own quirks, especially in supply. Find it. Use it. Make your own if you like. As your knowledge grows, also integrate common indications and contraindications.

But the key is to carry it. Paper, lanyard, laminate, whatever.

Then use it when you need it.

Types of Common Medications you'll probably need

As a suggestion, your Common Medication arsenal is likely to include the following. Naturally, certain Terms also have their own common Meds (Medications) that you should know, but generally:

- **Analgesia**: Common things commonly. You'll get a feel for how much to use as you go along, but commence with standardised doses at first, especially with paracetamol, NSAIDs, simple opioids and morphine. These are essential and generally everyone will look to you for them, from Nurses to Regs. This is especially applicable on Surgical Rounds and you want to set up your PRN regime early to prevent being inundated by calls of pain.

- **Antibiotics**: Again, very common ones for Medical and Surgical Rounds. Know especially common IV and PO drugs, e.g. ceftriaxone, metronidazole, gentamicin, azithromycin, Augmentin, benzylpenicillin, cefalexin, trimethoprim, amoxicillin, doxycycline, vancomycin, tazocin and flucloxacillin, so you can chart almost instantaneously as with the pain Meds, even pre-emptively when you know the indication.

- **Anti-emetics**: Have at least three types in your hand so you can throw them one after the other. Very important and much nicer for patients, Nurses and you. Consider metoclopramide, ondansetron (or another -tron) and prochlorperazine.

- **Nutritional/electrolyte supplements**: IV and PO – everyone's electrolytes are always deranged in Hospital so this is where *you* can make a difference. It's an issue that's (relatively) easy to manage but can have significant consequences if missed, so you should take charge of it early and vigorously (of course with Senior oversight).

    PO replacement is great and makes big differences in the long run, while common IV doses are rapid. Know also what fluid solution you are putting your IV electrolytes into. Your life is much easier if you know their dose and infusion times (often critical). Use the *Australian Injectable Drugs Handbook* if in doubt and update your Reference List. Consider especially potassium and CMP (calcium–magnesium–phosphate). Less acutely, remember vitamin D, B12, folate, iron and micronutrients.

- **Fluids (including blood products)**: Although there are often subtleties regarding the precise rates/amounts, you should know how to chart these at least and the common rates. Be aware of the common types of fluids (e.g. 0.9% saline, Hartmann's solution, 5% dextrose), common rates, indications and contraindications. Also, be aware of the various Blood products, including packed red cells, platelets and albumin. Blood products often need extra paperwork/logistical preparation, e.g. patient consent, notification of the Blood Bank and charting, so know your Hospital's policies early.

- **Aperients**: Obviously no one wants to be constipated, and being constipated in Hospital is twice as bad, so have a good number of these up your sleeve, starting with the PO agents and moving on to those administered PR. You'll often take charge of these too, though in some Surgical and Gastro (Gastroenterology) Terms and certain pathologies there are more subtleties in choosing agents, so (as always) run by your Reg.

- **Topical stuff**: Emollients/eye drops/creams, etc. – these seem so innocuous compared with the other treatments we use but are so common that it's much better just to get them done then and there. This is all about effective time saving and it's a luxury that's sometimes unaffordable to go back and chart Chlorsig. Also, these can make a lot of difference to the patient's comfort and condition, e.g. treating thrush with an anti-fungal or preventing skin tears with a moisturiser. So, knowing it then and there is of a great help too.

- **Puffers**: Common in any lung-related issue, so know this to prevent patients and you getting out of breath. Consider salbutamol and ipratropium spacer and nebuliser doses (caution in COVID-19). Many of the long-term Meds will be decided by Respiratory but the short term is yours.

- **PPIs (proton pump inhibitors)**: Everyone gets reflux. Especially in Hospital. Hence, know PPI doses both IV and PO for everyone's comfort. Often needed on Gastro Terms.

- **Other**: There'll be many other common Meds you'll chart, often Term specific. Build up as you go. Soon, you'll find you're keeping the best lanyard of all in your head through sheer repetition. But let the actual lanyard hang on you till then.

> **NB:** IF IN DOUBT, USE YOUR REFERENCE, E.G. AMH, ETG, MIMS, *AUSTRALIAN INJECTABLE DRUGS HANDBOOK* AND/OR SENIORS.

You can mostly decide in not very serious matters. Double check with your Reg for the more serious things or if you are concerned. In the beginning, it's best just to announce everything you do. Even when you're comfortable, checking is still advisable.

DOCUMENTS/FOLDER

Consider the following logic:

1. You'll find there's more paper than medicine on most days.

2. With lots of paper, you'll need somewhere to put it.

3. Always bring a folder (with forms in it).

Really, there's nothing worse than looking for random forms on a busy WR (Ward Round). You could delegate your student to do it, but (1) there are many clueless students (on these matters); (2) it's a waste of their time, which could be much better spent than form hunting; and (3) it doesn't really add to their learning, except that they now know looking for forms is painful.

You'll quickly get a feel for which forms are common. That is, the ones which are always wanted and the ones most painful to find. But, as a rule, if you ever need to look for anything once, take five or six copies of it. You won't feel the weight, but you *will* feel the weight of the stares of four Regs and Fellows while you search for that Consent form through fifteen different filing cabinets and twenty grids.

And, naturally, when you carry so much paper, the only way to keep organised and to prevent your documents from looking like they've been pulled from a scrap heap is a folder.

Storage clipboards/folders with a handle seem to work best, i.e.

- **Storage**: You can keep documents in it of all sizes without falling out, as well as pens, phone, food, etc.
- **Clipboard**: Holds the paper still as the patient's hand potentially shakes over the Consent form. Prevents Lists from flying before the speed gale of a Surgical WR.
- **Handle**: You can carry the thing with the most useless finger as your other four fingers do something else.

Now, in terms of documents, consider the following:

- **Scripts and S8s**: Patients are always discharging on the fly and at a wink's notice, so it's optimal that, even as the words of Discharge fall from the Boss's lips, your scripts fall into the patient's/waiting pharmacist's hands. It'll save many pagers in future and you won't need to walk back to give these out. Which sounds trivial, but won't be if it's twenty times, at each corner of the dodecahedral Hospital. Besides, Pharmacy often opens and closes at somewhat different hours so you don't want Discharge to be delayed because the patient couldn't get their scripts. Remember, anything can happen overnight.

  Again, S8s are critical, especially on Surgical Terms, since almost everyone gets an opiate of some sort, and that's one more thing you don't want to hold you up. Remember to stock up on scripts and S8s as you run low, e.g. as you walk past Pharmacy or on Ward stations. This may be less applicable if you have eMeds.

- **Med Charts**: Obviously not applicable for those with the luxury of eMeds, but for the rest of us not so technologically endowed, paper is the go and chances are, on every Term, especially Medical Terms, every WR will involve some change to the medications, if it be but eye drops. And there'll always be no space on the chart. Or the spares. Again, to avoid the painful search process, a stash of these is invaluable. However, be aware that these are the bulkiest of charts so carefully titrate carriage to need.

- **Fluid Charts**: As per Med Charts, but this is more the Med Chart of the Surgical Terms. Here, everyone's electrolytes are deranged or they are NBM (nil by mouth) or need Blood, so this document is essential, even used more than Med Charts often. Surgical patients also are usually Discharged before Med Charts expire. Besides, they're lighter so there's no excuse not to have a few.

- **Consent forms**: Absolutely essential on Surgical Terms and pretty useful on other Terms. The pace of Surgical Terms is often a sprint, and often a patient can be Consented just before Theatre, sometimes even on the table. That means they could be anywhere: ED (Emergency Department), the Wards, Radiology, the corridor to Theatres. And the last thing you want is to look for the form. So, always have a good stack about you as you may well need to consent five, six or more a day. On Medical Terms, it'll be mainly for blood transfusions, so fewer will be needed, pending the Term. On Geris (Geriatric) and Paeds (Paediatric) Medicine, it'll also help to have a few Substitute Consent forms as some of these patients may not have capacity to consent.

- **Outpatient Imaging and Pathology forms**: This is more for Discharge planning and is the same idea as scripts. Patients often need Outpatient Bloods (Medical Terms) and Outpatient Imaging (all Terms) so having these on you will again save time. Bring both in-Hospital and private Pathology/Imaging forms. Some Teams are very specific about where to send the patient. If you can provide all the patient needs even as the WR concludes, then as you continue your run all over the Hospital you can print their Discharge from anywhere and won't have to run back to give them this one thing, which has stopped them from going home some 5 hours ago.

- **Stickers**: Must get, especially for Discharges. Saves you writing an infinite number of patient details.

    Can be stuck onto Investigation forms, +/– scripts (except S8s – sorry), Medical Certificates, i.e. anything given to the patient. Can also be stuck onto Blood tubes (except Group and Holds), Fluid Charts and even on Med Charts (sometimes, and sometimes multiple times – check your local policy), so they're highly useful and time saving.

    Even if you know patients need nothing for Discharge, they'll always end up needing something. So always take a good half-dozen stickers on the fly, especially if you don't have time to do their forms on the WR itself. Less applicable if you're stuck on one Ward; however, the patient folder may be taken away by Nurses/Allied Heath/Pharmacy or you may be too lazy to walk, so get what you need while you can.

    Know how to print stickers. It may feel like a big effort (we'll show you how nonetheless). But it's a far bigger effort to write – some five times, on three different scripts and five different Outpatient forms – a twenty-letter surname and an address twice as long, an effort that doesn't much engage the cortex but very much engages the forearm muscles and your precious time for Discharges. So always keep a rich supply.

- **Photos**: We live in the digital age. Everything, especially communication, is much easier in the outside world. Make it easy in the Hospital world.

   Take photos of everything you need to reference later. This would include wounds (for review by Surgical Teams, with consent), various reports/letters (for every Team), electrocardiograms (ECGs) (for Cardiology) and Med Charts (for yourself so you don't have to run back and check later), and everything else that's *not* on eMR, etc.

> **NB**: ALL PHOTOS NEED TO BE TAKEN WITH CONSENT AND COMPLY WITH LOCAL POLICIES. DELETE AS SOON AS THE JOB IS COMPLETE.

   It's mainly a matter of resistance. The easier it is for others (and yourself), the quicker you'll get the answers and results you need. So, make it easy.

- **Medical Certificates**: Ideally, you'd print these out with the Discharge summary (see *Chapter 4*, section *Discharges/Useful documents to attach, but painful to do so*). However, this is not so easy when family members want a certificate. Then, you almost have to write it out, unless you do some interesting annotations on a re-printed Medical Certificate. Hence, carry at least one of these, so the family will stop hassling the patient to hassle the Nurses to hassle you for it.

- **Business cards**: When you're a Boss, you'll find medicine is a business too. And businesses need business cards. Patients often have no idea who the AMO (Attending Medical Officer) is because they see so many people, and AMOs not necessarily the most often. But a business card can be helpful, especially if given to the patient. So, bring these. They also help patients when they book appointments and they save you writing out the Boss's phone number and address repeatedly.

- **Overtime forms**: A controversial topic but what's uncontroversial is that you should always bring the form. Claiming is then physically possible (see *Chapter 10*, section *Employment Matters/Overtime*). Here, stickers are again useful as you can directly stick them onto the form on a late afternoon WR to prove you were seeing patients and were not, say, in the café. And remember to get the forms approved. Always follow strictly whatever protocol the Hospital has in place for them. It's hard enough to work. It's harder still to chase ancient money.

Medical Terms

Apart from the above, additional documents/forms are required on Medical Terms. Of course, various Specialty terms will again require other things, but you'll get a feel for those based on your own annoyance index.

You'll need more Med Charts for sure, for Medical Bosses are constantly tweaking medications. That's why it's a Medical Term. In fact, you need just generally more of all forms (except Consents/S8s) as you'll generally manage the patients for longer and more extensively medically than in other Terms and hence would naturally require more documentation.

Some other useful forms include:

- **MMSEs (mini-mental state examinations)**: Especially in Geris, every second person seems to need one, and the Boss wants one for everyone else.
- **NFRs (not for resuscitation forms)**: It's in Medical Terms that the Bosses most often sit down and discuss with the patient this pretty serious matter. A very common subject in Geris. Again, it's a bit silly if the Boss has gone through a very profound discussion and then the whole Team fluffs around directly after looking for a form.

Surgical Terms

As stated above, the pace is rapid, so the forms you'll need the most include Fluid Charts, Consent forms and S8/normal scripts.

Med Charts are less useful, but Outpatient forms are again quite common.

Bring Overtime forms (such a thing is very likely in surgery).

OTHER TOOLS

Besides the right forms and Medication Lists, here are some other things that are essential to navigate your minefield of jobs.

Always bring:

- **Stethoscope (steth)**: Apart from the steth being a pretty useful thing and almost the doctor's symbol, the Boss always wants to borrow it anyway, so it's as much for the Team as for you. Also, during Clinical Reviews, you look pretty dumb hunting for the plastic steth all over the Ward as if it was the Electronic Littmann Cardiology 33000. Also doubles as a tendon hammer (sub-optimal, true, but better than fictional).
- **Pens (preferably multicolour)**: These are obviously in hot demand from everyone under the Hospital roof and liable to get lost. Even so, a multicolour pen is very useful on extremely busy Terms. There'll be many patients, many jobs and many Rounds. Often, the Surg Regs will Round in between different Theatre Lists, apart from the morning WR, and you'll need to report various Ward happenings to them with Investigation results throughout the day as you walk in and out of Theatres. In Medical Terms, there'll be multiple Boss WRs, each with a new Plan.

    Hence, with multiple time points, the List becomes very confusing when you're unsure of which jobs are done and which are not, which raft of results to report and which have already been reported.

    Thus, the multicolour pen is very helpful, especially in distinguishing different rounds and to *focus* you on what to do with yourself. Make your own system. Start with blue in the morning, move on to green for the next round of reports and jobs, then red for the final round and black just for writing up the million things you need to write up.

    With a system, you can cross things off and only focus on one colour, while retaining one List for referencing everything and easily pick up anything that has been missed.

And all this for the price of a coffee. Thankfully, its effects will last longer.

- **Pen torch:** Helpful for PEARL (pupils, not the jewel) and looking for anything in a cavity. Needed during Death Certification. Also keeps your phone hygienic (it is not, contrary to public opinion, a flashlight).

- **Tourniquets +/- other cannula stuff**: You'll be throwing in cannulas left and right, and always the one thing missing on a foreign Ward will be the tourniquet. Rather than use a sleeve or torn bed sheets, have a stash of the professional's tools on you. Depending on the state of the Wards, you may also need stashes of dressings, bungs, gauze and tape. The cannulas are usually visible enough.

- **Official numbers: Provider, Prescriber and AHPRA (Australian Health Practitioner Regulation Agency)**: These are numbers you'll become very familiar with, very quickly, but, ad interim, a massive hassle to find if you're busy. Best way is to keep a note in your phone. Paper tends to get lost/grimy/illegible.

  - *AHPRA number*: Always needed for Term Assessments and Death Certificates (easy to get by searching for yourself on AHPRA; be worried if you can't find yourself).

  - *Provider number*: Every Investigation under the sun needs this one. Often only found in official correspondence with Medicare/official bodies.

  - *Prescriber number*: You'll know this one like the back of your hand, or phone for that matter, for you'll be prescribing all day. Found as above.

- **Other props**: Quite specific and as per the Term. Ask the Reg/prior JMO at the beginning if there are any other tools you need.

- **Contacts**: You'll be calling many people. Many times. So, to save time, collect contacts to save the use of Switch and the Switch wait time. You don't need them all on day 1. Collect as you go. Just remember to collect. If you've taken the trouble to find, save. See *Chapter 6*, section *Phone contacts* for the full list.

BAG

As you can see, there's quite a few things to carry now. Hence, consider…

A bag.

It seems to fix so many of the difficulties, in both Ward and life matters, in one stroke. Food, water, equipment, everything else you need, all in a larger version of your back pocket, without looking like a gluteus tumour. You'll find the bag probably saves you more time than a Surgical pace. You certainly need to walk less since much of what you need is knocking against your bum.

However, this is controversial. Some may consider a bag terribly unfashionable. But perhaps it's more unfashionable to be hungry, thirsty and in retention for 4 hours, while being unable to find anything useful and with pockets full of the useless. It's doubtful those states do much for your style and poise. But you take your own pick. Look good wherever you want to, inside or out, to your own feelings or to the back of some random's retina.

Of course, this is more for extremely busy Terms. In chill ones, you have time to fluff about and walk to almost everything, repeatedly.

We suppose it's mainly the trouble of carrying a bag that drives away most people. But the trouble of not having a bag may well be greater. A small one will do, and it may well prove a lifesaver on those busy WRs or, at least, have a lifesaver in it.

SCRUBS/UNIFORM

Hospital clothes

The JMO uniform is essentially the same as what you wore as a Medical Student: smart, professional, office-like clothing, generally appropriately conservative. If your style wasn't appropriate, you would've been informed of that during Clinical Days at Med School. So, by the JMO years, it's assumed that most need no advice on this. If in doubt, follow the lead of your Team, and it'll be difficult to go wrong (though we aren't suggesting you get a full suit and tie and the wheelie bag unless the Boss insists).

However, as a JMO, there's an additional uniform which is now accessible...

Scrubs!!! (Buy/get early)

Everyone likes buying scrubs. We suppose it makes us feel even more like a real doctor. However, there may also be *free* scrubs available for you – multiple sets (as you do need to change), yearly (scrubs wear out too). You can even buy extra sets at a rate quite inexpensive compared with those offered on many online markets.

After all, scrubs are your work uniform.

To buy/get

This is State dependent. Ask the Nurses, other JMOs, Medical Admin. Usually you can place an order online, measure yourself (there should be very explicit instructions on how), then order. Medical Admin may need to approve your order. Next year, you may also renew the order for fresh scrubs so you don't walk into the ED looking like you inherited them from your grandparents.

There is also a fair wear and tear option in case, somehow, your scrubs become destroyed (there are many ways in ED so we won't enumerate).

This way you no longer need to worry about anything, from colour shade to logo (you've probably never realised there were so many shades of green) for you'll have the State Health logo that'll be true enough wherever you work (if going to a new State, then new scrubs). And even if it's not quite the right shade of green/blue/other colour, it's the right shade of green/blue/other colour.

Alternatively, you can buy scrubs at the numerous websites selling them. Ask the RMOs (Resident Medical Officers) for the usual Hospital one. Just allow for ample shipping time unless you want to pay deluxe delivery rates the week before ED.

Do this early, even as soon as you get your staff ID. Stocks often run low so act in advance to present yourself in ED or After Hours like a pro. And there's no need to speak of how comfortable scrubs are compared with usual Hospital clothes. Scrubs are, well, clothes. The others can be straitjackets.

PAGERS

In silence there is peace.

These things can drive you nuts very insistently, very soon. Especially in your first busy Term. You may think you know about them, especially if you were given one in Med School (confess – it either never went off or it stayed in your locker). You don't.

They're probably the most temperamental, indestructible, oldest and loudest piece of equipment in the Hospital. And even when you've silenced them by returning the call, you haven't. For the person at the other end of the pager is almost always someone who'll be very insistent and commanding that you should sort out, whatever it is that they want you to sort out, right away. If it's busy, you could be paged while taking a page, and a good moment is when you can answer one page completely before another one comes in.

And, as said, pagers cannot be toned down. The cursed thing is so loud, and in your face, that you'll be paged even in your dreams, and certainly shell-shocked if you have no experience with them.

Despite their ubiquity, it's doubtful if anyone is ever really taught how to use them, or even given a manual or anything. We suppose that, since there are just three or four buttons, you're just supposed to figure it out (forgetting the iPhone probably has fewer buttons) or that you were so enamoured of them in Med School that you would've figured it out pre-emptively (though it really seems just a loud way of summoning you to work).

So, here are some pointers on how to use the things and, most importantly, not be driven mad by them.

General rules

- The Pause button = Options
- The Fat Power Button = Enter and Home
- Arrows = Arrows

In further detail:

- **Options**: Most are self-explanatory – press Options to get in, Arrow to scroll through and you keep pressing Options to go deeper into it. However, to choose an Option, often it's the Right Arrow or just Arrow, and not the Home/Power Button, which only seems to work when actually reviewing pagers (variable between pager models).

- **Never carry the things home**: And, if you do, turn them off. Often, people have no notion of time, not for doctors anyway, who are expected to be at the Hospital almost 24/7 and, most unfortunately, the things have a range of some 50 km. So, if you live within that distance from the Hospital, you may well be at home, eating a calm dinner, before the dreaded sound summons you to 'put in a cannula' or 'CrCl is low so reduce metformin dose' or something.

- **The beep**: We recommend setting the thing to vibrate so you're not driven insane. You'll definitely feel it massaging your belt or wherever you've strapped it to, so don't worry about missing it. However, what you won't miss is the PTSD from the constant Hospital war cry.

- **Power**: Get batteries from whoever manages you, usually Switch or Medical Admin.

- **Pager off**: One of most satisfying settings. The key is to go via Options and keep Arrowing or Clicking Options until it asks 'Pager Off?', in which case click right Arrow and not the Home/Power Button. Then enjoy peace.

- **To delete**: The second most satisfying setting, which, however, is often denied you. It is usually managed via Options→'Delete All'. But, if not working, it's usually due to unread pages. Hold the 'Arrow' key for about a minute to 'read' them all, then 'Delete All'. Note: You should read your pages.

- **Setting the time**: A mildly useful option to record the time paged and to track just how behind you are while wondering if the person has left the phone already (they probably have, probably right after paging even). Go to Options→Arrow until you reach Set Time→Click the Option button to raise the time, i.e. adjust it, then Arrow to go to the next time bracket→When done, press the Home key.

  This setting is useful as you can see when you were paged in real time instead of July 1980; however, sometimes it's too much trouble, especially in the age of the swipe.

- **Miscellaneous**: There are some other amusing options, such as 'Alarm' because there's nothing like being woken up by your pager, and 'Zoom In', which doesn't zoom (or makes the rest of the message illegible – 'Zoom Out' is more helpful), but know these main ones for general use.

Text pagers

Another interesting function of the pager is the text pager. One may query the usefulness of this function in the era of smartphones, but often strategic Hospital areas are strategically without reception, e.g. Theatres, ICUs, anywhere near the basement and, very often, your home Ward. This certainly avoids making pagers obsolete as those things always have reception.

Hence, though you're often at the receiving end of the text pager, most often from Pharmacy/Nurses, you can also make use of it, in many ways, which won't be delineated.

- **To send a text page**: Variable between Institutions so find out from IT. Often, it'll be somewhere on the Intranet offering Text/Web-based Paging→Login→ Add Pager Number→Send Message→Done. The receiver will see it's from you.

- **Reading a text page**: Go to the page→Press the Home button and keep pressing to read if there's any more of it. Else, go to the next page via arrow and keep clicking Home. Home shuffles through the whole page until the end, where it shows you where the number came from.

So, there you go, a little 21st century guide to a nearly 100-year-old piece of technology.

KEY POINTS

- Bring a Common Medications Reference List: with doses and ideally indications and contraindications, including analgesia, antibiotics, anti-emetics, aperients, electrolytes, fluids, puffers, PPIs, topicals and anything else common on your specific Term.
- Be aware of the procedure in charting Blood products: including Consent, specific rates, notification of Nurses and Blood Bank.
- Carry a folder/clipboard to store the myriad forms: including scripts, Med Charts, Fluid Charts, Consent forms, Outpatient Pathology/Imaging forms, patient stickers, Medical Certificates, AMO business cards, Overtime forms.
- Bring your stethoscope, many pens, pen torch, cannula equipment, Provider/Prescriber/AHPRA numbers.
- Bring a bag. To put all your stuff in.
- Wear scrubs.
- Learn your pager – especially the Off button, Delete All and scrolling through. Do *not* carry home.

THINGS TO DO

You may not be paid for this. But it will pay you.

Consider the following things to prepare physically and mentally before you enter the Term. Some may argue that these can be done in-Term. However, you want to be the best JMO, day 1. At least a functional one. So some things need doing.

- **Handover**: Refer to *Chapter 7*, section *Getting Handover*. One thing that definitely cannot wait till 'in-Term'. In Orientation week, this is easy as you'll be doing almost nothing else. Otherwise, start planning for it in the final week to final few days of Term. What else you need to do largely depends on what's handed over, so ask fruitfully and abide accordingly.

- **List set-up/proxies**: Refer to *Chapter 4*, section *Lists*. Pretty essential. Ensures a possibility of function on day 1. You can, at least, see the patients.

- **Documentation**: Refer to *Chapter 4*, section *Discharges* and section *Documenting/Ward Rounds*. Start changing the names of your auto-text to your new Term, Reg and Bosses. The WR must carry on at the habitual pace, new JMO or not. As for the Discharges, well, if you're fortunate, you'll have time to update your Template. Otherwise, it'll be an in-Term job.

- **Life Rounds**: Refer to *Chapter 3*. Ideal if pre-Term. Very possible to do in Orientation week. Possibly not done till a Boss. Try to make it earlier. Especially important if you have been seconded to a new Hospital.

- **eMR generally**: Refer to *Chapter 4*. As per your Handover. If you anticipate or are informed about major differences in ordering Investigations, documenting, Discharges or anything on the eMR system, update them now and re-orient your system. Scrambling *pre-* rather than scrambling *in-*Term does much for your speed and style. Especially important if you have been seconded to a new Hospital. You need to know how they do things there.

- **Meet/know the Ward**: Rather luxurious and implies that your present Term is chill. Can be done in-Term. But, if you have time, you should know how things work in your next Ward. This new Term may not be so chill. Find out where everything is, e.g. Med Charts, patient files, forms, scripts, cannula gear, printers, faxes, storerooms/equipment rooms and their codes, offices, e.g. yours/the NUM's (Nurse Unit Manager)/other Ward staff's, phones, computers, Blood chutes, Term-dependent special equipment, e.g. spirometer on Respiratory, and other facilities as per *Chapter 3*. Don't stress if you don't remember. This is just a feel for the Ward. Besides, you can ask. The Nurses know everything.

- **Meet/know the Team**: Refer to section 'People to know'. But, at the very least, get every contact you can. Almost all have phones. There is no excuse.

- **Read up**: This isn't an admin thing but knowing about the Term medically obviously helps. Not just for your learning (which is important), but for effective function too. Know about common things, e.g. common diagnoses, Assessment, Management, Procedures and other Term-specific things. Your Team's life and your own will be much easier and patient care will be optimised.

KEY POINTS

- Get Handover from previous JMO/give Handover to incoming JMO.
- Set up required Hospital Lists.
- Set up required auto-texts and Templates specific to the Term.
- Look after yourself – see *Chapter 3*.
- Adapt your eMR system to the new Term.
- Introduce yourself to the new Ward and Team – obtain contacts and understand general Ward functions. Find out where stuff is.
- Read up medically regarding the Term.

PEOPLE TO KNOW

We always want to see your best foot. Especially at the start.

As shown in *Chapter 6*, people are the most critical part of the healthcare system (in fact, of every system). You should try to know everyone you're likely to meet. However, there are a few people below (in no precise order) who you should definitely know prior to *or* very early in the Term to facilitate general smoothness of progression.

- **Term Supervisor**: Obviously critical. They'll be assessing and signing all your forms. Usually a Boss, sometimes their delegate, e.g. an AT (Advanced Trainee). Get to know who from Medical Admin and/or previous JMO.

- **Director of Training, e.g. DPET (Director of Prevocational Education and Training)**: Very important. Will look after you during your Intern/Residency. They're a chief point of contact for any issues you may be having. You'll probably be introduced at Orientation, else there'll be many other occasions.

- **Medical Admin**: Also very important. Determines your Hospital admin life, including Rosters, Term preferences, Leave and processing your pay. Remember to notify them early of *anything* you want to do, e.g. Terms/Leaves/Rostering/special requests, ASAP. You can't be too early. Do it even when you sign the contract. Also, confirm everything with email. Even if it's just a memo. You always want to leave a record. And you *must* follow meticulously all their admin and paperwork requirements. That makes it easier for them. Which will make it easier for you.

- **The Team and current JMO**: You obviously must know the Team and especially the outgoing JMO (see *Chapter 6*, section *Home Team*). They'll give you the Handover and all the tips/tricks of the job likely to determine your survival for the Term. Similarly, the Team is critical as you'll be working with them for up to the whole Term, or even longer. Find their details in the Team Rosters/Switch/Orientation.

- **The Ward Team**: Also highly important (see *Chapter 6*, section *Ward staff*) to ensure an optimal work environment in the coming Term. You'll meet most during the Term but you present as extra-organised and amiable if you know them beforehand.

- **People involved in your desired Training**: These include the Director of Training, Head of Department, clinicians involved in research/projects/audits and mentors. This is especially relevant if doing the desired Term. You'd want to know these things early, preferably even before the Term, so you can be involved in all opportunities and help yourself to get onto whatever programme you're aiming for. You also present as extremely proactive and keen if you get in touch with these people early. Also, opportunities, by definition, are sporadic, so the earlier you put up your hand, the more chance you have of catching them.

- **Signer of Overtime**: Also important (for your bank's health). Know early to avoid missing opportunities of getting these signed. Previous JMO knows best, +/– Medical Admin.

- **Help/support**: You'll need all sorts of this throughout your working life, whether from small things day to day to career-impacting decisions. The sources are variable between every Institution. Hence, pay special attention when such services are offered, especially in Orientation. There are nearly always employee support and career assistance programmes in every Institution. If unsure, you can search your Intranet; ask the Director of Training or their delegate, Switch, the relevant Department or Admin; or Google it. However, the key is to ask if you need it.

- **Medical Officers' Association**: Essentially one of the best places to meet your colleagues and fellow JMOs. You're all in this together after all. There is usually one in every Hospital and the extent they're involved in your Hospital life is variable, from advocating on your behalf regarding employment conditions to organising social events/lunches. Most do charge a fee for membership to fund their activities. Something worth considering.

- **Professional bodies, e.g. AMA (Australian Medical Association), MDO (Medical Defence Organisation), ASMOF (Australian Salaried Medical Officers Federation)**: Again, these are professional medical bodies that aim to represent your interests on a larger scale. AMA is the professional body for doctors and ASMOF is the union that helps especially with pay disputes. MDOs mainly offer medical indemnity insurance and help with legal issues. All of these bodies charge fees, so you'll need to weigh it up (though MDOs often offer free insurance to Interns/RMOs). Note: The Hospital also has indemnity insurance, but its focus will be the Hospital's interests and it's important for you to have your own legal representatives. Besides, as mentioned, MDOs usually offer free services to Interns/RMOs, so, within the limits of their fine print, you can potentially sign up to multiple MDOs and try them out before you start paying.

KEY POINTS

Know these people early in the Term/employed life (in no particular order):
- Term Supervisor
- Director of Training
- Current Team and outgoing JMO
- People involved in your desired Training programme
- Medical Admin
- Ward Team
- Overtime signatory
- Medical Officers' Association
- Medical Defence Organisation
- Sources of help/support
- Professional bodies

CHAPTER 3

The Term: Life Rounds

You, too, need to live.

Doctors, for all their being health professionals, ironically lead some extraordinarily unhealthy lives, both through poor personal habits and through compulsion, the one often leading to the other.

We are catheterising patients in urinary retention for 6 hours when we have been in retention for 10, and when ours is solvable without one (for now). We lecture patients regarding healthy eating, and then go ourselves directly for the fries and soft drinks at the canteen because of a whole day of profound abstinence. We tell patients to cut down on unhealthy drinks and caffeine intake, while we fuel our very consciousness with coffee. We educate others about good sleep habits when we sleep less than our screens. We talk about restricting screen time when our own lives are glued to phones or computers, for work or leisure.

The point is, it's not a great situation. But we'll try to make the best of it.

We're not here to lecture you. Do whatever you like. But know whatever it is you do will have consequences that must appear. The only question is time.

WHAT IS A LIFE ROUND?

We know you always dutifully go on WRs (Ward Rounds), willingly or not.

But have you ever been on an LR (Life Round)?

You spend some 50% of your waking hours, at least, at work, helping others.

Maybe help yourself a bit too.

You owe this to your own comfort, long-term wellbeing and general sanity, and you owe it to yourself to make life mildly less miserable. For let's face it, however much you may love work, it gets miserable. Very miserable. And very often too.

Miserable enough to want to quit Medicine and lay bricks for the next 50 years. (Not that there's anything bad about laying bricks, but we suppose, since you're a Doctor, you tended to prefer healing over bricklaying.)

And it's at times like these that you may need a certain confectionary, but chiefly those bodily comforts generally not denied the other citizens of the developed world. Like food. Water. And sanitary facilities. And some sort of apparatus to rest your gluteus. For, honestly, it's the lack of those that has made your mood terrible in the first place. And they're a very quick fix to restore yourself.

Hence, the LR.

But what is it?

Well, consider it as a Round on yourself, and the environment directly related to yourself, to sort out your life in the Hospital. A Round to ensure you're in a reasonably operating state. A Round designed to keep you 'BTF' (between the flags) when you exit the Hospital. A Round so important that, perhaps, you should go on it even before its recognised counterpart.

For, remember, your usual Round only looks after the patient you see, at that time. While the LR empowers you to look after *all* your patients, *all* of the time. And, unless your Hospital is getting a major upgrade, you'll only do this LR, once, each Term.

It will improve you marvellously. It'll allow you to become immensely more efficient and productive and, most importantly, a generally happier human being. And that happiness can only mean better care for your patients, when this full you in multiple senses, brimming with life and energy, comes to look after patients, rather than the empty (except in one undesirable way) apathetic you who is wondering what life is all about.

You should always do a LR. You'll do a million Medical ones. Surely it's permissible to do one at least for life.

Consider, thus, the tips below, which are completely practical and will hopefully pre-empt and save you much suffering that, ideally, you won't even know existed.

Of course, work is not five-star luxury. But, certainly, it can be tolerable.

By addressing some key domains, you should be able to pass your life in a very reasonable manner, even in a busy Term, and not require Admission to your own bed every day in a state that an MDT (Multi-Disciplinary Team) would not clear for Discharge.

AN EXHORTATION TO LOOK AFTER YOURSELF: JUSTIFICATION FOR THE LIFE ROUND

Some people may find it difficult to justify the extra time they spend on themselves. For we're all supposed to be so altruistic that our own needs seem immensely less important than the patient's.

This is a state that may well follow on from Med School, when no one knew what to do with themselves and would even enquire about occupying corridor space. Now, if you were like that even in Med School, when no one placed any demands on you, think how you'd be as a JMO (Junior Medical Officer), when everybody is demanding you do everything, and right now too. And amid all the pulling, the pushing, the stretching and the squeezing, naturally the first thing to be squeezed out is yourself.

Of course, you're not as important as the patient. Of course, you must get all these things done, irrespective. Of course, you must comply with all these expectations placed upon you. Because you're a Doctor, i.e. a reincarnation of Mother Teresa in a Medical setting.

No.

It's not true. And the chief reason is that it's not even really about you. In fact, it's about the patients. Of course, you're pretty important, too, but this exhortation is mainly for those who are pushing and stressing themselves into YZ (Yellow Zone) criteria. The others are already looking after themselves.

Amazingly, something that may not have occurred to you is that healthier JMOs means healthier patients. When you're fed, watered, relieved and looked after, you're actually more capable of looking after patients, rather than the hungry, thirsty, stressed you that so many constantly push themselves into.

Not only is it better for you physically, but also mentally. You may think that with a BSL (blood sugar level) of 2 you'll be able to function. Unfortunately, you won't be able to function. You'll likely need others to exercise their functions on you. That is, the MET (Medical Emergency Team) with an infusion of dextrose and IM glucagon.

In fact, you're not capable of exerting yourself so excessively, much as you may think you're able to. It's great to be able to tell everyone that you can handle it. But it's far worse to tell them that you can when, really, you can't.

And even if you can now, you won't in the long term. And it's the long term where we'll need you to be. And at the end of the day, everything is about patient safety. And it simply isn't safe for you to exert yourself so.

When you're tired, hungry, thirsty and weaker in mind and body, you not only stress yourself but you also make poorer decisions, you're rushed, your judgements are without judgement, you miss a thousand things that it would be impossible to miss in your homeostatic state (we know we're asking a lot, you probably haven't attained homeostasis since entering Med School), you're harder to work with, you become shorter and sharper and, all in all, you're compromising patient care.

So, look after yourself. This exhortation may not be needed for the general population. But it's a special cohort, Doctors. At times, you could even say a mad cohort.

So, for those who are so very guilty about it, whose altruism is genetic: remember, you're not looking after yourself for you (though you're doing that too), but you're looking after yourself for the patient. Because healthier Doctors means better Doctors and, as in all other trades, all those seeking help for their health look askance at a Doctor who is sick, a supposed master of health.

For people may well not trust the builder whose own house is in tatters, the tailor who has holes all over his clothes, the barrister who is being sued in all directions and so on. For the Doctor, your own self is your house and one of the safeguards of trust in yourself.

Help yourself to help others.

Astonishingly, mind and body go together. If you're well physically, you will naturally lay firm foundations to being well mentally. And as Doctor-ing is often more head work than hand work, you'll definitely need a clear head to clear patients of their Issues.

AN EXHORTATION AGAINST EXHAUSTION

It's the mentality that needs changing.

That you must get it done.

The fact of life is – you'll never get it all done. That's just a fact. There'll always be more work. Even work that's not your own. And when you do all of it, more work constantly walks in the door. It's called patients (in the most respectful, and yet most pragmatic, sense).

Hence, the existence of working hours, a testament to the system's recognition of two great truths.

First, that work is endless.

Second, that, unfortunately, people have to eat and sleep or they won't come to work tomorrow.

Consequently, the system has created a time for work and a time for rest.

And you should respect that. You must be able to let go. And hand over.

Hence, the most important thing is to do the amount of work you can, in 1 day. Not 2 days, 3 days or a week's worth. One day's worth. And then leave the next day's work to the next day. And how do we know how much is 1 day's worth of work? Very easily. One shift's worth of it.

There's a culture of doing everything. That you must do it. That it's unfair on the After Hours person. That your Team is relying on you. All those things are true.

But yourself? Where are you in all this? Oh, never mind me. I can handle it. No, sorry, you can't handle it. You may be able to today, tomorrow, in a week or even in a year. But not forever.

Why not?

Well, you're like a machine. In fact, you are a machine (in a way). Like a car, say. Just alive.

And a very expensive machine car you are too. We're not talking prestige or any of those unquantifiable things, but in actual cost. It has cost a fortune to make you, for yourself, for your family and for society too. At least 20 something years of education and all the resources and time from many people along the way to get you here – family, peers, mentors, Doctors, other staff, patients and society.

And, now you're here, society is expecting your service for all that effort. And as current laws are going, some 50 years of service. At least.

But, despite all the effort that went into making that great 'you' car, suppose you always drive it on dirt roads, don't maintain it, never wash the thing, don't know what a service is, never pump the tyres, always run it on nearly no oil, forever scrape the tank's base and park it constantly over the salt spray, is that responsible to that 'you' car? To everyone who made that car?

And yet that's exactly what you're doing when you try to do 10 days of work in 1 day.

Don't.

Sure, there'll be constant demands on your time to get it done. Everyone will want you to do something, now. That pressure will always exist.

But there's so much that you should not be under the pump for. So much that doesn't need to be done, *now*.

It may be relieving to some for you to do it, now. It may relieve their anxiety. But you come to work not as a temazepam. You come to help patients, and stay alive yourself. Hence, keep calm, triage, prioritise and ask your Seniors if unsure.

Do *not* work yourself to collapse. You would be doing a disservice not only to yourself but also to all the contributors to where you are now, to your future patients, to all the lives you're going save, to society, to your own circle of family and friends, and to the long-term health system.

It's ok if everything is not absolutely perfect. Just do your best. No one can ask any more.

And remember that, whatever happens, there's always a tomorrow. And what we need is teamwork, not heroes. For team workers are heroes in the long term, for they're there for the long haul. While heroes often aren't.

PRACTICAL TIPS

Mindset

The most important thing is the mindset. Often, busy Terms are basically survival Terms. Hence, you must go into survival mode.

And what's survival mode in Hospital?

Sit when you can, eat when you can, drink when you can. That pretty much summarises everything about the LR.

You have no idea how much your function improves after PO 600 mL H_2O STAT. And how function deteriorates when you're dehydrated, hypoglycaemic and in retention.

People often think 'I will do this once I finish this.'

Stop.

You'll never finish 'this'. Because once 'this' is finished, something else will turn up. And something else. And something else.

But that food, water or toilet won't turn up, ever. Nor a new kidney 40 years down the track. So sort yourself out first. Because only then will you be able to sort out the rest.

We have Nurses doing 2- to 4-hourly Obs (Observations) on patients and calling YZ for patients left, right and centre. The fact is that you're probably in YZ criteria right now.

Below, we'll talk the practicals.

Facilities

Always scout out all the nearest facilities prior to a Term starting. You won't have time after it starts.

Find out the nearest toilets (a toilet Round if you will) on your level and perhaps a few other places. Don't grudge that time looking, especially when you have time to wait. There are times when you can't.

Scout out staff rooms, kitchens, fridges, microwaves, taps, canteens and water fountains. Nurses, cleaners, admin, etc. are a great well of knowledge for this as they've been here a lot longer and know about these things.

Scout out non-awkward rest portals too, somewhere you can get some quiet time from all the craziness. A few minutes there can really improve your mental health. Libraries are often great places but it depends on the Institution.

Ask for lockers. Medical Admin usually knows, or the Ward staff. There's a lot of stuff, surprisingly, that you'd rather dump here and not carry to and from work daily.

All this preparation will give you a possibility for relief when there's none to be found. All through the day, there'll be scattered minutes of semi-freedom. This will enable you to utilise them and recharge yourself.

Food

Everyone knows about being hangry. But everyone forgets the effects of hangriness when busy. Don't you forget.

Breakfast and lunch are the most important meals. Breakfast is not in working hours so do what you like, so long as you eat it. But, as for lunch, its importance lies in making the rest of the day mildly more tolerable. As for dinner, everyone likes it, which is fine, but since you'll be unconscious shortly anyway, what difference does it really make?

Thus, always, always have your lunch. Even if you have to stay back as a result. It's entirely worth the delay. For food refreshes like almost nothing else, save water and sleep. The first two are possible. There's not much chance of the last at work.

Yet, it appears that the biggest obstruction to food, however, is not the will but the way or, rather, the access. People do feel hungry. But people don't always have food by them. Nor is there always time to sit and eat. As a result, reducing barriers to access is critical.

The best way is probably to carry food on you. Don't bank on sit-down lunches. Eat on the go. Every mouthful counts. As you pursue your crazy life, at least something is mashing in the pylorus.

The half-hour break that is in our Contract is often in words only. However, with food on you, there are always random moments, and you can eat *and* Discharge on the fly. And those calories will carry you a long way.

Keep some snacks too. This will depend on your own metabolism. Again, we won't preach. Some say high protein, some high sugar, we say whatever keeps you going. JMOs always tend to lose weight on busy Terms so that can work to your advantage or not. But it's far better to eat a reasonable amount during the day than binge at night and fast perforce during the light. You'll certainly support the PPI industry but it'll do you no favours, especially as you're not really using that much energy when you sleep while your tanks are empty enough in the day when you really need it.

Knowing where fridges, cupboards and microwaves are helps make your own food more palatable.

Naturally, everyone knows where the café/canteen/vending machine is, but, as always, your own food has the potential to be much better and is usually less expensive.

Food in fridges and cupboards often belongs to somebody. However, there's also food there which truly belongs to nobody in particular but is highly edible. We will say no more.

Also, if you become immensely desperate, sometimes there are wandering trolleys.

Water

Water is absolutely essential. Don't forget to drink.

A common fallacy is that you think you can cope with being thirsty. You can't. There's a reason people die within days without water, and yet may last a month without food. And each day is only mini-weeks and months, hours and minutes being their new dial.

Water deprivation is more insidious than food deprivation. When concentrating, you often forget about thirst. However, you become slower and more confused and the brain fog comes upon you much faster. Think about the relief you get when you do have water. It's almost a new day, better perhaps even than a nap.

So always hunt out taps and water fountains and stock up whenever you can. Here's the advantage of a bag. While others have to go and search for their bottle or cup, for, however close it is, it's always far, yours is on your back pocket and you can stay hydrated even on a WR. Alternatively, know where cups are. The cupped hand is not always suitable. Especially when you remember what said hand has been doing.

Try to drink every few hours. As said, you'll forget about being thirsty. But your body certainly doesn't and will make you pay in hours of stupefaction.

Relief

No, we don't mean the Term, we mean the room. Make time for it and put it ahead of non-urgent Jobs. You're more efficient when you don't need an IDC (in-dwelling catheter).

And even on the WR, you're permitted to respond to the callings of nature. Being a higher-order animal should mean being better able to look after yourself, not worse. Of course, try to find a less awkward moment, but when it needs to happen, make it happen. Consider periods of waiting, Boss/Reg phone calls, excursions for legitimate purposes, e.g. trips to Radiology or transitions between Wards. Announce the fact if needed. This is one thing, however distant one is from JMO years, people will understand.

Sitting

Sit everywhere. Your knees'll need orthopaedic intervention after 10 hours of standing, so find every opportunity to sit down.

Watch all the Regs. All of them sit when they can, something they know from long, and likely painful, experience. As for JMOs, you probably can't sit at the patient's bedside. But we're sure there are always places to sit, e.g. convenient railings and ledges. You don't need us to tell you where. Just look for them.

And, of course, when you're away from the bedside, always do Jobs sitting. Concentrating JMOs unconsciously and unnecessarily stand for hours on end even after the WR is over. There are no fights to the death. You don't need to be the last standing. Even if you're on a WOW (Workstation/Computer on Wheels [COW]), sit. They have brakes. You need them too.

If you're absolutely in a desert, then the wall itself will do. There are always plenty of those.

Walking computers

Pushing the WOW is hard, especially when trying to type, avoid obstacles, peer through and/or around the screen and chase after the Reg who is running away from you as if you have the plague, all at the same time. Get the Student to steer. Or, even better, turn the screen. The screen readily rotates, so the edge, and not the face, faces you. Alternatively, lower the whole WOW's adjustable stand. But don't stoop. Irrespective, you must have clear vision ahead. Last thing you want is to run over a patient with the WOW and cause an iatrogenic fall, while you type about a patient who had a fall.

There is also usually very stiff competition for WOWs through the Ward. You often share them with Nurses, Allied Health and other Medical staff and it can be impossible as you transition between Wards to find a new one. Pending Hospital policy, if allowable, take your WOW for a round trip through all the non-home Wards and especially to the ED (Emergency Department), where the fight for WOWs is even fiercer. You'll avoid that fight. Just remember to bring the computer back or face dire consequences. Also know where the battery recharge station is for spare battery packs and recharge before your WR.

KEY POINTS

- Life Rounds: A Round designed to seek, source and maintain the necessities to keep you fully operational.
- Look after yourself, irrespective. You are extremely important. Only if you stay alive can you save others.
- Your mindset must be of survival and conservation of energy.
- Do not delay bodily functions.
- Sit when you can, eat when you can, drink when you can, get relief when you can.
- You are more efficient when you are healthy.
- Locate facilities early, e.g. toilets, kitchen, locker, water fountains.
- WOW screens can be rotated so you don't run anyone/anything over.

CHAPTER 4

The Term: IT

The cyberspace you must master.

We know. We all hate it.

The thing that we must all use. The thing that doesn't load. The thing that never works. Not, at least, the way we like. Sometimes not at all.

Well, hopefully, with this guide, you'll be able to look at it as little as possible, and yet get the job done. Which is what you want, right? Ideally, it'd all be automated so you wouldn't need to look at it, and can actually be a Doctor.

But, until we have Skynet, that isn't happening.

So, the next best thing is to build a system so you can look at eMR as little as possible – smartly, not hardly. And then, effectively, you'll almost have Skynet, only one that does the job and doesn't kill everyone in the meantime.

You would've had eMR training so we'll mainly build on that knowledge with tips they usually don't show in training.

It's always recommended that you contact IT for everything. We know there's no time. However, time invested in your tools will always repay you a thousand-fold. And there's no tool so useful – and if ill-used so frustrating – as eMR.

 NOTE

The below assumes that most of your hospital's functions are computerised. For those mainly relying on a paper-based system, consider:
- Collecting/pre-filling frequently used forms (in accordance with the principles below).
- Pre-writing notes on paper.
- Know all the paper file quirks.

- Be very good friends with Admin (who know all these things).
- Purchase of custom stamps for commonly used texts, e.g.:
  o Your name and provider/prescriber numbers
  o Common investigation/management sets with boxes beside them to tick or cross out
  o Stamps aren't usually expensive. Your time is.
- Await eMR's coming.

NB: THE NAMES BELOW ARE THE GENERAL GIST, AND CAN VARY BETWEEN HOSPITALS. SIMILARLY, NOT ALL FUNCTIONALITIES ARE AVAILABLE AT ALL HOSPITALS. CHECK BEFORE YOU USE.

MINDSET

Let the computer be the secretary. You are the Doctor.

Fast and correct should be your motto.

How is that even possible?

Why, computers.

Why aren't they Doctors then?

Well, they may very well be eventually, but the main reason they aren't – and, for that matter, that they haven't taken over the world (yet) – is because they mainly do repetitive things fast and accurately while humans like to imagine that they can adapt to situations. Now to prevent ourselves from becoming obsolete, you need to turf all repetitive actions to the computer and do the actual Doctor part well.

Yet, we're so often buried in the former that it leaves little energy for the latter. That's why you need to build a system for yourself (or borrow another's) so that you don't need to do any of the dumb, repetitive things, which you're liable to get wrong anyway, and focus on the things that require your real judgement, which you may still get wrong but you're the best we have so far.

Automation.

That is the mindset. Make the system pull the hard yards. Make yourself monitor. For monitoring is immensely easier than pulling the hard yards. And you can definitely monitor many more yards than you can pull. Yet if you have a well-built system, all the hard yards it pulls are yours, and you can thus look after many more patients while simultaneously achieving a higher standard of care.

Automation will be your lifesaver. There are an infinite number of repetitive things we need to do. If you do all of them, you'll drown. If they're done for you, you'll surf. We will go through many examples below. But you're on the ground. There'll be other circumstances. This is the principle to deal with all circumstances.

Thus, whenever you find yourself doing anything repetitive, you should immediately be thinking how this can be automated. Kill repetitiveness. That is your only advantage (and fast waning too) over machines. And only then will it leave you time to do the things that cannot be automated, i.e. looking after patients and tailoring your management to their unique clinical condition.

Remember to consider automating everywhere, but chiefly in Documenting, whether paper or electronic. For this is an immense portion of your job, and, if that's well sorted, you'll free up that immense portion of your job for true clinical training.

Below, we'll show you all the common aspects of eMR you'll navigate, and hopefully guide you to the easiest, and yet most accurate, way to do all that needs doing, so you can get off the WOW and actually see patients, and be a better Doctor instead of a better typist.

KEY POINTS

- Automate absolutely everything where possible.
- Use the machine advantage.
- All repetition has potential for automation.
- Your job is rigorous monitoring and analysis.

LISTS

You need to know what to do. And who to.

This is first as you can't really go anywhere, do anything, without a List. This is the guide of your day and, often, of your Hospital life.

So use this well, and you'll have taken the first step to sorting out work.

SETTING UP A LIST

Very important. Needed on every new Term, especially if your Regs haven't been proxied and have more than likely forgotten the inside of eMR (or are an overseas locum, who may well be a Consultant Cardiologist but will need to Consult you about this List business). Or, even worse, they may have never had an auto-populating List and you wonder how they got to week 7.

And now they're stretching out their hand to you, in slow motion, waiting for the List to be put in their hands.

Now is the time for you to act. So make that List.

1. Click 'Patient List' (top Toolbar)→A List will pop up.
2. Press the Spanner in top left→A pop-up will appear with two columns.
3. Press 'New' button in bottom right→A whole bunch of stuff appears that looks scary and complex.

But it isn't.

Really, it's just grid coordinates. There are two columns again. All the ones on the left are merely categories, the grid coordinates, which, combined, give a correct permutation for what List you like. On the right are specific selections, e.g. which Consultant, which Ward, etc.

You can do anything really, but, generally, people will only set up Lists for three reasons:

1. Home Team (usually based on Consultants [Bosses])
2. After Hours (based on location)
3. Custom (based on yourself and added manually).

The point of most Lists is, again, automation. Auto-populating. So that you don't need to find them or miss them through the whole Hospital. So that patients you need to know will appear of themselves on your List, and disappear when you don't need to know about them. The below will show this.

After Hours

As After Hours is about Ward cover, you need Ward Lists. So when someone calls you about Ward Level 5, East Wing, Bed 7D, you know exactly who that is without fluffing about for the patient's reference number.

Hence, set up Ward Lists of each Ward you're covering. For Regs, a whole of Hospital List is useful, as are Ward Lists you commonly Consult at. Pretty easy to set up.

1. As above.
2. Double click 'Location' for the 'Patient List Type'→Two columns appear.
3. Keep expanding the 'Locations' folder on the right column until specific enough.
4. Choose the Hospital→Choose the Ward.
5. Go to 'Discharged Criteria' (left column)→Various options appear on the right→Check 'Only display patients that have not been Discharged'→Click 'Finish'.
6. Move that Ward List from 'Available Lists' to 'Active Lists' with the arrows. You now have a List of the whole Ward.

Home Team

For the Day Team. So you know who *your* patients are. A little more complex. But the key is Bosses, i.e. the List is a sum of all the patients that all your Team's Bosses are looking after. Hence:

1. As above.
2. Double click 'Provider Group' for the 'Patient List Type'→Two columns appear.
3. In the right column→Check all the Bosses your Team has.
4. Now click 'Locations' (left column)→'Location List' appears on the right→ Check your Hospital (right column). Remember that this is for inpatients only; avoid clicking 'Clinics' unless you see them there.
5. You may also need to go to 'Encounter type' (left column) and check 'Inpatients' only.
6. Go to 'Discharged Criteria' (left column)→Various options appear on the right →Check 'Only display patients that have not been Discharged'.
7. Name your List at 'Enter a name for the List:'.
8. Click 'Next' if you wish to proxy people (see section 'List maintenance').
9. Done: You now have an auto-populating List of patients who are all under your Bosses. Your List will now self-update at will and patients will of themselves appear and disappear from it as soon as they are Admitted or Discharged.

You can also fiddle around and choose 'Medical Service' (left column) for Medical Terms with only one Team, e.g. choose 'Endocrinology' as the 'Service' and follow the above scheme instead of 'Provider Group' or any other method as you require.

The only problem with this List is that you can't add or take away any patients from it. Hence, patients you may have TOC'ed (taken over care) are painful as you must wait for the Ward Clerk to update the system (may be days), and Discharged patients are annoying as they vanish (you must alter 'Discharged Criteria' to 'Discharged in the last XXX days' to find them again, another painful task). Also, Consults can't be added to the List, which is a pain for Regs. Hence, consider the following.

Custom List

The easiest List to set up and you can add or delete patients from the List at will. However, it won't do anything unless you do something to it, i.e. no automation at all. To generate:

1. As above.
2. Double click 'Custom' for the 'Patient List Type'.
3. Enter a Name and hit 'Finish'→Done.

The possibilities with this List are infinite. You can use it as your Team List by copying all patients from the auto-populating one across and you can add patients to it for whatever purpose, e.g. Consults, After Hours, Follow-up. You can also remove them if you no longer need them. Only thing is you need to maintain it.

Consultant List

Bosses will mostly expect a List to be placed in their hand, even as they materialise. Regs will give a heads up, e.g. 'Boss is Rounding today', which is code for 'get their List ready'. Unfortunately, your normal List won't do for it'll contain the patients of many Consultants, about whom the materialising Consultant knows nothing except their own. And they don't want to trawl (nor will you when you're a Boss, enough done as a JMO [Junior Medical Officer]).

You could set up a List for each Consultant. But, if you have ten, that's troublesome.

Instead, first sort the List based on Location, then Consultant (click each column heading); then simply highlight, right click and select 'Hide' for all patients not under the Rounding Consultant.

Done. You now have your custom Consultant List, ready at every moment, regardless of what odd hour they round.

LIST MAINTENANCE

You need to maintain your List. You may want to change things, add new Bosses, fiddle around with the order of columns, etc. There are three buttons here to do stuff to your Lists.

1. **List maintenance ('the spanner')**: Chooses lists. Pops up two columns: 'Available Lists' and 'Active Lists':
   - Left/right arrow makes the selected List 'Active' or 'Inactive'. 'Active Lists' appears as a tab on your 'Patient List' screen, i.e. the ones you'll often refer to. 'Available Lists' are ones you don't need for now, e.g. List of prior Terms.
   - Up/down arrows shuffle the physical order of your 'Active Lists'. For prioritising/aesthetics.
   - Also used for making new Lists.

2. **List properties ('the pointing finger')**: Changes lists structurally:
   - Adjusts the 'Properties' of the List you're now in. Will bring you back to the page where you first set up the List to modify if needed, e.g. changing 'Discharge' criteria to find a Discharged patient with no Discharge papers. Not much used, unless structurally changing the List, e.g. adding a new Boss.
   - **Proxying**: Lets other people, e.g. Regs, use your List. Click the 'Proxy' tab on top→Click 'New'→Find the Reg under 'Provider' (last name first)→ 'Access' is mostly 'Full'→Grant access for a reasonable time→Click 'Apply' and 'OK'→Remind Reg to transfer it from their 'Available List' to their 'Active List'.

3. **Customise columns ('the red/yellow pen on a paper')**: Changes list aesthetics. Quite useful to include different pieces of patient information and customise your columns. Quite self-explanatory too: move active and available columns with the arrows then shuffle them up or down using the blue arrow as in 'List maintenance' above:

- Click and simply add categories that you want and delete what you don't. While on the left, you can organise column order by up and down arrows and at last save.
- Useful columns to include:
  - Room and bed (for where to go in the WR)
  - Patient Record Number (everyone wants it)
  - Name (duh)
  - Age (especially for Consults)
  - Admit Reason (though you should know)
  - Attending Physician (who to call)
  - New Results (useful in future, to check when new Results are available).
- All else is relatively extra, of little use and only takes up space and ink.

Other functions to play with: Access these via right click on the individual patient row. You can hence 'Add to a Patient List', 'Remove Patient from List' (only in Custom Lists, not auto-populating ones), 'Sort' or 'Hide' (very useful when counting patient numbers as number of patients hidden tells you how many patients you have; also good to hide patients who are on the List but, for some reason, you don't manage; also thus reduces depression).

PERSONALISED LIST/EXCEL LIST

Copy your List to Excel

On a busy Term, there isn't much time to write, let alone type. Then there are Regs or Bosses constantly shouting out Plans, then directly walking off, unlikely to repeat themselves and perhaps forgetting that the average writing or typing speed of any normal human isn't likely to exceed a hundred words per minute.

Hence, as the Plan is the most important part, a compromise is always to get that down first. But there isn't much space for it on the usual eMR List. And, even on normal Terms when you're not typing-sprinting, you still don't want to read all your 'Progress notes' all over again to enact the Plan.

A good way to set up Lists *with* space for Jobs is to copy the whole List to Excel (highlight in eMR and Ctrl+C). The whole table takes very readily to the Excel cells and will distribute properly. The trick is always to paste to the first cell, column A (or always in the same way), but, even though this column remains blank each time, don't delete it. Next time, still copy into column A (the empty one). This keeps the formatting. If you neglect this, your formatting will keep deranging itself.

After that, format it (*once*) into a way you like, with enough room to read the thing and two free columns: one for Results to note and the other for Jobs to do. You may delete the 'Admit Reason' if you have time and write up some actual Diagnoses and Past History of patient. 'Landscape print' is preferable as this leaves more space to write.

Printing (landscape forever)

Use landscape double-sided print. Not just to save paper – it's less depressing to carry a List that somehow fits on one page double or triple sided than to carry a three-page List.

To see if landscape print fits, go to the 'Print' tab, then come back to the usual cells; dotted lines will appear denoting the printable space. Then shrink your List to that space. 'Wrap text', cut 'Attending Consultant', shrink font – do whatever you need to do to fit the List into the margins to improve mood.

Save

Remember to save this perfectly formatted document for tomorrow. When you've spent all the effort of shrinking the size of the Boss's name, the patient's name, 'Wrap text' left, right and centre, deleting 'Consultant' everywhere, etc. and, in general, shrinking everything until it's barely legible, just to leave enough space for your two or three columns to write up Jobs in hurried, size twenty font hand-writing, you really don't want to do it again.

Patients will change but that's fine. You can simply delete the whole thing. But because you've formatted it correctly, once you copy tomorrow's List into the document, and delete the excess columns not needed in the List, it'll auto-format and save you doing it again. Therein lies the importance of pasting the whole thing to the cell A column but not deleting that empty column in cell A; for some reason, it preserves the format of the whole.

Here's also the importance of the columns' order as you'll want to delete adjacent useless columns. Usually have it roughly in the order of Location, Patient Record Number, Patient Name, Age, Attending Consultant, Admit Reason, other columns +/– adjust to your own circumstances. That way, you can still have extraneous columns in eMR, while they're readily deletable in your Excel List.

Hence, you'll now have a rapid, useful List for yourself each morning. Often enough, Regs will jump on board with this List as it gives them space to write stuff too instead of minimising to size three font to match the space of the printed List, or doing all this swanky origami folding and no longer being sure if you should be ordering the Abdo CT for this patient or the one below.

However, Bosses are mostly old school and like the usual printed List. Besides, they don't do that much List writing, so print them one of the usuals.

> **NB:** THIS IS AN EXTRA JOB, SO USE AS NEEDED. THE EXCEL LIST IS PRIMARILY USEFUL ON BUSY DAYS TO ACCOMMODATE AND ORGANISE THE MOUNTAIN OF JOBS FLOODING YOUR WAY. THE ORDINARY LIST WILL LIKELY DO ON THE CHILL.

ROUNDS LIST

What is a Rounds List?

This is just your regular List, only with customisable columns that can display certain Results/Investigations/patient numbers you choose, for all your patients.

How and when to use

Very useful mainly when you have large numbers of patients who you're not familiar with and, unfortunately, don't have time to be familiar with. For, the chances are, they'll leave before you've quite registered them on your List, let alone when you're aware of their whole story. Quite common in high-turnover Surgical Terms, where your chief role *is* turnover.

Here, you need to keep things flowing or, rather, jetting along, while, at the same time, making sure nothing is missed and no one gets seriously ill. And if something *is* missed, not necessarily to treat it yourself but rapidly to identify and notify your Seniors to treat it.

However, if you constantly go through things one by one, again and again, you may get 'red' fatigue (too many deranged numbers), and hence may miss things through sheer exhaustion of energy and time. Especially when you have forty patients.

Consequently, you need a quick way to sweep through the parameters and quickly find issues, and no way does this better than the Rounds List, which compresses all critical patient Results into one document for you to peruse.

Essentially, the Rounds List is a great way to *mass monitor multiple critical patient numbers* and rapidly identify derangements in key areas. With a correct set-up, you can effectively see the Temps, HR, Sats, Hb, WBC, CRP, Br, eGFR, Cr, etc. – whatever numbers you want – for *all* of your patients in one glance. Plus, the system auto-flags for you the deranged ones.

This can be very useful as you can instantaneously identify changes in the parameters of every patient, without trawling and without shuffling through all of eMR. Hence, having immediately flagged at-risk patients (if the Rounds List is well set up), you can immediately swoop down your focus on them and begin appropriate Management. This is almost ideal as it combs out most issues in one go, without you looking for them, and the remaining ones you can find as you go along.

Another good use of the Rounds List is that it can quickly show you the numbers you need to monitor daily and, as long as you know the previous result, you know the meaning of this one and can act accordingly.

Limitations

- **No trends/changes**: A number is just a number; to use it, you'll need to know the baseline. However, that you should know already, for, after all, this List's main action is to pinpoint.

- **Correct parameters chosen**: You must know what you're looking for. The Rounds List won't show derangements in parameters you haven't set up. Don't be lulled into a false sense of security if your Rounds List is pristine. The Rounds List is no substitute for clinical judgement and monitoring. It's the coarse comb. You're the fine comb.

- **No subtotals**: The List only documents the latest result, and not subtotals, so it is of limited use for drain outputs (though daily outputs are still helpful).

- **Single-point parameters:** Hence, it's best used for Assessment scores, Bloods and Obs. And, even then, it's a good idea to know what has been happening to monitor trends.

- **Set-up**: Mildly painful. But the pain is more than liberally paid off by saving you the pain of trawling through thirty or forty different Obs and Bloods and getting red fatigue at only 8 a.m. Also allows you to monitor patient numbers without a computer.

- **Can't print**: Screenshot and print in *Word*.

Setting up

Ok, we lied. The Rounds List is pretty easy to set up; it's tailoring it to the desired Investigations/Observations that is hard.

Click 'Rounds List' (next to 'Multi-Patient Task List', a List you'll be very familiar with)→Choose the List you want a Rounds List of→A window will appear→ Check 'Select all' and dropdown, then select 'Assigned'→'Rounds List' will appear and auto-populate.

All the columns are moveable and shrinkable so do it just like in Excel for printing space issues.

To get the parameters:

1. Find the far-right column and expand its size as in Excel. The Results will appear here so give it space.
2. Go to the top of the column and right click→Select 'Insert Column' (where you want the column inserted).
3. You may also 'Delete Column' via the same process.
4. Now start expanding folders and choosing the Results you want. As there are lots, see below to get the common ones. Find the others PRN.
5. Click ALLOCFSETS→Then ALLRESLTSECT→Then ALLSERVSECTS→Then you reach a few choices:
   a. Laboratory: All Lab Results are here, so merely expand and choose. In terms of sections, this is pretty obvious, e.g. Biochem under 'Blood Chemistry', FBC, etc. under Haematology and so on. However, if in doubt, simply go to the usual 'Results' tab and it tells you the test result's classification, e.g. 'CRP' is under 'Immunology' and 'WCC' is under 'Haematology'.

b. Patient care: These have all the Nursing Obs data. The one most useful for you is 'Observations'. Use 'Measurements' for daily weights (when patients are weighed), 'Vitals' for Obs (you'll need to find out which arm BP (blood pressure) is taken by trial and error), and the others as needed, e.g. urine output, drain output. Scroll through to find the one parameter you want.

c. Other two folders aren't much use.

d. Too many Results/parameters: There are *lots* of Results. This makes your parameter hard to find. So scan carefully. To make it easier, expand all necessary folders then keep clicking the first letter of the desired test, e.g. 'C' for CRP until 'CRP' appears. This will save some eye strain.

6. Once the parameter you are looking for is highlighted/chosen→Click 'Next' and choose how far back in time you want to look for that result. Useful if you don't want to see faraway Results as it'll stay blank and you'll be sure that the Results you see are recent.

7. Click 'Next' again, enter a 'Header' or name for the column (be as short as possible), then 'Finish'.

8. You now have an auto-populating List of all the patients with your wanted parameter, e.g. you now know everyone's CRP instantaneously or, at a glance, who is febrile.

9. Screen print and print from *Word* via landscape.

The most effective thing about the Rounds List is that you can see who is sick, right now. Of course, you should still look through everyone, but you can triage your time much better if you can at once identify the sick, tachy, febrile patient at 7.30 a.m. rather than at 11.30 a.m. when you've finally got through your forty-patient List.

HANDOVER/MULTI-PATIENT TASK LIST

This is a List primarily for After Hours and allows for the fact that patients can deteriorate at any time but Doctors happen to need sleep and lead a life of some sort out of work too.

Essentially, this is the electronic List of all patients in the Hospital who need *something* overnight/during the weekend, be it monitoring, repeat Reviews/Investigations/Management/etc.

If you have a patient you're concerned about, but don't want to stay back till 10 p.m. when the second trop is due (just kidding, no one expects you to stay back), you can hand over to After Hours to chase and allow you to sleep while not missing something, like a NSTEMI.

Likewise, if you're After Hours, this lets you know who is sick in the Hospital and to be ready.

Going home and giving people work to do

To do this, go to 'Ad hoc'→Look down the long list until you see 'Medical Handover'→Select 'Medical Handover Summary Form' and 'Chart'.

This'll bring up a whole bunch of stuff. Key areas to enter are the 'Situation' (the actual problem) and 'Recommendation' (what needs to be done). You should fill out the other parts too but keep it relevant to the actual Handover task. Check the other yellow boxes as appropriate.

After that, you'll need to call the After Hours person and personally hand over if it's important. Sometimes people don't look at the List and thus things get missed. But this is less likely if you call them. If it isn't that urgent, you can simply chart it.

Please give sufficient contingency Plans, especially if you're asking the After Hours person to check Imaging and Bloods. Remember that the After Hours person knows nothing about your patient; consequently, they would appreciate knowing what to do after the Results have come back, whether positive or negative.

As with most Consult forms, the act of bringing it up most usefully stops you from looking at the History, or the rest of eMR, as, clearly, you should've committed it to memory already. So, if you haven't got an eidetic memory, copy that History into *Word* before you actually start the Consult. Then you can copy it into the Consult form.

Finding work to do because you're at work while people sleep

1. Go to 'Multi-Patient Task List'→Click 'Handover Tasks'/'Handover' tab and peruse Jobs→Click yellow tab/square next to each patient Job to signify completion.
2. To modify your Multi-Patient Task List, you can call IT or right click 'Departmental View', i.e. top bar in grey→Select 'Customise Patient View'→ Pick your location, by either Hospital or Ward→Go to side tab 'Time Frames' →Select 'Generic Time Frame'→Then put in the range of times you want to see Jobs for.
3. Remember to click 'Save' under 'Location Filters' unless you want to repeat the above process each time.
4. Log in and log out and refresh if it doesn't auto-update for you.
5. Click the Jobs to see what needs doing.
6. Start triaging then doing Jobs.
7. If the Handover form doesn't appear→Go to Patient Profile and pretend you're charting a Handover→The Handover form should appear, filled with the instructions→Execute.

TASK MANAGER: JMO JOBS LIST

Old school Hospitals often have a big book at the front of the Ward where Nurses put in Jobs to do and JMOs cross them off. That system, though handy, doesn't sit well with our electronic millennium.

Hence, Task Manager, the eMR version of that fat book.

Set-up

These should be set up before you start each After Hours.

Set up one List type for each type of After Hours shift there is.

Go to 'Task Manager' (same column as 'Patient List')→On the left column→ Click '+' sign ('New List')→Choose Facility/Hospital→Choose Ward(s) you cover →Click 'Refresh' sign (Generate List)→This will populate the jobs in your area of cover→Click 'Save' sign→Name it→List will be saved in future.

With all the Lists saved, you can simply click on whichever shift type you're working, and the Jobs List will populate automatically for you.

Use

Mainly self-explanatory.

- **Acknowledge**: To acknowledge the Job. That's nice. Sometimes the Job disappears off the List. Quite unhelpful when that happens, especially if not done yet.
- **Complete**: It's done. Useful for the next shift. Do this, so they don't have to waste time trawling through a whole lot of done Jobs. Nothing more frustrating than looking for a Med Chart for 10 minutes only to find it's already been recharted. Or cannulating someone difficult then finding they have one on the other arm.
- **Cancel**: Useful for your shift. There are a few categories including 'Completed by other staff' (very often), 'Duplicate order' (unbelievable number of times, especially at shift changes), 'No longer required' (your call), 'Patient deceased' (self-evident) or 'Patient refusal' (you don't want to be charged with assault).

The 'Cancel' function does help your sanity as, without stirring, you can cut a three-page List down to one and you'll be under much less pressure. Use as per your judgement. You can also call the ward directly to find out the necessity and status of many things.

Filter

This List can be filtered, by clicking the column headings.

- 'Priority' and 'Required By' columns can help to prioritise; however, judge for yourself.
- 'Task' helps group all related jobs so you can clear them in one stroke, e.g. Med Charts/cannulas.

- 'Patient Information': 'Location' is the most useful so you can streamline your walking and clear jobs in one walk, one Ward.

> **NB:** INTERESTINGLY, ALL THESE ORDERS ARE ACTIVATED JUST LIKE YOUR USUAL ORDERS SYSTEM FOR INVESTIGATIONS, I.E. 'ORDERS' TAB. YOU CAN SEE THE NAMES OF THESE ORDERS TOO. YOU MAY CHOOSE TO USE THIS SYSTEM INSTEAD OF THE 'HANDOVER TASKS' TO HAND OVER JOBS, E.G. 'DOCTOR ORDER–CHECK BLOODS', 'DOCTOR ORDER–CHECK IMAGING'. WRITE AN EXTENSIVE COMMENT, HOWEVER, TO DETAIL WHAT YOU WANT DONE AFTER THE AFTER HOURS DOCTOR, FOR EXAMPLE, 'CHECKS BLOOD' (REFER TO SECTION 'ORDERING INVESTIGATIONS').

EMERGENCY DEPARTMENT: WHEN NOT IN ED

When you're not in ED, it's often necessary to do much ED stalking, especially when ED has called your Team about a patient but not Admitted them yet in eMR.

Virtually only ED has *FirstNet*, the ED computer system; when they haven't told you the patient's record number/your writing is illegible, instead of going to ED, you can see all ED patients still in *PowerChart*.

Go to 'Patient Dashboard' (same bar as 'Patient List')→Click 'Emergency Medicine'→Choose your Institution→Click 'Emergency Dept.–All Patients'→ See 'List of all ED patients'→Stalk on.

If you need a new ED List, simply close the opened dashboard as if you were going to close all of *PowerChart* and, when you next open the Dashboard, it'll have refreshed.

Now you can see all the ED patients you need to, without calling or going down to ED.

> **NB:** THERE IS SOMETIMES AN OPTION CALLED 'TRACKING LIST' IN THE SAME TOOLBAR AS PATIENT DASHBOARD (THOUGH IT IS SOMETIMES HIDDEN UNLESS YOU PRESS THE DROPDOWN), WHICH OFTEN IDENTICALLY REPLICATES THE *FIRSTNET* SCREEN. HOWEVER, IT MAY CAPTURE ALL THE EDS IN YOUR HEALTH AREA SO YOU NEED TO FIND YOUR ED AMONG THE MANY.

JOURNEY BOARD

You know that big computer board you see hanging in many Wards?

You can see it on eMR too!

Whatever.

Though, sometimes it's useful, especially if you know what the symbols mean, and it's most helpful in terms of Allied Health matters. Use/don't use as you like. The main help is that you can see what the rest of the Ward knows about your patient's progress and when patient transport is coming.

First, to see it, you must have the Ward Lists created. Then, go to 'Journey Board' (in the same bar as 'Patient List', click down button if you can't see it)→Click 'Select a Ward' (top-right corner) and choose the Ward.

Same deal as for 'Patient Dashboard', i.e. to see another Ward's Journey Board, you have to close the whole window then repeat the above process.

Now you don't have to go to the Ward to look at it (though it's doubtful anyone has).

KEY POINTS

- Setting up a List: Know the procedure, especially for Boss based, Location based and Custom.
- List Maintenance: Know the key functions, i.e. how to choose which Lists are displayed (the spanner), how to alter List properties/how to proxy (the pointing finger) and how to customise the columns (the pen on paper).
- Personalised List/Excel List: Know this procedure to create a more informative Handover and reminder List for yourself. Copy List to Excel →Format to printable area→Delete excess columns→Save for tomorrow →Repeat.
  o Use when busy.
- Rounds List: Use in high-turnover Terms. Displays select Results of all patients on the List in one go to allow for mass monitoring of critical Results of many patients. Know set-up procedure (see section 'Rounds List/Setting up').
- Handover/Multi-Patient Task List: A Handover process from day Doctors to After Hours Doctors. Know how to add patients for review and how to review patients other clinicians have requested reviews for.
- Task Manager: JMO Jobs List: Another Handover process but with less clinical information and universally utilised by all HCWs (Healthcare Workers), including Nurses and Pharmacists. Your Job book. Know the set-up process and how to clear Jobs from your Task List.
- ED: You can see ED patients (without being in ED) via Patient Dashboard or Tracking List.
- Journey Board: Can be viewed without going to the Ward via the Journey Board tab; Ward Lists need to be set up in advance.

FINDING STUFF

Or, rather, failing to.

We are always looking for things.

Old notes, reports, Consults, Investigations, Clinic documents, etc. All of which are critical for patient assessment *now* but are never found.

In fact, we waste an extraordinary amount of energy and life not in doing things but in looking for things to do things, somewhere in that labyrinth called eMR. Somehow, everything is all there, somewhere. But it seems that whoever designed the system had the Minotaur's maze for information in mind rather than accessible Medical records. So here is some string to hopefully lead you out of there before you're devoured by frustration.

There are three systems of documentation that we will discuss.

POWERNOTES

Use filters.

PowerNotes is usually recommended as the first port of call in Documenting, to find and to input. For some reason, it seems the fastest of the systems, so that usually implies the best. All the rest pretty much have no big advantages over PowerNotes except perhaps the Search function in Continuous Docs, so optimise PowerNotes and you'll rarely need to use anything else. Yet, while it's the best, there are some strange, counterintuitive quirks. If you know them, function is optimised; if you don't, it is ruined.

PowerNotes is pretty self-explanatory and you'll get basic training anyway. Literally, scroll and read. Everything is chronological. Remember do *not* widen the left side contents too much, or it'll look weird and you'll need to scroll to see the author. To fix, simply narrow it till it gives your usual format.

Documenting tips will be in Documenting. Here is all about reading. So, the main rule is, of course, …

Filters

Always use Filters. There's nothing worse than trawling through twenty thousand Nursing notes informing you that the patient is still maintaining their airway but missing that one critical note from Cardio re TOC (improbable) or Rehab saying they're taking your patient, please prepare everything and you didn't.

The chief default Filter is Physician notes (gives you *only* Doctor entries), which helps a little. But not much. So here are some other essential ones to prevent cross-eye through sheer trawling and how to set up.

Set-up

1. Click the '...' button next to the dropdown tab on PowerNotes. It'll bring up a giant box with lots of boxes.
2. Click 'New' at the bottom right for a new Filter, or go to the existing Filter in the dropdown to modify it.
3. Ignore most and just go down to bottom left ('Select the Document Types you want to see') and check the types of notes you want to see.
4. For further personalisation, look through the whole thing yourself but usually that's enough.
5. Give the Filter a name, then press done. Once selected in the first dropdown tab from before, you'll now see all and only the types of notes you filtered for.

Filter types needed

- **All Allied Health**:
  - Social Work, Physio (Physiotherapy), OT (Occupational Therapy), Dietician, Speech Pathology, Podiatry, etc. Each needs its own Filter; also create a combined Filter for all of Allied Health so you don't have to change between Filters.
  - They give very essential input. Also, it shows whether they've seen the patient or not.
  - Check 'Progress Note–[type of Allied Health]', then check everything else related to them. It's a long list, just scroll. At least you'll just scroll once, not an infinite number of times.
- **Operations**: *Essential* on Surgical Terms for obvious reasons→Check 'Operation Report'.
- **Discharges**: Pretty helpful to see the prior Discharges and hence the PMHx (Past Medical History) and Medication Lists. These are often comprehensive and correct if recent→Check 'Discharge Referral–[various types]'.
- **ED notes**: Sometimes, it seems that patients have always lived in Hospital, there being no end to the 'nexts' pressed and you have no idea of their initial presentation. The 'ED Case History' helps with that, to confirm that they weren't actually born there→Check 'ED Case History/Discharge Referral'.
- **Others**: Use on a PRN basis. Also Term dependent. But the main idea is that you know how to set it up. Now just check the appropriate 'Note' type you want, e.g. Mental Health, and you will instantly get it.

Now if the above doesn't work, it's usually because the Filter is still too coarse. This is especially true when looking for specialist Medical/Nursing notes, e.g. Consults you need to find that are meshed in a million Medical notes, Wound

CNC (Clinical Nurse Consultant) notes that are meshed in a million Nursing notes. Or particular people you need to find to see if they have any input but don't fit in the other categories or aren't usually checked, e.g. Neuropsychologist.

However, there's a solution. Filters are, after all, blunt instruments. For the scalpel of Filters, know the specifics and use the ...

'ONLY' function

1. Go to the dropdown tab.
2. Click 'Only'→Click the tab next to it and filter by 'Author'/'Contributor'. Yes, this requires people to know people's names, an effort it's true, but not quite as effortful as trawling through three hundred entries to find the one note with the last forgotten bit of the Plan.
3. You can also filter by 'Note Type' and this almost obviates the need for the above Filter set-up as it shows you what types of notes, e.g. Medical, Pharmacy, Physio, are available for this patient, so it serves the double function of filtering the desired note type *and* knowing if someone has seen your patient or not, i.e. if there are no OT notes, then OT hasn't seen them yet.
4. Other 'Only' options are available but the above two are most useful.

So PowerNotes is pretty comprehensive, but, sometimes, things are still not there. So, for the next step ... .

KEY POINTS

- Chief system used.
- Set up and use Filters based on note type/class→See section 'Set-up'.
- Common types include for each Allied Health type, ED notes, Discharges, Operations/Procedures.
- Use the 'Only' function to display notes from one person or note class.

CLINICAL DOCS

Trawl.

Not a bad system, but complex and hard to click through so many folders. Based mainly on continuous folder expansions. Most things are in the 'Progress notes', including Allied Health. However, many procedural reports, e.g. Endoscopy and Echo (Echocardiography), are here and nowhere else.

Otherwise, various Specialist/Clinic reports/letters may well be there, if you trawl, but very hit and miss. Use more in desperation or if you know something is always there. Also, it tends to have *everything*, so if it's on eMR it should be here, somewhere.

Most usefully, use the Filter (bottom left):

- **by Type**: i.e. Progress notes, ED reports, etc. The default. Keep expanding folders and keep looking. You'll just have to keep reading the folder headings and guessing. Letters and Consults sometimes strike gold.

- **by Date**: Self-explanatory. Particularly useful if you know someone has written something recently, but their note is not anywhere else. Looking through the recent dates should reveal it.

- **by Encounter:** i.e. Presentations to Hospital; may be useful to look for frequent flyers.

- **Performed by**: i.e. By author; useful as you can see everyone, literally everyone, who has ever written for the patient.

- **by Status**: Not much use, unless you're looking for notes you haven't signed.

Simply click on whichever you want to use. Another very useful function is…

Patient data from other Public Hospitals (without faxing)

Another interesting function is the eHealth Record, found under Miscellaneous Documents. Enter it by opening the 'Image' attached to it like in a Radiology report. This opens another window and often shows much patient data from *other* Hospitals. Under the Patient Summary, Imaging and Pathology tabs, you can often find Discharge Summaries, Imaging and Pathology performed at other Hospitals, often not in your Network. Can be very useful especially if there are no data anywhere else. However, it isn't always complete and may not have many Progress notes, but it's much better than nothing. My Health Record can also be so accessed, and its use will be greater as it's increasingly integrated into the health landscape.

However, if you still haven't found what you are looking for, consider Continuous Docs … .

KEY POINTS

- Comprehensive but difficult to find things.
- Keep expanding the folders.
- Use its Filter function→Categories as shown.
- eHealth Record function sometimes allows access to records from other Health Districts.

CONTINUOUS DOCS

Searchable.

The most useful thing about Continuous Docs is the use of the Search function, which allows you to comb all of eMR instantaneously.

It's the top-left little binoculars.

You can literally search the entire eMR. Which is extremely useful and saves an infinity of trawling energy.

However, the most irritating thing about this system is many things:

- You can't copy out of it unless you double click and bring up a new window.
- It's confusing at times where each note runs up to (strange yellow highlighting that lags).
- tHe dAte PeOpLE haVE sEeN ThE pATiEnT Is cONfUsInG: Usually top-right corner but variable sometimes when constantly 'updated'.
- Slowness.
- Not all notes are by default there, and you must adjust the Filter to Admission date to capture all the notes.

However, the chief redeeming feature of search sometimes justifies it all. By simply adjusting the time Filter, you can capture notes from the Stone Age, and then, by using the Search function and typing key words, e.g. Gastro or *whatever* it is you're looking for, Continuous Docs will search through *all* the records, even if the patients saw the Cardiologist when Stonehenge was being erected. If it's on the eMR, Continuous Docs will find it.

Otherwise, other redeeming features are the Filters, including:

- 'Document Type', e.g. for Allied Health.
- 'Designation', for Doctor, Nursing, Allied Health.
- 'Encounter', for each Admission/Service.
- 'Author', self-explanatory, especially if you know everyone's names, though beware if the Boss sees and you were expecting the Reg, hence missing the Boss.
- Others: self-explanatory.

All are handy to use, *but* all thwarted by the limited time frame that Continuous Docs retrieves notes from *and* the inexplicably long time it takes to get any more. Similarly, most of its functions are already duplicated in PowerNotes, so you really don't need to wait.

However, a critical thing is some key Specialties, e.g. Palliative care and Rehab sometimes use it exclusively. Hence, you must check Continuous Docs else it'll appear as though they've never seen your patient when they actually have. And you'll Consult them again and again and both will think the other needs Psych input.

KEY POINTS

- The only readily searchable eMR database→Click the binoculars symbol and enter key search terms.
- First, maximally expand the time Filter to search for what you need.
- The usual Filter system can also be used.
- Permits continuous scrolling.
- Otherwise functionality and dates are clunky.
- Used exclusively by some specialties so check this.

OFFSITE DATA

You often need data about patients who are not onsite. It's generally easier and better to find that offsite data than repeat the Investigation on the patient. Yet, sometimes, only barely.

For some reason, in the world of smart watches and the 'Cloud', Hospitals still insist on using 18th century technology. Fortunately, we don't keep an aviary, but we're still using fax machines and pagers. So bear with it and try to be efficient despite these intrinsic obstructions.

First, certain decisions usually hinge on the information you're tracking. Hence, with all the below, in the interests of speed, *always* ask for a verbal report of whatever you want unless too complex/long *or* you *must* have written authority before enacting the decision. Just get the information, and make/enact the decision. There's usually only *one* thing you're really looking for. Get that, document and commence. The IT gods alone know when the fax is coming. So long as it does, it won't stuff up your day. Waiting might.

GPs

There'll be a thousand things you need to chase from the GP so you need to keep this sharp and fast.

When talking to them, give the patient's name and DOB (date of birth) (there is no Patient Record Number) and ask for a Health Summary/Medication List/anything else you want. Some practices want you to fill out some form. Usually this is not needed so try to speak with a Doctor or Nurse there who usually actually knows what you require. Remember that the reception are usually administrators and don't have much idea about the things you want, while the others have worked in Hospitals long enough to know the frustration of getting offsite data.

Always have your own fax number handy (best to save it in your phone).

Most of the time you don't need to speak with the GP unless you absolutely need to, e.g. actually about the patient (they and you are both busy and it'll usually mean a hold of some 20 minutes that you can't really afford on a busy day), and a Practice Nurse can help you too if you just need documents. You can also ask them to take a message if non-urgent/non-critical Handovers/notifications.

Besides, you really can spare the GP that sort of admin. They've done already enough in their time. Just let them practise Medicine now, please, as you'd like to when you're a Consultant of any sort.

Private clinics

Same as GP. The main thing is to track down which rooms the patient goes to (ask the patient) as the Specialist often works all over the place. You don't want to go room hopping as your ears wander all over Sydney and finally find the patient files after 2 hours of multiple holds. Information is definitely not synchronised between practices so if the patient can tell you where to go first, it'll save you much trouble. Patients usually know which suburb they had to trek to.

Always get as many letters/Clinic notes/Investigations as possible in one go. You don't want to call back. Try not to wait at the fax. Even if they say they'll fax it now, it won't come now. Ask someone always there (usually the Ward Clerk) to keep an eye out for it.

But, before you start, if there's a recent Admission, look through the patient's old paper files (the fat folder bundle that follows the patient everywhere). Request it from Medical Records if it hasn't come up (Ward Clerk can help). Probably, the JMO before you has already done it all, and it'll be much easier to flip through that than wait for unknown fax machines.

Hospitals

Always ask for Medical Records and they'll fax through quite readily, though it may be very hard to reach them at all. Get the direct number from their Switch. Medical Records usually knows and can get whatever you need.

The Ward Clerk may also help to call if the holds are impossible. They often have fifty lines attached to one phone and can afford one hold the more. However, give very precise instructions about what you want. That is, written down, verbatim.

External Imaging

This can be obtained from a PACS (Picture Archiving and Communication System) coordinator/Computer Administrator, who possibly can upload it for you onto the system. There's sometimes a system you can login to but ask the PACS person for details. It also helps if the patient brings their CDs with their images. Alternatively, private places can generate the images for you on disc and you can give it to your PACS to upload it. The report is often readily faxed over from private Imaging centres.

External Pathology

Usually extremely rapid and helpful as they're trained Technicians who know what clinicians want. Faxing is rapid and emailing Results is also possible.

However, as said, get a verbal first. When asking, give headings of Results. Nobody will know where eGFR is, but say 'It's under biochemistry, under the creatinine' and the most non-Medical person can still find it. If you're frequently consulting these Pathologies (i.e. more than once), contacts should be saved.

Some Pathologies also provide an online look-up service where, once registered as a Doctor with them, you may search their entire database at will for patient Results. This will save the call and the fax. However, each Pathology is different, so check with the largest and most common ones. Also, you may have to be a Consultant and you may need to pay.

KEY POINTS

- Always get a verbal report when possible.
- Check that the correspondence hasn't already been chased by the previous JMO if the patient has been recently Admitted.
- Know the standard procedures of GPs, Specialist clinics, other Hospitals, external Pathology/Imaging.
- Know where the patient has actually been to, e.g. location of Specialist rooms.
- Have your own fax number/email handy.
- Get every single Investigation/letter you can in one go.
- Ask your Ward Clerk for help.

OTHER PLACES TO LOOK

In spite of all the above, there may still be difficulties, still some nooks and crannies you haven't cleaned out with your massive Search brush. Here are a few other combs to scrape out the last, most resistant information scraps.

- **Other Hospital's Patient Record Number**: If the patient has been to another Hospital, at times, it helps to search the Patient Record Number of the other Hospital (often on the Discharge Summary of that Hospital) to get the full Admission Notes. If the patient didn't bring their Discharge, you can search their name and DOB and that may bring up Encounters with other health services. Comprehensive access to external Admissions data is often invaluable as the Discharge Summary may not be complete or the patient doesn't have it.

- **Encounters**: Every interaction the patient has with the Hospital is recorded as an 'Encounter'. Sometimes patient information disappears because the incorrect 'Encounter' has been selected, especially of various Orders you may've placed. To amend this, choose the right one, i.e. click 'Patient/Encounter Information'→Click 'Visits' tab→Choose the most appropriate 'Encounter'. It's filtered by date and if an inpatient or not as well as by Medical Service (often meaning who's responsible for the patient then), e.g. ED or Cardiology. When double clicked, the system will offer to change the 'Encounter' and, after that, new information may appear. This is especially useful to see if certain 'Orders' (pending Investigations) were placed as these will not appear in incorrect encounters.

- **Patient Information section**: This contains all the information regarding contacts, including the patient's NOK's (next of kin), family's, GP's, Nursing Home's, etc. As above, go to 'Patient/Encounter Information'→Switch between the 'Patient Details' and 'Patient Contacts' tabs, and all the data will be there. To find if the patient is private or not (an often enquired for piece of information), go to 'Encounter Details' tab and it'll show either 'Uninsured' or list the Insurer or DVA (Dept Veteran Affairs), etc. under 'Financial class/Health Fund'.

- **Patient Schedules**: Sometimes, patients/Bosses will ask you for appointment times that were previously booked. If in the same or linked Hospitals, this can show up on eMR instead of calling. Click 'Patient Scheduling'→You can see all the appointments booked, including even Theatre bookings.

- **Form Browser**: Sometimes used by various Clinics, e.g. Pre-admissions. Its structure is odd (like an expanded contents tree) but just glance through and double click what's relevant. Nurses tend to use it more but occasionally useful data not found elsewhere are there. Copy data out of it via right click or double clicking→Expand the info into a new window, then copy.

KEY POINTS

- Patient Record Numbers from other Hospitals.
- Switching Patient Encounters.
- Patient/Encounter Information section for personal details/insurance status.
- Patient Schedules for appointments.
- Form Browser for various Clinic notes, e.g. Pre-admission Clinic.

HOME SCREEN (AKA PATIENT SUMMARY)

The most important page. Use wisely.

This page is the heart of the eMR system. All the strings of *PowerChart* are in your hands on this one screen. Whatever you need to do can almost *all* be initiated here. It's also the fastest page to load.

With these virtues, speed and comprehensiveness, it's the one page you should optimise the most for maximal benefit and minimal eMR gazing.

The amount of life we lose in waiting for eMR is astronomical. It's probably the single biggest killer of Doctors, after lifts (hence stairs). The sheer amount of existence that goes into that void is heartbreaking, so the less you can die there, i.e. whatever is the fastest, the better.

The 'Home Screen' is useful both for acquiring information *and* for initiating interventions. So, ideally, the rest of eMR will become as obsolete as possible.

So please take the trouble to set this up. If you have a well-set-up 'Home Screen', life will be so much easier, Results viewed so much faster, Jobs done so much quicker, Documenting so much smoother and everything just better in general.

The Home Page's three main functions include:

1. Orders
2. Documents
3. Results.

In fact, those are the three most important things you use eMR for. And those three must be optimally customised in the 'Home Screen'.

Optimising the 'Home Screen' primarily lies in what to keep expanded (to get info at a glance) *and* how to use the quick links for the functions. These will be discussed here generally, and the exact methodology will be shown in the relevant sections. In brief, always have expanded the following.

> NB: THE BELOW IS THE MERE SET-UP. HOW YOU'LL USE EACH OF THE ABOVE FUNCTIONS WILL BE DETAILED IN THEIR OWN SECTIONS. AND AS YOU USE, YOU'LL SEE HOW STRUCTURE RELATES TO FUNCTION, EVEN IN THE IT WORLD.

ScratchPad Orders

Order everything here. For some reason, the Orders tab is stroke-inducingly slow while the ScratchPad has everything you need, so long as you know (or can guess) the name of the Investigation. All you do is search for the test in the 'Search' bar, and match to the closest.

There are a few small quirks in terms of precise naming, e.g. 'Pelvis X-ray' rather than 'Pelvic', the latter will turn up nearly nothing and you'll think Radiology is broken, but these you'll figure out pretty quickly.

Here, there's no searching in endless columns, no trawling through endless rows of tests, just the ones you need, now.

And, for even better organisation (see section 'Ordering Investigations'), you won't even need to search and all your favourite tests will be just a click away.

For those with eMeds (electronic Medications), a similar methodology can be adopted for common Medications and Fluid Orders; however, much more care is needed as these are Managements you're instituting – there's much more variability and fine-tuning, so be aware. However, the process is just as fast.

Document Launcher

Get 'Progress Note–Medical' *and* 'Discharge Referral' by directly clicking from here in the purple subsection. It instantly generates the document you need, ready to input data. This saves some five or six other clicks compared with via PowerNotes and the associated deathly wait times and confusion. Use it.

Vital Signs/Observations

Obs. Good to eyeball. Shows a few data points back.

Lines, tubes and drains

Keep this expanded to keep track of what's in your patient. Not always accurate, but at least if there's an IDC written, you'll remember to look for the real IDC. And if it can come out.

> NB: TO KEEP EXPANDED, GO TO THE TOP RIGHT CORNER OF TAB YOU ARE INTERESTED IN→CLICK '='→CHOOSE 'DEFAULT EXPANDED' →DONE. YOU CAN ALSO PICK COLOUR THEMES IF YOU'RE BORED.

The following are useful, but don't expand them, including.

Clinical Notes

Rapidly shows, without going to PowerNotes, who has written anything for your patient. Good way to rapidly eyeball for Consults made. However, will blot out Document Launcher (which is much more useful) if expanded, so don't.

Pathology Results

Shows last three Bloods. Usefulness ambiguous. Good for a quick eyeball.

Medical Imaging Results

Useful to see all the Imaging the patient has had. You can click on it to instantly bring up the report.

KEY POINTS

- Use the ScratchPad Orders system for *all* your ordering, including any Investigations/Medications.
- Set up shortcuts (refer to section 'Ordering Investigations') early so all your favourite Orders appear here and make ordering 'click and go'.
- Keep the Documenting subsection expanded to launch new documents rapidly, especially 'Progress Note–Medical' or 'Discharge Referral'.
- Keep certain Results subsections expanded to see at a glance, especially Obs/lines/drains output.

VIEWING INVESTIGATIONS

See and observe. Quickly

Quite self-explanatory mostly and will be taught in eMR training. However, a few tips in addition:

- **The right tab**: *Always* click the relevant tab for Results, i.e. Pathology for Bloods, Medical Imaging for scans, Microbiology for bugs and Patient Care Results for Nurse-inputted data. Don't trawl All Results or Diagnostic. Again, it's about focus. You only have limited focus daily. Let the system focus for you. Minimise trawling.

- **Scroll**: Scroll to the far left for the most recent Results. Sounds obvious, and yet … . People have done your Bloods, you just need to see them.

- **Searching individual Results**: You can display only one specific result by clicking the '…' button next to Flowsheet just under the Results row of tabs at the top. Then type in the Result type you're looking for, e.g. weight, and it will display all entries in that Result. Reliability fluctuant.

- **Navigator**: Next to the list of Results there's a contents panel called Navigator with all the categories, e.g. Blood Gases or Coagulation Studies. Very useful to jump between Results, especially if you know the category of the Result, e.g. CRP under Immunology. Mostly self-explanatory and saves scrolling/ trawling.

- **Tear Off**: Often you need to input the Bloods/other Results into your notes. So you dance between windows in *PowerChart*, opening and closing your Progress notes. Time wasting. Some people just do it in *Word*, but impractical if you're running on a Surgical WR as you can't save.

  Use the Tear Off function. Whatever page you need to refer to (mostly Results), click 'Tear Off' next to 'Change User' and that screen will 'tear off' into another window. Re-size so you can read your Progress notes and Results windows simultaneously. Then, just read the Results on one side and input on the other, so you don't need to memorise the WBC, Hb, CRP, eGFR, Cr, HCO3, urea and all the LFTs in one glance *or* click back and forth fifteen times to get all the numbers.

  An alternative method is to open *Notepad* alongside and transcribe the Results there, then paste across. We don't really recommend you do all your notes there (though some do) as you lose the benefit of your auto-texts, and, as you're frequently interrupted and jump between computers, you could accidentally lose all your notes as there's obviously no 'save' function in *Notepad* linked with the whole eMR.

- **Patient Care Results**: Deserves a special mention. Others are self-explanatory but this one has much data you need but do not know where it is. Consider:
  - **Weights**: Under 'Measurements' (much needed in Cardio and Renal).

- **Obs**: Under 'Vital Signs'. If your Reg insists that all numbers need inputting, copy numbers here into your notes. Saves to-ing and fro-ing between 'BTF Observation Chart' and 'Progress notes'.
- **All Nurse-inputted data**: This includes *many* things, so just look. Names are self-explanatory. Consider AWS (alcohol withdrawal scale) score, BSL (blood sugar level), ketones, urine output (especially from IDC), stool chart (under 'Bowels'), Neuro Obs, drain/stoma/other outputs, GCS, UAs (urinalysis) and so on. If in doubt, ask yourself if the result was recorded by a Nurse. If yes, it'll be here.

- **Inputs and outputs (and other Nurse-inputted data)**: If it isn't under Patient Care Results, check 'I-View ', 'BTF Observation Chart' and 'Advanced Graphing' (all along the same column of tabs as Results and Patient Summary):
  - **I-View**: Anything with a 'tick' next to it means data are present. Again the Contents is on the left and self-explanatory. 'Bedside Tests' has UA and BSLs, 'Tubes and Drains' sometimes has outputs. But for most input/output data, go right to the bottom of Contents to the 'Input and Output' tab and it'll expand a new set of Contents and show all Input/Output data, e.g. IV fluids received, stool chart, urine output, etc. Also use the ticks to guide you.
  - **BTF Observation Chart**: Mostly has Obs in it and trends. However, sometimes also has weight and UA. Just scroll down to the bottom.
  - **Advanced Graphing**: Near the bottom of the main contents. Useful for visual people as it graphs daily input and output so you can see graphically if balance is achieved and the proportions of each contributor, e.g. what volume was IV fluids, how much was PO intake, how much was urine output, how much was drain output. Also available under I-View under the 'Input and Output' tab.

- **Trends**: You can graph your Results, and even against each other. Check the box next to the Result you want to graph (check multiple if you like), then click the 'Graph' button on the top left (next to the green magnifying glass) and you get graphs for each Result to see the trend over time.

- **Extra info**: If you right click a given Result, you can get extra information about it, including 'Order information'. Choose the relevant button, e.g. 'View Order Info' or 'View Details' or 'View Comments'. Things like who/when/where the Investigation was Ordered is often found here. Additional interpretation data and comments from Pathology are also here.

- **The Eye**: Click the Eye, i.e. 'Bookmark', top left, next to the green magnifying glass to have 'viewed' the Results. Probably best do this under 'All Results' tab.

    Why?

    Because now you get instant updates if new Results (especially ones you've been waiting for) have come.

    How?

    In your normal List, there's one column with a clipboard in it. If there's none, this implies that there are no new Results. As soon as a new Result comes, it reappears (when you hit 'Refresh' in the top-right corner). Hence, this is only useful if you constantly 'view' or 'bookmark' for all your patients once you've viewed the Result.

The main limitation is that you can't filter the type of Result the clipboard appears for, i.e. all new Results including a new Nursing note or a new BSL will activate it. However, it is still potentially useful, but requires daily maintenance. You can also achieve the same effect by clicking the 'clipboard' in the List, which will bring up a new window of all the unread Results. You can click the 'Eye' then. However, this window is often slow if there are lots of Results (e.g. with newly Admitted patients), so do this in the 'Results' section, then you can do it from the clipboard thereafter.

This method is one of the optimal ways of getting minute-by-minute updates of the patient's Results and appears impressive, without the trouble of running constantly through every patient's eMR file. You want to be the first to know. This way, you will be.

- **The green magnifying glass (the 'seeker')**: For eMR veterans. Once you've used eMR enough, you know instinctively where everything is. You know exactly which row CRP will be, where TSH is, which column HbA1C will be under. But it's far back in time and you can't be bothered to scroll. Solution? You can click the 'seeker', which will bring up a mini-map/aerial view of that tab, with blue/pink bars for all the normal/deranged Results. Simply click where you know your Result will be and 'seeker' will instantly take you there. Nifty but you need experience.

RADIOLOGY

Lots of tricks which you'll pick up, especially if you want to do Radiology (even more when you're using their fancy programs as a trainee). Also depends on how much you look at the images. However, you'll focus mainly on X-rays and CTs. Also note sometimes different programs are used to view images and there may be variability to the below, though the general principles and functionalities are the same.

General (including X-rays)

Pretty much play with all the buttons along the top (hover over a button if you don't know what it does) or right click and choose the relevant option. But generally:

- **Contrast/brightness**: Hold right click and slide mouse up/down for brightness, left/right for contrast. Useful for emphasising certain parts of the image if you're not sure, e.g. a consolidation.
- **Zoom**: Hold the scroll button and slide up/down. Useful for zoom, especially fractures.
- **Toolbar elements**:
  - **Self-explanatory**: 'Double triangle' sign for rotate/flip, 'magnifying glass' for zoom, 'angle' sign for calculating angles, 'Reset' tab to reset your changes, 'arrows' to shuffle between images.
  - **Black square/black square with divider**: How you want to view your images for comparison, e.g. side by side or top and bottom.

- **Reverse clock sign**: Shows Historical Exams, i.e. past scans.
- **Brightness sign**: Which window you want to view. Explained later.
- **Ruler sign**: Generates a ruler on screen so you can measure stuff.
- **Right click elements**:
  - **The obvious**: Zoom, Flip/Rotation, Historical Exams (for all past scans).
  - **Window**: Very useful as it focuses on the density segments for given tissues, e.g. Chest/Lung Window for Chest CTs as low-density resolution is the focus as lungs are less dense and Abdomen Window for Abdo CTs as it's more dense. Mostly for CTs but useful in X-rays. Another useful feature is 'Invert' as it shows the negative image and sometimes lights up consolidation and other pathology very well. Always try it.

CTs

Your Radiology and Surg Regs probably know much more about these so pick their brains. However, generally:

- **Click Pause button** when scrolling through the CT: Prevents bumpiness when scrolling.
- **Click Play button** to 'play' or auto-scroll the whole CT. If you need to send a video to your Reg.
- All above general rules still apply.
- **Look at all views**: Axials may be classical, but Coronals are great, especially with Chest/Abdo. Sagittals are also useful, especially in CT brains/spines.
- **Check phases**: Scroll down the list of CTs on the left panel and check the phases, e.g. non-contrast, arterial, portal venous. They all show different information and different elements light up. This is Pathology and System specific, so ask your Regs. Just be aware it exists and try to look through each.

KEY POINTS

- Always jump to the correct Results subclassification tab to focus your attention, e.g. choose the relevant tab using the Navigator.
- Use the Tear Off function to simultaneously view Results and input your Progress notes.
- Patient Care Results (or similar equivalent) includes *all* Nurse-inputted data and many important Results, e.g. weight, bowel chart, BSLs, GCS, UA, ketones, outputs.
- Use I-View, Advanced Graphing, Obs chart as alternative sources to find these.
- Use the 'Graphing' function to obtain trends of the Results. Can graph multiple Results against each other.
- Use the 'Eye'/'Bookmark' to record having 'read' new Results.
  - o Instant update any time a new result appears.
  - o Needs daily maintenance to mark 'read'.
- Radiological images – many tips to view/extract the images; see section 'Radiology'.

ORDERING INVESTIGATIONS

Your favourite Job.

A big part of your life is Ordering Investigations. And though, of course, you should all be using great care and diligence in Ordering the Investigation, tailoring to the clinical scenario and appropriately requesting tests to clarify the clinical picture and only order those which will alter your clinical Management of the patient, etc. etc. or so the book says; the fact of life is, you're Ordering the same Investigations again and again, most of the time.

And whatever's said about the actual judgement, it's indisputable that the actual process of Ordering is the same. And sameness = minimise = automate.

Hence, to shorten the process maximally (ideally telepathically, but if not that currently), there's only one golden rule in ordering Investigations.

Always use the ScratchPad (almost)

That is, always order from the Home Screen. For some reason, the Home Screen seems to have the processing power of the whole eMR system and leaves probably 1% of the RAM for everywhere else, all else being so slow by comparison.

So, to prevent more life being wasted on waiting for eMR (along with all the other mortal hazards of being a Doctor, including waiting for lifts, waiting for Echo reports to appear on the system, finding WOWs, looking for charts and waiting for coffee), Order everything from the Home Screen.

Follow the tips from the Home Screen section, but only for uncommon tests, i.e. search and Order.

However, for *common* tests, there's an even better way.

A way to order thirty Bloods in as many seconds (depending on how long your password is and how trigger happy you are with the mouse).*

A way where there's no need to fill in every yellow box every time (which obstructs you until you put something in it, like a baby bird's mouth), e.g. choose 'No' to 'Clinician collect' again or put in the time or who knows what else.

A way which allows one click of the big button called 'Order', sign for it and the Job is done.

How are we to harness this way, *the* way? (Fear not, we can hear you shouting through the pages.)

Very easily.

Just follow the instructions below and you'll soon be able to complete the Investigation Orders even as the words fall from the Senior's lips, or even slightly before then.

PRINCIPLES

Use Favourites.

This is the way. You must use the 'Favourites' function.

What is Favourites?

Essentially, it's a prefilled Order, set up how *you* like it. Every test saved as a 'Favourite' will be ordered in exactly the same way as it was saved and needs only your signature to complete.

Once you've correctly set up this system, Ordering Bloods, Allied Health Consults, and various swabs, urines and Imaging will no longer be the nightmare time vampire of 4.45–7.45 p.m.; it'll be almost instantaneous and certainly subcortical.

You'll no longer need to look for the test. You'll no longer need to fill in all those details again and again. For each Blood. Of each patient. You won't need to put in your pager for the nth time.

Just click, sign and done.

---

* In no way does this advocate blind ordering of tests. Of course, always take into careful consideration the clinical necessity when you order any Investigation. CRPs cost >$100 each.

Below we'll show how to set up the 'Favourites' in such a way to make even Ordering Bloods for fifty Surgical patients over the weekend faster than saying the tests, and how to effectively organise your 'Orders' so that every common Investigation is at your fingertips.

SETTING UP YOUR FAVOURITES

1. **Get tests**: Search for the test(s) you want to 'Favourite-ify' in ScratchPad.

2. **Order**: When all found, click the 'Sign' button (top-right corner; looks like an envelope with a number indicating the number of tests ordered). If you haven't set it up before, it'll take you automatically to the classic Orders page (after entering data into the 'Clinical History' box, etc.).

3. **Input data**: Now, for once, and once only in your life, you'll need to input all the things they ask for, manually. Do it *exactly as you normally want it, daily*.

   This'll be how it's prefilled for you, every time, forever more.

   If they're the same class of tests, e.g. Blood, also highlight (click and drag) them all and input once for their common fields, e.g. 'Clinician Collect, Y/N' or 'Date/Time'. Note this dragging doesn't help if different types of tests are selected together, e.g. FBC and Wound Swab, so use 'hold+Ctrl' and select the same classes. Also, remember to leave blank the sections which *need* adjusting *each* time, e.g. 'Patient Weight' for MRIs.

4. **Add to favourites**: Now, highlight the tests in your List of Orders that you want to put in one folder/category (click, hold and drag)→Right click→Select 'Add to Favourites'. This will bring up a 'Favourites' window.

5. **Generate folders**: Click 'Create Folders' and create various useful categories (common ones detailed in section 'Folders/categories') and place those selected tests in the appropriate folders.

6. **Repeat**: Repeat the process for different rafts of tests or simply select a created folder to put a new test into it.

7. **Start ordering**: You are *done*. Go to Home Screen, where Investigations is expanded under the ScratchPad search bar, and you'll see all your folders or tests right there, with one big 'Order' button next to it. Enter the folders as needed.

   Now, each 'Favourite' test will be ready, one click away, and you need only input the 'Clinical History' or the variable data, but with *every* other field pre-filled and ready to sign.

8. **Sign** and **Order** away

> **NB**: YOU CAN'T ADD GROUP AND HOLD TO YOUR FAVOURITES FOR SOME REASON.

FOLDERS/CATEGORIES

Now, though the 'Favourites' system is very streamlined, organisation into folders is critical. You'll have many Favourites, maybe thirty different items which are very common (Orders systems work for *all* Investigations, including Radiology- and Nursing-involved Investigations, e.g. urine MCS, as well as Medications in eMeds), besides various rarer tests you'll order again and again in various Terms, e.g. Autoimmune Screen on Rheumatology.

Now, since the 'Order' tab on the Home Screen is limited in size, you can't fit that many there. And you don't want to scroll through a hundred different ANA, ENA and dsDNA tests looking for the daily FBC Orders.

Hence, arrange all your tests into folders, each made of rafts of tests you usually order together and, since you can easily fit some ten or twelve folders there, this will ease the screen squinting and finger work. Then, click and order away.

We suggest the following categories.

Bloods

Common Bloods

The ones ordered all the time, every Term, and After Hours. Good to keep relatively steady so you don't have to keep changing them as you move across rotations. Plus you can stay in one folder when ordering dailies. For example, FBC, EUC, CMP, LFT, CRP, APTT, INR, troponin, BSL, blood culture, Add On tests, β-HCG (more in ED and mostly in women), amylase/lipase (mostly ED also), VBG (often ED), ABG.

Geris Bloods

Most will go through a Geris rotation and most Consultants seem to want these at some point of the Admission or in Consults. So this is useful in the Term and in ED when Consultants ask for them as you Admit. For example, TFTs, vitamin B12, folate, iron studies, vitamin D (+/− syphilis antibodies).

Specialty-specific screens

Obviously Specialty specific, so no rush to set these up unless you're doing that Term. However, very handy once set up, especially when you're Consulting that Team. For even as they bombard you with their standard screen, you can check them off on screen.

The below list is a general, non-exhaustive suggestion so tailor to your Terms and Reg tastes. There's much crossover so think what's appropriate. Also, everyone probably needs the normal blood set.

- **Haemolysis**: Blood film review, LDH, reticulocytes, unconjugated bilirubin, haptoglobin, direct antiglobulin test, G6PD, ANA +/− other autoimmune tests, CD55/CD59/PNH testing.
- **Thrombophilia**: Anti-cardiolipin Ab (antibody), EPG, IEPG, protein C, protein S, homocysteine, anti-thrombin III, prothrombin genotype, factor V

Leiden genotyping, lupus anticoagulant, activated protein C resistance +/– autoimmune tests.

- **Rheum/autoimmune**: ANA, ENA, dsDNA, rheumatoid factor, cryoglobulin, ESR, C3, C4, IgG subclasses, ACPA, uric acid +/– viral.
- **Gastro/liver**: Faecal calprotectin, ceruloplasmin, serum copper, iron studies, viral, autoimmune, e.g. ANA/IgG subclasses, anti-smooth muscle Ab, anti-microsomal Ab, anti-mitochondrial Ab, alpha-1-antitrypsin, serum paracetamol, urine drug screen, toxicology screen, anti-liver kidney microsomal Ab, cancer screen (e.g. AFP, CA19-9).
- **Renal**: Autoimmune, EPG, IEPG, ASOT, anti-DNAse B, CK, anti-GBM, PLA2-R, serum free light chains, urine protein/albumin creatinine ratio, urine protein, urine creatinine, urine electrolytes, urine osmolality, osmolality.
- **Viral**: Hep B core Ab, Hep B surface Ab, Hep B surface Ag, Hep C Ab, Hep A serology, Hep E Ab, Hep D Ab, HIV 1 and 2 Ab, EBV, CMV.
- **Cancer Bloods**: CEA, CA125, CA 19-9, CA15-3, AFP (α-fetoprotein), β-HCG, Chromogranin-A, PSA.
- **Endocrine**: ACTH, cortisol, metanephrine (plasma and urine), plasma catecholamine, HbA1C, C-peptide, fructosamine, vitamin D 125 dihydroxy level/25 hydroxy level, TFTs, TRAb, thyroglobulin, sex hormones.
- Etc.

This arrangement not only makes ordering the infinity of tests easier but also helps your learning, for, by sheer reviewing and grouping, one learns they're together and strengthens the association in the mind between certain tests and pathologies.

Every place will have its own little quirks, just know them or ask the Reg to tell you and then create the 'Favourites' folder for it. It'll save much time in the Term and out of it.

Nursing Orders

Another very common raft of tests is Nursing Orders – tests which require help from Nurses.

Includes Investigations of every type of body fluid which is sampled without any major intervention; namely, swabs, poo, wee, sputum, wounds, stomas, fluid from other orifices, etc. You get the idea.

Again, you can standardise the format (yes, it's almost always 'Clean catch urine') and ready them all under a folder that can be called 'Urine/Poo/Swabs' but you may wish to name it something more edifying.

Again, these are just like Bloods, very common, and if you can order at will, it'll save much time.

These include specifically:

- **Poo**: VRE screen (nasal and rectal), faecal bacterial screen, *C. diff*, faecal ova and cysts and parasites, faeces viral screen.

- **Wee**: Urine microscopy, culture, sensitivities (virtually everyone who walks into Hospital), and a lot more but Specialty specific, usually Renal or Urology, e.g. urine microalbumin/creatinine ratio and urine cytology, and urine Biochem of all sorts, e.g. urine sodium, glucose, protein, metanephrine, etc.

- **Phlegm**: Respiratory rapid nucleic acid detection (aka rapid viral/flu swab), respiratory virus RNA detection (longer version of previous), sputum culture, culture swab nasal/pharynx/tonsil, acid-fast bacilli.

- **Surgical**: Wound swabs, body fluid crystal examination, body fluid culture. (Leave 'Body site' and 'Specimen type' blank so it'll be all-purpose. And it's indeed very versatile. Look at what it includes. You'll never be at a loss.)

- **Other orifices** that are swabable: Eye culture, ear culture, etc.

- **Miscellaneous**: MRSA screen (you'll be hassled about these).

> **NB:** IF YOU CAN'T REMEMBER ALL THESE, JUST SET THEM ALL UP AND YOU WON'T NEED TO.

Essentially, the list includes every orifice a probe can reach, and as each secretion of the body is swabable/culturable/investigatable, you just need to get a feel for what's common and make it easy to access.

> **NB:** THESE TESTS OFTEN CAUSE FRUSTRATION AS IT'S A MYSTERY WHEN THEY'RE DONE, IF AT ALL, EVEN IF THE ORDER FORM IS PRINTED, PUT IN THE FOLDER/SOMEONE'S HAND, HANDED OVER AND DOCUMENTED IN THE NOTES. BUT, REMEMBER, A LOT OF NURSING IS SHIFT WORK SO THINGS MAY GET MISSED, ESPECIALLY IF YOU HAND OVER AT THE TRANSITION BETWEEN SHIFTS OR TO THE NURSE NOT LOOKING AFTER THE PATIENT. SIMILARLY, PATIENTS TEND NOT TO PEE/POO ON SCHEDULE. JUST CHILL AND KEEP TRYING.

Allied Health

Before a patient is for Discharge, you'll find there's someone(s) other than the Boss who must give the nod. Allied Health. You may fix the patient Medically, but if they can't walk that's not much of a cure.

Sometimes known as the SWOT Team or PSWOTD (Physio, Podiatry, Social Work, Speech Path, OT, Dietician), you'll find that you often need their help, usually at least one group for each Specialty and all of them in Geris. But you need to ask fast, as their schedule fills up quickly. Again, you'll need to build a similar rapid system to Order their Consults. For though your 90-year-old NOF (neck-of femur fracture) may need PT, without the Order no one will know.

Again, similar rules, try to input as much as possible that is generic or very common, e.g. pager number, and save these Consults in their own folder. You can even input the reason for referral as usually it's one common one and you can adjust it if necessary. Besides, you can always put the tailored version in the 'Clinical History' as required. As for urgency, it's usually Discharge dependent. The closer they are to Discharge, the more urgent. Hence, if you get in early, you don't need to be.

That said, try to put in the Order only when the patient can engage with Allied Health. Not necessarily entirely cured, but can engage. It's hard for the tubed patient to demonstrate how they usually make tea to OT or mobilise with PT.

- **PT (Physio)**: For everyone who needs to walk. And has trouble. Main thing to remember is if the baseline is very poor, e.g. sling hoist, or exceptionally good like an Olympian and they just had a UTI for 3 days, they probably won't benefit much from PT. So try not to Order it then. Also good for chest physio, if the patient needs help passing secretions.

- **OT**: More complex, as they cover many roles, but if the patient needs equipment, has difficulty doing daily ADLs or needs cognitive/functional Assessments, they'll probably need OT. However, generally don't Order OT for nursing home patients. Check your Institution's policy. To get Rehab, often needs support from at least PT and OT (documented).

- **S/W (Social Work)**: If there are social risk factors, e.g. homeless, vulnerability, and/or the patient needs Services at home, S/W can deal with the situation. If they need any sort of nursing home placement or when you hear a lot of acronyms such as ACAT, TACP, RACF, NCAT, etc., S/W is essential. If they need some sort of support outside of Hospital, S/W can help. If they're very high-functioning, well-supported and generally extremely contented human beings with every aspect of life, save this gallbladder or pneumonia, S/W probably won't be helping much.

- **Dictician**: Stuff to do with food. You are what you eat and though most of us would probably benefit from such a Consult, still, it's often essential for patients where diet is one of the main therapies or heavily affected. Many Cardio, Gastro, Renal and GI Surgical patients require such education. Often Reg initiated, but you can suggest. Dieticians also are good at various feeds, especially in Surgery and Geris, such as NG/NJ/JJ/TPN feeds.

- **Speech Path**: Often Nursing initiated, called any time that someone looks like they might choke. You should look out for it too, i.e. anyone at risk of aspiration or has swallowing difficulties probably warrants such an Assessment. Also helps with communication Issues, e.g. post stroke. Consider Neuro, ENT, Respiratory and GI causes for at risk patients.

- **Podiatry**: Anything to do with feet. Consider diabetic foot ulcers.

There are more Allied Health disciplines but these are the common ones. How often you need the others is Term and Institution dependent. If you Consult them more than twice in the first week, build a 'Favourite' for them for, chances are, you'll need them many times more.

Imaging

This is the other bread and butter of Jobs and, like Bloods, can be standardised. It's mostly not worth Favourite-ifying all the Imaging, for most you'll use only on a few occasions as Imaging is highly anatomy dependent. But for common ones in Term, it's certainly still worthwhile.

Again, highly Term dependent, but, as a minimum, have the following:

- **Chest X-ray**: By virtue of being in Hospital scores you one. Besides, as pneumonia, APO, CCF, perforation, COPD, pneumothorax, etc. are so common, this is definitely the top test. Also useful for confirming NGT/PICC/etc. placement.
- **Abdo X-ray (supine and erect)**: There's much constipation, SBO, LBO, etc. in Hospital and this helps with the Assessment.
- **Pelvis X-ray**: Falls are common. Broken hips are also common.
- **CTB (CT brain)**: Everyone with anything neurological seems to get one, so in ED and on Wards, especially Neuro, this is a high-demand test. Also for people who fall on heads on warfarin.
- **MRI brain**: Easy to order but hard to get.
- **CT AP (CT abdomen pelvis)**: For anyone who has something wrong in the tummy region, whether we are sure of it or not. Basically half the Hospital and most of ED.
- **CTPA (CT pulmonary angiogram) +/− VQ scan**: 'PE, could it be PE?' is always the question asked. Now, you'll know. Very common in After Hours, and Respiratory and Cardiac Terms.
- **Abdomen ultrasound**: This is similar to CT AP, and often in Gastro or Surgical Terms. Often for gallbladders and livers.
- **CT BCAP (CT brain, chest, abdomen, pelvis)**: Often used for cancer staging.
- **Echocardiography**: Essential in Surgical and Cardio Terms, the latter for obvious reasons, the former to assess for fitness for surgery. There are more criteria you can't prefill here, but something is better than nothing.

The critical thing in Imaging is, of course, the History and differentials you give. Hence, the money is in the 'Clinical History' box or calling/going to Radiology. So standardise the Order form. As Imaging is so time dependent, anything that speeds up the Order process will help you get those scans. Make these as ready to Order as Bloods and your scan is one step closer to getting done.

MODIFICATIONS

As mentioned, your 'Favourite' should serve you fine 99% of the time. But there are, occasionally, modifications. You're at a MET (Medical Emergency Team) call and there are no Blood collectors. MRIs with different weights. Getting Physio for a reason other than 'Mobility'. Your Bloods need to happen at a specific time, not 5 a.m. And so on.

So you need to change things … .

Modifying a Standard

In other words, changing a one-off. Same way as usual, except click 'Modify' instead of 'Sign' after you click the ScratchPad 'Sign' button. This will take you back to the standard 'Orders' page and you can modify whatever needs modifying. Even if you forget to press that button, but remember later, simply cancel when you actually need to sign for it and that'll achieve the same effect.

Modifying the Standard

This is in cases where your whole standard Order needs to change, e.g. when you're changing Term and the pager changes or you're in ED and everything becomes 'Clinician Collect'.

This is one of the only times you have to go to 'Orders' (sorry, we lied when we said never).

Go to the 'Order' tab→Click 'ADD'→Under the 'Star' button→Click down arrow →Click 'Modify Favourites'→Now you can add or delete stuff as needed.

Unfortunately, you can't directly modify the 'Favourite' you've already saved, so you'll need to delete the old 'Favourite' and recreate it via the whole process as per section 'Set-up'.

BLOOD RULES AND MYTHS

Since Ordering Bloods is another one of the profound things that JMOs do, and it occupies a proportionately large part of our time, we think it warrants some extra rules and myth busting to make this section as smooth and as little time draining as possible. So consider the following…

Myth: Weekend Bloods can be done via ScratchPad

This is semi-true, semi myth. There are two ways about this.

Using the standard Orders system

Enter the 'Orders' tab as if you were going to order Bloods. Usually→Click 'Star' for 'Favourites' and when you've found your 'Favourites' List of Bloods, just click the blood order, e.g. FBC, over and over again for however many days/times you need.

For example, if you need to order 3 days' worth of Bloods (or more, e.g. a public holiday), just pretend to order 1 day of Bloods, click through the set of tests you need, then click right over them all over again.

And keep going.

And going.

Just keep count in your own mind how many clicks you've made. The system will look like it's not responding (no uncommon thing for it). But it is. Just slower than the average speed of a speeding turtle.

For while it seems like nothing's happening (the Order itself will highlight, lag and look like it isn't responding), the system is actually recording the number of clicks you've made and adding them on accordingly. So keep count yourself and don't over-click or second guess yourself. Just keep cycling through the tests with the clicks.

When you're done, and the system finishes thinking, click done. And now the key thing is the sequence you've clicked everything. If you've done it in daily cycles, all you need to do is to highlight the whole lot of 1 day's set of Bloods (which will be adjacent to each other) and change the date of collection. For example, if ordering FBC, EUC, LFT, INR, click them in that order three times then highlight each set and change the dates to, for example, Saturday, Sunday and the Monday after.

If you've done it in a weird order that's confusing, then you'll have to confuse yourself further and modify the days of collection one by one or segment by segment.

But otherwise, through repeated clicking, i.e. reordering the one test repeatedly, in the right order, then separately altering the dates, you can sign once and the weekend is ready to go.

This'll save you ordering then signing three to five times, depending on how many public holidays are in between.

Using the ScratchPad: Modified

You can sort of use the ScratchPad, but it requires some organising. Suppose you're in the folder where you want to Order Bloods repeatedly. Go and click Order against the Bloods as usual. But, then, click the folder name in the directory of the ScratchPad itself (top of the ScratchPad Order section). The folder will reload, and you can click Order all over again. And again. Then, 'Sign' for it as usual, click 'Modify' instead of 'Sign' and it'll bring you to the standard Orders page for you to adjust the dates as above.

If you did click 'Sign' by accident, the system recognises too many repeat Orders so will try to force you to 'remove' all of them. Don't. Click 'Cancel' and it'll automatically bring you back to the standard 'Orders' page and you can continue as above.

This method requires you to similarly memorise how many cycles you've gone through, but slightly longer memory, so use as you prefer.

Myth: Your Bloods get randomly cancelled for no reason

While it may seem that way, that doesn't actually happen; even if it effectively does, there's a protocol reason for all those cancellations.

Go to the 'Orders' tab→'Dropdown' menu→'Completed Orders' or 'Cancelled Order' or 'Active Orders' which have been marked as 'Cancelled' and find your fugitive Bloods→Right click and click 'Order Information'→Go to the 'History' tab and it'll show you all the actions on the Blood Order, including the blood collector and reasons for non-collection.

You'll find some useful insights into why things were cancelled, including blood collector missed (rare enough), patient absent (more common) and duplicate Orders (even more common).

One of the most useful reasons is 'Patient Refusal' as this alerts you to chat with the patient and emphasise the importance of having Bloods taken (pretty common especially in Paeds) instead of trying to stalk down the blood collector, cross-examining them on why Bloods were not done on your patient for the fifth day in a row and being met with a 'Can you read?' response.

Myth: You must adjust the blood collection time to tomorrow mane 5 a.m. else Pathology won't collect

You generally don't need to adjust the time. For, whenever you Order, it'll automatically go to the next Blood round available (*not* just cancel), e.g. Orders after about 1 p.m. will go to next day (if you have a midday round).

> **NB:** WE HAVE CALLED PATHOLOGY. AND IF YOU DON'T BELIEVE US, CALL PATHOLOGY (DISCLAIMER: INSTITUTION DEPENDENT; CALL PATHOLOGY TO TRIPLE CONFIRM).

It's very worthwhile to confirm these details as it'll save you much trouble in future.

Many of these matters may seem rather trite and petty. We mean, how long does it take to click a date and write 5 a.m.? But for anyone who's been on a busy Term, when it's 7 p.m. and you're exhausted by a day of Clinical Reviews, Theatres/Clinics, extended WRs and Jobs, and you've been here since 6 a.m., then you realise you haven't Ordered Bloods for the next day.

For forty patients.

And you need to click through the date and times for each one. It will seem less trite then, but simple satisfaction to merely hit five buttons and sign, rather than adjusting for each person, and the accompanying agony as you click and fluff around for each patient, times forty, through incoordination secondary to sheer exhaustion.

Myth: 'Add Ons' happen even if the blood was taken in the last century as there's a giant blood place where they keep all blood forever

A related myth is that you can 'Add' an infinite number of 'Ons' to just one Biochem tube, so long as you keep *PowerCharting* it.

The fact is, you can only 'Add On' so much and for so many days after. Usually, try less than 48 hours. But to be sure, especially with important tests, always call Pathology to confirm if it can be added on at all. Better to know early than find out 5 days later that your 'Add On' was cancelled. Also, some tests can only be 'Added On' in shorter time frames and with special conditions, e.g. blood place on ice in foil, so check.

KEY POINTS

- Always use your Favourites section to order all common Orders (Investigations to Meds).
- A Favourite = all standard parameters/variables of the Order are already customised + prefilled to your standard specifications = one click + signature will place the Order.
- Anything you commonly Order or routine sets of tests, e.g. Liver screen should all be rendered into Favourites→See section 'Folders/categories' for classes.
- Set up your Favourites at the earliest opportunity→Instructions in section 'Setting up your Favourites'.
- Categorise all your Favourite Orders into logical categories, e.g. Regular Bloods, Imaging, Allied Health, Special blood sets, such as Autoimmune Screen, Common Medications, Nursing-assisted Investigations.
- Favourites can be modified→See section 'Modifications'.
- Weekend Bloods can be ordered via ScratchPad as long as you keep clicking the directory folder to refresh the folder→See section 'Blood rules and myths'.
- There's a limit to 'Add On(s)' for blood.

eMEDS

eMeds is increasingly rolled out through various Hospitals and will likely supersede paper Medication charts in time. You will receive extensive training in eMeds and it may also be subtly but significantly different between Hospitals.

The key is to stay focused during the training and make notes as needed as well as know where the manuals/IT support is if you need to reference it.

The aim here is not to teach eMeds (you'll have whole modules, online and in-person, on that), but to note areas you need to pay attention to as well as small tips to assist with smooth usage of the program.

Consider the following key functions.

ORDERING MEDICATIONS/FLUIDS

The process is essentially identical to Ordering an Investigation, so the same rules apply.

When entering the Medication in the search bar under 'Orders', often prefilled Medication/Fluid options appear with common doses/amounts. Select the one which closest resembles your intended Order. Note there is no need to type the whole name. A part (of even multiple words) will generate suggestions, e.g. 'sod chl' will generate 'sodium chloride 0.9% 1000 mL continuous infusion', one of perhaps a dozen options.

After choosing the most appropriate Order, check and modify it to the Order you want to chart. Apply the doses/rates, etc. you want. Most of it is self-explanatory. However, take particular care with 'First Dose Date/Time' as this indicates when you want to give the first dose (often important and can be adjusted for a future time). You can also use the 'Priority' function for STAT Orders. Also take care with the 'Stop Date/Time' as this allows you to pre-emptively plan for Medication cessation, especially antibiotics. As you would on paper charts, try to plan a regime in eMeds with these methods.

Favourites for Meds/Fluids is harder as each patient's requirements are different. However, note the 'Common Medications and doses' section as you can often save these as your Favourites. Common analgesia, antibiotic, anti-emetic, aperient, PPI, fluid, electrolyte/nutritional replacement regimes can be saved and applied almost instantaneously and as readily as your blood Orders. However, always remember to check before you Order. Modify as needed. This is a treatment, an intervention, not an Investigation, so much more care is needed.

If a Medication is very special, you may have to Order it under 'Unlisted Medications'.

MODIFYING MEDICATIONS/FLUIDS

Same process as modifying a regular Order. Go to the 'Medication List' tab and right click the Medication you want to modify. Mostly, 'Cancel/Reorder' is most useful to modify. If in doubt, you can cancel the Order completely and just restart. All other options are self-explanatory, e.g. 'Cancel/Discontinue', 'Suspend' to temporarily stop a Medication, 'Resume' to resume it, 'Reschedule administration time' (quite useful if you'd like to change the standard administration time of a Medication), 'Order Information' (for the information), 'Convert to Prescription' for potential Discharge Medications. You can also copy the Order by right clicking then 'Copy' if you're applying one Order multiple times, e.g. fluid bags.

VIEWING MEDICATIONS/FLUIDS

Can be viewed in Medications List, MAR (Medication Administration Record) and MAR Summary.

Medications List

Good to modify the Medication.

MAR

Good for seeing all the active Medications and when given (a small piece of text with dose correlating to time) and what will be given (in independent tab-like boxes or tiles). You can also cancel one-off doses of Medication by right clicking the tiles of Medication not yet dispensed and 'Chart Not Done' with the appropriate reason.

Change the dates you'd like to view by right clicking the top grey bar with dates and select 'Change Search Criteria' and apply the dates you'd like. Then, sidewards scroll at the bottom of the page to the date you want to view. The little arrows at top left/right can also increase/decrease times viewed by 1 day forward or back, e.g. you can choose to view 3 days of Medication dispensing or 2 days.

You can also change the administration time of Meds here by right clicking the Med itself on the left column, and selecting 'Reschedule Administration Times'. A pop-up will load with dosing options; you need to put in the new schedule and choose a dosing timetable you want, especially regarding when the next immediate dose is.

MAR is also useful for classifying Medications. On the left column, one can apply:

- **Time view**: Default application. Self-explanatory.
- **Route view**: Sorts all Meds by route given, useful for many things, e.g. knowing if any IV Meds remain so IVCs (intravenous cannulas) can be removed ASAP, Discharge planning (e.g. teaching patients to dispense new SC (subcutaneous) Meds) and other such practical/logistical considerations.
- **Therapeutic class view**: Sorted into many classes, including anti-infectives, anti-neoplastics, cardiovascular agents, CNS agents, coagulation modifiers, hormones/hormone modifiers, nutritional products, metabolic agents, etc. These can be further expanded into the finer pharmacological classes. Excellent way to check the Medication types that patients are on (especially if there are many home Meds) and summarise the patient's current Medication situation according to their Issues and focus on areas which need addressing, e.g. checking for DVT prophylaxis and anticoagulation, existing antibiotic regime, existing cardiac Medications. Uses are evidently endless.

MAR Summary

Best for seeing the history of all Medications dispensed. Regarding adjustment of the time frame and views, follow the same rule as in section 'MAR', i.e. you can sort into time/therapeutic/route views and adjust for the time frames you'd like to view. You may need to expand the 'Views' bar at top left to 'Show Views'. Also displays ceased Medications. You cannot modify the Medications.

OTHER KEY FUNCTIONS

There are many other functions of eMeds that are mostly self-explanatory. When the patient is Admitted, you need to document their Medications under 'Document Medications by History' and continue/modify/cease their home Medications under 'Admission Reconciliation'. When the patient is Discharged, a similar reconciliation of Medications will occur where Medications to continue/modify/cease/convert to prescription will be clarified in the 'Discharge Reconciliation'. A similar process is observed on Transfers.

You need to know how to prescribe Common Medications, e.g. warfarin, insulin, patches, fluids, electrolytes. You should also be aware of how to prescribe various standardised Medication plans, e.g. DVT prophylaxis or asthma exacerbation treatments. These are Hospital dependent and you need to learn them on the job. However, they are very handy as they include prefilled sets of Medication Orders, and you only need to select those you need. You need to know how to taper Medication doses (click the Taper sign and follow instructions). There will be other Hospital-specific bits and pieces.

Learn these from your Seniors, your peers, your IT. And learn them soon. For, at any time, you may need them.

KEY POINTS

- Apply the same principles to Ordering Medications/Fluids as for Investigations.
- Use similar Favourites categories as those stipulated earlier in *Chapter 2, Things to bring/Common Medications and doses.*
- Tweak settings to your specific preferences, e.g.
  o 'Priority' function for STAT Orders
  o 'Stop/End Time' to time a cessation of Medication, e.g. antibiotics
  o 'First Dose Date/Time' for first-dose timing.
- Orders can be copied if giving multiple times, e.g. Fluids bags via right click desired Order→Select 'Copy'.
- MAR view classifies Medications via various methods, e.g. admin time, drug class, administration route:
  o Can also cancel doses and modify regular administration schedules.
- MAR Summary view gives the History of actual Medication administration. Also can be classified.
- Consider the availability of Medication sets, e.g. DVT prophylaxis set, including TED (thrombo-embolus deterrent) stockings, heparin, enoxaparin, etc., or asthma exacerbation set, including weaning salbutamol regime, ipratropium, corticosteroids, etc.

DOCUMENTING

If it isn't documented, it didn't happen. Really? Yes, really.

Another irritating but very important tick box of your job is Documenting. Unfortunately, it's just one of those things in life which, though you dislike, you have to do, like taxes (unless you're a tax consultant). And it absorbs a tremendous amount of time. Probably half your job. At least.

We all know how to type. However, we don't really want to type. Especially the same things.

Again.

And again.

The good news is you don't actually have to type, for the majority of cases.

You're not writing a novel. You're writing a WR. And, usually, many things happen the same way, day in and day out. Hence, there's a way which you can both document and not document. Or, rather, someone else documents most of it and you just need to check their work. Who is this magical person (for perhaps you're thinking it's an eternal Medical Student) who doesn't make mistakes, doesn't ask questions when you're trying to hear the Plan and doesn't disappear after the round?

Templates.

The auto-text from which, with a quick key/code, beauteous, error-free prose flows.

But, just like your Student,* you need to train the Template. And, once trained, the Template is a thousand times faster, more accurate and more consistent, and is in constant attendance.

And, even better, you only need to train it, once.

The importance of Templates can't be overstated. In the electronic era, where everything must be written down, you can easily be buried if you don't avoid repetition. Nurses use it. Allied Health use it. Consultants use it in their Clinics. The world at large uses it. You should use it.

Suppose you were a Boss now, and you had a Medical secretary and a Dictaphone, you'd still need to tell your secretary how you'd like things done, at least once. And you'd still have to dictate each letter, forever more.

What if, after you taught the eMR system, this system could potentially be much faster than a secretary, act almost instantaneously and save you even the effort of dictating?

And yet this system is available to every person with a login. Only take a little time, a little thought and look forward to a personal assistant that will always be reliable, fast, correct and need no pay at all.

The new eMR.

Now this only works for two reasons.

First, Documenting is everywhere, from JMOs to Consultants.

Second, common things happen commonly (as is well known). And so, common Documenting happens commonly too.

Apart from slight differences, many scenarios, from the History, Examination and Investigations to treatments and Procedures, are almost exactly the same, time and time again, so, very quickly, you'll know most matters like the back of your hand. And you'll wish, instead of writing the same things for the nth time, that it would appear with the thought.

---

* Please note that we are in no way advocating that Students become Documenting automatons, or making any comparison between them whatsoever.

Now until true neural-to-computer interfacing happens or an ever-present attendant is around, that won't happen. But it can come close. Very close.

Templates.

You can use them anywhere. We include a common list below, but be creative. Tailor it to your job. You know what's most frustrating. Here's your chance to make it not so.

The main principle is anything which you type repetitively, consider Templating.

Anything where the format is the same and only set data points need changing, Template.

Anything with sameness, Template.

Anything that requires typing more than once, Template.

Templates can be long or short. Whole report formats can be Templated. Short phrases can be Templated. Paragraphs of common Assessments can be Templated. Even words can be Templated. 'Ophthalmologist' is liable to incorrect spelling. 'Eye' is not.

And as you cumulate, eventually, with a few key strokes, a few data points inputted, a few lines amended, you'll construct whole reports at a rate that even the fastest typist, for all their clatter of keyboards, cannot reach.

Common JMO Templatables could include (each detailed in relevant sections):

- Discharges
- WRs
- Short Common phrases, e.g. 'BO' for 'Bowels opened' or 'E&D' for 'eating and drinking/tolerating a normal diet'
- Consults/approvals
- Protocol-based reviews, e.g. IVC review, post-transfusion review
- Record of Procedure performed, e.g. IDC inserted
- Common Histories (relevant negatives, adjust if positive) for each body System, e.g. Neurological, or common reviews, e.g. Falls
- Common Examinations (relevant negatives, adjust if positive)
- Common Investigation sets, e.g. thrombophilia screen
- Common Management sets, e.g. hyperkalaemia (modify to situation)
- Combination of the four above Commons into sets to match common scenarios
- ED Case History/Discharges
- Beyond JMOs: case by case but adaptable to Consults, Operation reports, Procedural reports.

However, this list isn't exhaustive. Templates can be extended into whatever Specialty you pursue, whatever job you have, whatever your rank. For, everywhere, there'll be History, Examination, Investigations, Management and Procedures.

And, everywhere, they'll repeat themselves. And, where they do, Templates can be used.

> **NB:** TEMPLATES ARE MOST USEFUL WITH RELEVANT NEGATIVES AND NO PATHOLOGY. AS KNOWN, HAPPY FAMILIES ARE ALL ALIKE, UNHAPPY FAMILIES ARE EACH UNHAPPY IN THEIR OWN WAY. SIMILARLY, NORMALITY IS ALL ALIKE, WHILE PATHOLOGY IS PATHOLOGICAL IN ITS OWN WAY. FORTUNATELY, NORMALITY IS FAR MORE COMMON, AND WIDESPREAD, THAN PATHOLOGY. HENCE, BY TYPING THE PATHOLOGY, AND AUTOMATING THE REST, YOU'LL FIND THAT THERE ISN'T MUCH LEFT TO TYPE.

So, follow the principles above, and method below, and watch your Documenting automate as you become the Doctor, instead of writing about Doctor-ing.

KEY POINTS

- Aim for maximal automation and Templating.
- Use everywhere, stretching from as short as common phrases, such as 'observations stable afebrile', to entire reports, such as Discharge Summaries. Some examples are given below.
- Template everything that is ever repeated.

TEMPLATING METHODOLOGY

Hopefully, we've enticed you to make Templates your chief right arm in Documenting. Yet there are a few key methods to maximise their effectiveness and minimise their errors. Consider doing the following.

Create them

You know they're useful. But you just can't get around to it. Well, get around to it. They're very easy to make.

Literally highlight your text→Right click→Select 'Save as Autotext'→Brings up new window→Enter your shortcut code in 'Abbreviation' (what you type to activate the auto-text)→Your highlighted text is already in the main body, you can modify now as needed→Click 'Save'→Done.

You now have whole tracts of instantaneously generated text at your command. By typing the 'abbreviation', the saved text will instantly be summoned and shave hours off your documentation.

Remember, always err on the side of excessive generation. It won't hurt if you make a few extra/useless Templates. It will if you must keep typing infinitely.

Use them

Remember to use them. It'll be clunky at the start. But it'll soon fly. Make that mental effort to use the auto-text instead of typing. It'll be habit soon enough. On the flip side, avoid Templates obstructing you. The best method is capitalising the Template keyword or adding a symbol before it, e.g. '#'. You can thus avoid triggering the Template's generation when you just want to type the word itself, e.g. '#FOLLOWUP' instead of 'follow up'. Also reminds you to use the Template as suggestions will appear as you type the first letter.

Read them

It's tempting to Template and go. But don't. Always read through it carefully. You've already saved the time typing. Read what you've 'written'. This will prevent 99% of errors. Don't grudge the reading. This ensures accuracy and prevents you from writing something stupid, e.g. the intubated patient who you examine as 'alert and orientated'. The system may type fast, but it doesn't know if what you've written doesn't make sense. You do.

Update them

Templates become unsuitable, especially with different circumstances, e.g. new Terms, new Regs, etc. Anytime you feel you're constantly tweaking the Template, update it. It's easy.

When in the Documenting window, simply click the third button from the right, which shows a small document with a red arrow to a larger document→aka 'Manage Autotext'→Search for your auto-text by entering the 'abbreviation'→When you find it, click 'Edit'→Edit the text as you like→Click 'Save'→Done.

Your auto-text is now updated.

Add to them. Delete parts of them. Modify. The effort is always a hundred times repaid.

Error-proof them

The biggest pitfall with Templates is incorrect documentation due to generic use of the Template without thinking. We advocate three methods to prevent this.

1. **Read it**: Mentioned above.
2. **Build in fail-safes**: Whenever there are options or choices in your Documenting, always leave '_' blanks. Clicking F3 automatically jumps to them in eMR, or you can use Ctrl+F in any other program. Then, you can simply indicate the option/direction you want, e.g. positive or negative, yes or no, '_fe/male' to remind yourself to indicate whether male/female. The point of the fail-safe is to force your attention on areas of Documenting where you *must* make a decision. This makes a Template both versatile and error proof. Essentially, it turns your Documenting into forms which are mostly filled out. You just need to fill in the final yes/no. And with well-placed '_' blanks, you'll be reminded to *look* for what's needed as well as document accurately. Your attention is thus focused only on areas of the document needing your input and not wasted on

extraneous details. Hence, centre your fail-safes around their precise place-ment and use them as a compass to guide your documentation and even assist your Assessment.

Remember especially to place '_' before every multiple optioned Template, e.g. '... on behalf of Dr _ X/Y/Z'. You'll be reminded to pick one, and not include all of them.

Another benefit of this fail-safe is it prevents you from writing something inaccurate if you forget as the blank will render the phrases null and nonsen-sical if you don't input appropriately. However, you'll never forget because ... (see next point).

3. **F3/Ctrl+F check**: Documents can get long and you're often doing them inter-mittently. To trawl through the whole thing is hard. However, you don't want to miss any blanks or have your fail-safes trip you over. Hence, when about to sign off, click F3 or Ctrl+F for your 'blanks' items, e.g. '_' or other symbol. This automatically screens your whole document and identifies anything you've missed for you to instantly address. And it's virtually 100% accurate.

Borrow them

We understand that effort is a great barrier to many things. Hence, reduce that barrier. Inherit Templates from previous JMOs, who are mostly more than happy to help. Share and apportion Template creation with colleagues. Remember to use in-built system auto-texts. This is variable between Hospitals, but, often, the system can input system data directly with certain keystrokes. For example, 'T' in certain fields auto-populates today's date, 'N' populates current time, '.VitalSigns' populates the patient's latest vital signs in beautiful format. '.Weight' or '.Allergies' populates the current weight and allergies. '.' or '/' followed by various denotations can populate extensive pre-existing Templates with current eMR data. As these are not universal, the best way is to ask/call IT, especially at Orientation, to sim-plify your life ASAP. Alternatively, test out these functionalities yourself to see what's most suitable for you.

Keyboard shortcuts

We include these here as they will make your Documenting life (especially edit-ing) considerably easier. You should master shortcuts, else the JMO years will be very long, especially in front of the WOW/COW. Many Windows/Office shortcuts do work, with exceptions. Notable ones to use include:

- **Home/End button +/– Shift**: You always want to change something at the beginning or end in your documentation. Avoid the arrow or mouse's search and get there now. Also, you always want to delete whole lines of text. Use 'Shift+Home/End' for instantaneous modifications.

- **Ctrl+arrow +/– Shift**: So your modification is in the middle of the line? Just waiting for the cursor to move as you hold the arrow key is painful. 'Ctrl+arrow' skips between words. Much easier. Add 'Shift' and you can highlight specific blocks of texts to edit.

- **Windows sign + arrow (four directions)**: Changes the Window size. 'Up' arrow for maximise, 'left/right' to shift window to occupy left or right half of screen, 'down' to shrink and two 'downs' to minimise. Useful for typing data from two windows and quickly alternating.
- **Escape**: Sometimes closes various open Investigation reports.
- **Page up/down**: Gets through reports quicker.
- The raft of other common shortcuts, e.g. MS Office ones, Ctrl+A (Select All), Copy/Cut/Paste, etc., Alt+Tab.

Below, we will discuss each of the key types of Documenting and how each can be made faster, more efficient and accurate, starting with the chief document you go through daily, the Ward Round.

> **NB:** AGAIN, IF YOU DON'T HAVE A FULLY COMPUTERISED MEDICAL RECORD SYSTEM, YOU CAN STILL MAKE USE OF THE TIPS HERE INCLUDED. REMEMBER, WHEREVER YOU NEED PRINTED DOCUMENTS, INSTEAD OF SAVING IN eMR, SAVE ALL YOUR TEMPLATES IN A MASTER WORD FILE. THIS IS ALMOST AS EFFICIENT AS ALL YOU NEED, INSTEAD OF A BEING A FEW CLICKS AWAY, WILL JUST BE A USB AWAY. EVERYONE (LIKELY) HAS WORD OR SOME SORT OF WORD-PROCESSING PROGRAM, IF NOT eMR.

KEY POINTS

- Create Templates ASAP→Highlight text, right click and select 'Save as Autotext'. Follow instructions in the text.
- Make using Templates a habit.
- Always review your documents/Templates for errors.
- Update/revise them as circumstances change, e.g. Terms, via 'Manage Autotext'.
- Leave '_' blanks or build in options, e.g. male/female in your Templates to allow for selection of options and reduce chances of errors.
- Move between '_' blanks with the F3 key in eMR or Ctrl+F outside it.
- Borrow/inherit/share Templates from your predecessors and colleagues.
- Use routine keyboard shortcuts to assist in Documenting→See section 'Keyboard shortcuts'.

WARD ROUNDS

Who cares who was at the WR so long as the patient is treated? Ah yes, medico-legal does, who, by the by, never reads any of your notes until something blows up. Then, every comma will be scrutinised. So how to beat those odds, when you, who must write everything, every day, are pitched against those who don't need to write or read your documents except that one instance you didn't write?

Templates (as mentioned).

Only an automated system that minimises error rates is sufficient against any patrol.

The WR is one of the chief forms of interaction with the patient and all other HCWs. It's also official. It, like all other Documenting, is a legal document. Nurses won't do certain things unless you document. Hence, WR documentation is extremely important, as it's the centre of communication from the Team to everyone else regarding the patient's care. So you need to get it right, and quickly.

You'll get a feel very quickly of what the Team wants written. And if you don't get a feel, the Team will tell you. And as soon as you know, set up the Template immediately.

Every Team has its particular quirks about what it wants documented. Again, ask. But some general guides (and Templates) are below for *every Term*.

XXX [Your Term's name] **Ward Round – surname 1, surname 2, etc.** [Surname of everyone who was there, in order of seniority, including yourself]

Progress
[Progress]

On Examination (O/E)
[Obs]
[Other Exam findings]

Plan
[The most important part]

Now is where everyone starts to get different.

Surgical documentation

Usually short. The above is almost complete +/– you can note what sort of Operation the patient is getting/got, day X in the first line. In addition, Surgeons often want to know various inputs/outputs, especially of drains/stomas, temperatures and days of antibiotics. Other things will be Term specific; however, they're often more keen to know than necessarily documented, though, of course, this is surgeon dependent.

The most important part is the Plan, which you should pay meticulous attention to. The entire Surgical thought process is not often transcribed as Surgeons want to get to Theatre and they have only 1 hour to see fifty patients. Hence, they're unlikely to detail to you everything they've been looking for and essentially just tell you what to do. So, document as much other stuff as you can, but be absolutely certain the Plan is clear. If the Plan isn't clear even to you, make sure you ask.

Surgeons always walk super-fast, so you'll have a disadvantage there, especially while you're pushing the WOW in dress shoes while they're in comfy crocs and are pushing nothing, apart from you psychologically.

However, get as much as you can out of them on the WR, shout after their departing shadow when needed and, if still unclear, just march into Theatre. There, you have the advantage for they're scrubbed and glued to the table (so to speak), with immense difficulty even in opening doors to escape you, while you're quite mobile and can pester them with questions that they'll just have to answer to get rid of you. Yes, they may make you wait, and may become annoyed. But that's much better than a wrong Plan and a sick patient.

Hence, relatively easy if there weren't so many to write for, so keep it sharp.

Medical documentation

More extensive and detailed. Consider the following:

XXX [Your Term's name] **Ward Round – surname 1, surname 2, etc.** [Surname of everyone who was there, in order of seniority, including yourself]

XXX-year-old male/female admitted for XXX with a background/complicated by XXX

Progress
[Progress]

On Examination (O/E)
[Obs]
[Other Exam findings]

Investigations
[Pertinent Ix]

Issues/Impression
[Main Impression or Issues List]

Plan
[The most important part]

In detail

Opening

> ### XXX-year-old male/female admitted for XXX with a background/complicated by XXX

Often, many Seniors would like an opening statement giving the context of the patient. You should do that with Surgical Rounds too, but the patient's stay is usually too short to forget, the turnover is too high and you really don't have time, so you'll have to make do within the limitations of reality.

However, in Medical Rounds, as you mostly spend more than 2 minutes per patient, it's presumed you'll have time to note these things.

Usually, you can copy from the day before to each new day's note, just as a fresh reminder for your hundred-day stay patient, why they're still here. In case you've ever forgotten.

Progress (what happened)

This is the History. Here, you write down everything that happened on the WR, including the patient's answers to your questions, your answers to the patient's questions, concerns, complaints and other happenings observed, e.g. overnight reviews, acknowledgements of Consulted Teams (always have '_ *input noted with thanks*' via auto-text key) and other salient happenings.

The style will be variable. You'll develop according to your own style and the Team's. Some may want verbatim; others want you to synthesise what the questions were pointing at, e.g. 'No infective symptoms' versus 'No cough, coryzal symptoms, fever, pain, diarrhoea, nausea/vomiting, dysuria'. Some may want both. Satisfy your Team.

Consults and the Admission Note (i.e. first meetings with patients) tend to have longer documentation. It'll often appear that a Long Case was done with the full History of the Presenting Complaint, Past Medical History, Family History, Social History (SHx), Examination, Investigations, Impression/Issues, Plan. Good to set up a Template for these cases also or use the ED Template.

Subsequently, 'Progress' will shorten and only detail daily matters.

On Examination (what was seen)

Variable depending on the Reg's Examination style. However, you should have a generic Template for a normal general Examination and possibly some Term-specific ones if the general one doesn't work, e.g. a Neuro Examination Template (Table 4.1).

Table 4.1 An example of a General and Neuro Examination Template

General Examination	Neuro Cranial Nerve Examination

• Alert and orientated
• Peripheries warm and perfused
• Mucous membranes moist
• JVPNE (jugular venous pressure not elevated)
• HSDNM (heart sounds dual no murmurs)
• Chest clear
• ASNT (abdomen soft non-tender)
• BS (bowel sounds) present
• Calves SNT (soft non-tender)
• Nil peripheral oedema
• Nil cellulitis/rashes apparent
	• CN (cranial nerve) II, III, IV, V
	  o Visual acuity intact: (–/–)
	  o PEARL (pupils equal and reactive to light) and normal accommodation
	  o Nil diplopia
	  o Extraocular movements intact
	  o No nystagmus
	• CN V, VII
	  o Normal power in mastication muscles
	  o Normal power in muscles of facial expression
	  o Normal sensation in V1, V2, V3 in domains of _
	• CN VIII
	  o Hearing grossly intact in L/R
	  o Rinne's test:
	  o Weber's test:
	• CN IX, X, XI, XII
	  o No tongue or uvular deviation, no fasciculations
	  o No hoarseness of voice
	  o Normal power in trapezius
	  o Normal power in SCM
	  o Normal strength in muscles of tongue

Neuro Upper Limb Examination	**Neuro Lower Limb Examination**

• Neurologically grossly intact
• Nil obvious abnormalities on inspection
• Tone normal L/R
• Upper limbs power:
  o Shoulder abduction Left/Right= 5/5
  o Shoulder adduction Left/Right= 5/5
  o Elbow extension Left/Right= 5/5
  o Elbow flexion Left/Right= 5/5
  o Wrist extension Left/Right= 5/5
  o Wrist flexion Left/Right= 5/5
  o Finger abduction Left/Right= 5/5
  o Finger adduction Left/Right= 5/5
  o Finger extension Left/Right= 5/5
  o Finger flexion Left/Right= 5/5
• Upper limb reflexes:
  o Biceps normal L/R
  o Triceps normal L/R
  o Brachioradialis normal L/R
• Coordination:
  o Nil dysmetria L/R
  o Nil dysdiadochokinesia L/R
• Sensation: Normal in all domains assessed, including:
	• Neurologically grossly intact
	• Nil obvious abnormalities on inspection
	• Tone normal L/R. Nil clonus
	• Lower limbs power:
	  o Hip abduction Left/Right= 5/5
	  o Hip adduction Left/Right= 5/5
	  o Hip extension Left/Right= 5/5
	  o Hip flexion Left/Right= 5/5
	  o Knee extension Left/Right= 5/5
	  o Knee flexion Left/Right= 5/5
	  o Ankle extension Left/Right= 5/5
	  o Ankle flexion Left/Right= 5/5
	  o Ankle plantar flexion Left/Right= 5/5
	  o Ankle dorsiflexion Left/Right= 5/5
	• Lower limb reflexes:
	  o Knee normal L/R
	  o Ankle normal L/R
	  o Plantar normal L/R
	• Coordination:
	  o Nil dysmetria L/R
	  o Nil dysdiadochokinesia L/R
	• Sensation: Normal in all domains assessed, including:

Etc. *(You can incorporate other Templates for detailed Examination of other Systems as required)*

This is essential as the vast majority of Examinations will be normal, or only have slight abnormal elements. This normal Examination Template will save you much time as you can simply modify the abnormal elements (if any) while the remainder are valid. This will save you writing 'no dysdiadochokinesia' fifty times every day. It's also useful during your own independent Reviews for you, presumably, will look for everything on your Template.

As mentioned, delete the unneeded. Which is far easier than typing the needed.

Always include Observations first. Some are happy with 'Obs stable afebrile' (which you can Template with the keys 'obs'). Other Regs want each number, in which case just copy from the Patient Care Results +/– add a heading before each result. In ICU, where there may be no numbers in eMR, have auto-text setting up each vital, e.g. 'HR=_ RR=_ BP=_ Sats=_ Temp= _' and read off the monitor and their big charts. Alternatively, use ICU Templates, e.g. Airway, Breathing, Circulation, etc.

Investigations (what was tested)

Mainly on Medical Terms. Include here all the key Investigation findings, including Bloods, Imaging, Pathology, Procedural reports, Microbiology, etc. You can usually insert the Conclusions of the reports verbatim here.

If there are certain Investigations the Team monitors daily, Template them with '_' for numbers, e.g. 'ALT_, AST_, GGT_, ALP_, Br_'. Again, use the Tear Off function to avoid constantly switching windows and read and copy the numbers.

Issues/Impression (what we think is happening)

Medical Round favourite. Similar to your Issues List in the Discharge, only some may not pan out and some may not yet be in play. Think of it as the daily Discharge. Tells you the various matters that needs addressing, helps keep track of them and prevents you forgetting.

This isn't always easy to work out, as it requires you to synthesise the clinical picture and essentially figure out the various Diagnoses related to the patient.

Hence, try yourself first. Place the Issues in sequence of importance. Use your Medical knowledge to work them out. This mainly centres around either Diagnoses or matters you need to fix, e.g. Hyperkalaemia, or any other 'matters' of significance, e.g. social Issues/advanced care planning. Then get the Reg to check. Practise this, especially if Physician inclined, and, eventually, you too will be able to generate fifteen-point Issues Lists at a glance and hopefully treat all aspects of the patient.

Once an Issues List is generated, you can copy to each following day, and update/modify accordingly depending on the clinical course.

> **NB:** SOMETIMES, REGS PREFER THE ISSUES LIST AT THE TOP AFTER THE PEOPLE ATTENDING THE WR, SO TO GUIDE THOUGHT DURING THE WR AND ALSO HELPFUL FOR MET CALLS SO NO ONE IS TRAWLING. TAILOR AS APPROPRIATE.

Plan (what we're gonna do about it)

Mostly the same as standard. Key thing is, as always, get everything and be specific. You can bold and underline important parts (may or may not work). Some Seniors are specific and want each part of the Plan to correlate directly with the Issues above. Comply with their customs. You can also ask the Seniors who have specific customs to check your note. Better to get it right, now. Also, try to anticipate the Plan where you can, and put question marks where you're not sure or need their confirmation. This reminds you to ask them for clarification and also provides a good learning opportunity as you can see what they're looking for (mostly what you missed).

> **NB:** EVIDENTLY, THE ABOVE CAN ALL BE TRANSCRIBED TO THE SURGICAL WR; HOWEVER, LIMITED BY PRACTICALITY. SOME PEOPLE DO COME IN EXTRA EARLY JUST TO BEAUTIFY INTO THIS FORMAT AND PREP NOTES. YOU COULD ALSO PERFORM IT DURING THE DAY. UP TO YOU.

KEY POINTS

- Create standard format WR Templates.
- Heading: XXX WR – (list of attendees' surnames).
- Opening line: XXX-year-old male/female admitted for XXX with a background/complicated by XXX.
- Progress: All that happened of note during the WR, including patient interaction, other HCW interactions, overnight occurrences.
- Examination: Exam findings. Template standard Examinations and specialised Examination sets, e.g. Neuro.
- Investigations: Use the Tear Off function to record Results, Template parameters if monitored daily, e.g. LFTs.
- Issues: Aim to develop yourself and check with a Senior. Good learning opportunity. Also update Issues daily.
- Plan: Aim to develop yourself and your Senior will modify. Potentially correlate directly with Issues above.

OTHER DOCUMENTATION

There's much else happening apart from the WR. Hence, the general rule is:

Document everything

You must do this. This not only makes sure that everyone is on the same page, that everyone knows what's happening, but also ensures you're responsible *only* for things you're responsible for, and not responsible for things you're not responsible for. We are dealing with people's lives here. It's a serious matter. As a JMO, you make few decisions and nearly no critical ones. It's of paramount importance that people know what actually happened or is happening.

Hence, if something happens, or you're required to do something, document. Brief is fine. Pretend you're the ABC reporter of your life. Be entirely passionless and simply note down what happened. (Remember: Just Medical things please. We don't want to hear how great your lunch was. Or the hunger from the lack thereof.)

Hence, document when you have (non-exhaustive):

- Authorisations/requests from your own Team/Consultant for decisions, especially in Treatment.
- Consulted/discussed something with other Teams and their Plan (both what they ask you to do and what they'll do): see section 'Consults/After the Consult'.
- Updated or attempted to update other Teams/Consultants and their responses (especially in After Hours).
- Gained approval from Radiology/other Special Services.
- Updated/consented/attempted contacting/discussed anything with the patient/family.
- Patient Reviews of any sort (see *Chapter 8*, section *Clinical Reviews*).
- Performed a Procedure, e.g. IDC (see *Chapter 8*, section *Organising After Hours: Jobs/Types of Jobs/Other Procedures*).
- Any significant patient interaction.
- Any significant interaction with other HCWs.
- Attended any meetings (mostly with families).
- Tried to deal with anything difficult, e.g. failure to reach other Teams, Radiology or patients and their family. And the number of attempts.

For sensitive matters where the wording is very specific and bears special significance, it's best to try first, then ask your Seniors to check. They're usually happy to, for accurate record-keeping and medico-legal reasons. Certain things must've been discussed with the patient. Patient responses need to be recorded. The degree of detail is variable. They'll gauge how specific they want to be.

The main thing is not to fail your duty of care to the patients. The next most important thing is to write down that you haven't failed. Doctors often feel the one is sufficient, but, actually, the other is almost as needed. In this chronically busy and high-stress environment, people are often too preoccupied with what they're doing to notice what you're doing. And unfortunately, after things happen, if you didn't document, it didn't happen.

So, make sure everything you've done and discussed with others is clearly noted. It doesn't have to be an essay, a line or two will do, but it'll certainly help you very much if anything ever does go wrong. And it may well prevent things from going wrong by alerting those who can prevent it from going wrong to act.

The critical importance of documentation is that it formalises everything and, where things don't happen as expected, it shows that you've tried your best, you've fulfilled your duty of care, but, unfortunately, the fates weren't on your side.

If people could sue the fates, they would. But, in default of that, they'll sue you. And so, to prevent that, do what you should and document, and let the fates have their due.

We know you've been doing the right things. Now just let everyone know that you have.

KEY POINTS

- Everything, everything must be documented. See the list in the text.
- Documenting is of medico-legal consequence.
- Must be accurate and timely.
- Discuss with Seniors if unclear in any aspect, e.g. level of detail/key points.

ATTACHING EXTERNAL DOCUMENTATION/MEDIA

You sometimes need to attach information outside of eMR, into eMR. This mainly includes pictures or text (which you don't want to type again).

Suppose you wanted to show a Specialty Surg Reg a wound, but they're at another Hospital with no reception. Or you've received a twenty-page GP fax, with lots of important information, but you don't want to type twenty pages. What then?

There are rapid ways of attaching both into eMR without breaking your fingers or cursing the phone towers. We'll consider the methods for both pictures and text.

Text you don't want to type again

So long as it's printed text, it's easy. Forget about handwriting. There's no true OCR (optical character recognition) yet, and, even if there was, it wouldn't work for Doctors. Hence, consider the following (remember to always clarify and comply re local document transfer/encrypting/privacy policies and obtain consent where needed. Also delete from your devices once functions are complete):

1. **Photograph/scan the document**: Scan is best for optimal clarity. Most Hospitals have a scanner.
2. **Put on computer**: Scanners often send directly to your staff email. Ask the Ward Clerk if unsure. Then download.
3. **Text extraction**: Now you'll either have a PDF or Image of the text. There are many programs and websites that can extract text from it, most of which will be blocked. For the computer savvy, you can try carrying a suitable program on a USB and hence extract as you normally do (make sure it complies with local policies). For everyone else, just use Microsoft *OneNote* (which is *not* blocked and is mostly installed).
   a. **To use OneNote**: Open it→Copy your image/screenshot/PDF into *OneNote*→Right click image→Choose 'Copy Text from Picture'→Paste somewhere→You now have a bunch of text which includes what you want.

4. **Get text**: Take out what you want and transfer it to your 'Progress notes'. You've now avoided typing immense amounts of text and auto-transcribed it directly to eMR.

Pictures you want the world (of Consulted Regs) to see

Pictures. Or a thousand words. Of first stuttering inadequacy then merciless grilling. You pick. If the former, consider the following. You know the latter.

1. Get Consent, then the photo.

2. Transfer photo to Hospital computer.

3. Copy photo to *Word* and shrink to a small-ish size (else eMR will crash).

4. Directly copy into Progress notes as if you were copying text.

Done. You now have pictures directly uploaded to eMR and saved the words.

> **NB:** AGAIN, CHECK LOCAL POLICIES RE UPLOADING TO eMR AND PHOTO TRANSFERS

KEY POINTS

- External text, e.g. Specialist letters, can be attached into eMR via scanning then extracting text from the PDF/photo.
- External images can be pasted into *Word* then into eMR text boxes.
- Always check and comply with local policies re consent/document transfer/encrypting rules.

EMERGENCY DEPARTMENT DOCUMENTING

Similar rules apply as above. The main difference is ED has two documents that you should develop Templates for that are slightly differently from those for the Ward.

ED Case History

Here is where you perform the initial patient Assessment.

The Documenting is pretty similar to the Discharge Summary main body, i.e. Template the headings of History Presenting Complaint, Past Medical History (+/− Medical versus Surgical History split), Family History, Medications, Allergies, Social History, Examination, Investigations, Impression and Plan. There's little to Template within the headings as each patient is different, apart from standard Examination Templates. You may have an opening line Template of '_-year-old male/female presented with _ on background of _' just to set the context.

You may also have various Templates for System Screens, e.g. raft of questions relating to Infections, Cardiac, Neuro, Respiratory, Gastro and other Systems, e.g.

Nil pain

Nil fevers

Nil chills/rigors

Nil cough

Nil coryzal symptoms

Nil new rashes

Nil nausea/vomiting

Nil diarrhoea/changes to bowel habits

Nil dysuria

Nil recent overseas travel

Nil sick contacts

for a brief infective screen. Also helps to remind you to ask for things if you've forgotten. Modify if any are positive. These are also useful as you conduct Reviews on the Ward. Hence, consider your own History-taking skills and Template them, ideally for each of the common Systems and for common scenarios, e.g. Falls.

Prior to seeing the patient, as you note trawl, you can also commence your documentation and pre-load especially the Past Medical History. Helpful as may guide your Assessment.

ED Discharges

These are much less extensive than the Ward Discharges as the patient likely remains with you for less than 5–6 hours, either going home or to the Ward. Hence, you'll generally write all that happened to them in ED rather than having much of a Template. There isn't usually an Issues List and all is included in the paragraph or two you write to the GP. Those with many Issues have gone to the Ward.

Hence, simply discuss their progress in ED and Template the Plan as usual as per Discharges. Subject to personal habits, but you can then attach the patient's ED Case History at the end so the GP/Specialist has a better idea of the clinical course in ED. Some place this between the opening paragraph and the Plan; others puts it at the end of all. Suit yourself.

Feel free to use the Discharge Summary Introduction (see section 'Discharges') transposed across, amending 'Place' to ED and there isn't an Admitting Consultant usually. The progress you'll type case by case and the conclusion is likely similar (especially as they're going home).

> ### KEY POINTS
>
> - ED Case History: Template standard headings, e.g. Presenting Complaint, PMHx, Family History, Meds, Allergies, SHx, System Screen, O/E, Ix, Impression, Plan.
> - Generate Systems screen Templates.
> - ED Discharges: Unlike Ward Discharges, mainly prose detailing the patient's ED progress instead of Issues.
> - Rest is similar to usual Discharge.

EXTERNAL REFERRALS

You'll often be required to write referrals to various Specialists/Clinics/other Service/other Hospitals.

Unfortunately, eMR doesn't get involved here as the destination is almost always external. Also, a Discharge Summary, though required, is usually insufficient.

Hence, to generate these most readily, create a *Word* Template, saved on a USB you carry, preferably with your Institution's letterhead for extra spankiness (inherit from previous JMO or ask Ward Clerk/IT). This is also for any official-ish letter you need to write, e.g. various Doctor's letters, etc.

Also, you can set up a Template in eMR for the actual wording with F3 blanks and copy it across to *Word* to print. Here, however, are most of the actual details you'll need to type.

Consider the following eMR Template:

> **Attention to:** [whoever's attention you want]
>
> **Re:** [Subject matter of referral]
>
> **Patient name:**
>
> **DOB:**
>
> **Patient identification number:**
>
> **Gender:**
>
> **Address:**

Contact details:

[No need to Template the Patient details, you can copy directly *all* the above from the Discharge Summary's Patient Details Fields at the top. If there isn't a Discharge, generate it, save it empty and copy it. They'll need a Discharge eventually.]

Dear Dr _ [name of Specialist/Clinic/Service],

Thank you for seeing _ [name], a _-year-old _male/female referred from XXX Hospital for _ [insert medical condition/reason of referral].

[Now include, briefly, pertinent, relevant medical details and exact reason for the referral. This will be variable for each case. You may choose also to copy across Past Medical History/Medications. You can also generate a more detailed Template if referring always for the same reason and if the Specialist wants things in a special way.]

We look forward to obtaining your advice for the ongoing management of _ [whatever it is]. Please find the Discharge Referral attached for your perusal [if they wanted it].

Kind regards

Dr XXX [Your name]

XXX [Your Term] Intern/Resident/SRMO

XXX Hospital

Phone Number:

Pager:

Provider Number:

On behalf of Dr XXX

Provider Number of Consultant:
[If you know it. Not always essential]

This Template should do for most. Be tactical in how many Templates you construct. If you're referring often and mainly to one of two Clinics/Specialists in the Term, then Template specifically for them. Else, a general Template will do.

These referrals aren't usually long, i.e. less than a page, and are more an administrative tick box so Specialists can begin seeing the patient from a Medicare perspective. Hence, a brief outline of their Admission with the reason for their referral, with the pertinent findings, is often sufficient; of course, pending Specialist/situation. As always, fulfil their specific requirements. Much information can be copied from the Discharge or they can be sent the whole Discharge.

KEY POINTS

- Use the suggested Template and generate specific ones if often referred to.
- Find the Hospital-specific letter head and print (paper form) or copy onto it (electronic form on Intranet).

DISCHARGES

Bane of existence

Yes, we all hate them, and in the midst of our crazy life, WR to 7 p.m., repeat Boss Rounds, Nursing staff constantly asking you to do various things, families wanting updates every 20 minutes, Patient Flow calling you to send people home, and your pager screaming its head off like an unfed fledgling, why yes, in that midst, you have to do these very important pieces of paperwork that may well never be read, not even by the 'Dear Doctor' to whom it's so tenderly addressed.

Now is there a way to do them, and yet not be done by them?

After the experience of more than a thousand Discharges, we feel there's really only one way.

Templates.

But what we will show here is not any ordinary Template. We'll show the Template that'll be as close to the automatic Discharge Summary as it can be for now, while we use an eMR system that feels like it's from the time of 'Space Invaders'.

As mentioned, perhaps when Skynet happens, we'll have auto-programmed Discharges. Only downside, perhaps, is no people to write them for.

Key principle

The key behind a rapid Discharge is preparation.

Everything is about preparation.

The scenario will always be something like this. It's 4.30 p.m. (Ideally. Perhaps it's 7 p.m.) Suddenly, the Boss appears and would like to do a quick Round. And the net result of said quick Round is that the Boss has decided the 200-day Admission, who you inherited from your predecessor twice removed, who has had two ICU

Admissions, three Theatre visits, perhaps twenty Issues, and who you have personally seen perhaps twice, is for Discharge.

Today.

Right now.

And their Discharge cannot be posted. Because it's a nursing home. And you never post Discharges to nursing homes.

And the NUM (Nurse Unit Manager) has caught the word and has already swooped upon you, saying things like 'We need beds'. And, of course, the eternal question: 'Are the Discharge papers ready?'

No. They're not ready. Nothing is ever ready, until you make it so.

We will show below, when confronted by the above, how, first, not to get a systolic of 220 mmHg and, afterwards, how to send the patient, today, right now, without staying till the night shift is leaving.

METHODOLOGY

Have one. Anything is better than none.

In the ideal world, everything is set up for you, but this isn't the ideal world, it's the real world and nothing will ever be set up for you. Unless you set it up for you. Your system. Your Templates. And though there'll be much adjustment and constant updating, it's worth it in the end. Though the first Discharge may take three times as long, all the rest will only take a fraction of the time and you'll benefit endlessly henceforth.

So consider the following Plan for a smooth and effortless Discharge.

1. **Master Template**: Optimally, you'll inherit some sort of Template from your buddy JMO and adapt it, but if you don't, make one. Now. Render it as generic as possible. You'll almost never use this Template in native form, but it spawns each Term's Template. Know how to use it rapidly (shown later) and what to adjust each Term.

2. **General Term Templates**: You may wish to have a slightly more tailored Master Template, one for each of Medical, Surgical and ED Terms. Optional, and sometimes worthwhile as each broad Specialty shares characteristics.

3. **Term-specific Templates**: Create the Term-specific Template ASAP, optimally day 1 of Term, or even in the prior Term if it was chill. Detailed later but update the Bosses, the Specialty, the Hospital (if you've changed one), the Sign-off, the Generic Plan and any other Term-specific details. If you're covering multiple Teams, set up one for each. There are always bits that are different and it's more than worthwhile to have a new Template. Remember, the effort of setting up a Template is far less than correcting every time into infinity.

4. **Auto-text**: Create as much auto-text as you need. Err on the side of excess. Remember the principle of automation. Avoid sameness. Automate sameness. Anything you need to type twice, automate. Details to follow but an infinite number of things are (or almost) the same, from Issues, to Medication regimes, to Plans, to various common phrases, e.g. 'Please follow up with Doctor [XXX] in [XXX]…'. Auto-text-ify all of them as soon as you type them once.

5. **Start early**: Start Discharges ASAP, even on the day of Admission. Plan for Discharge on Admission, as Patient Flow often repeats. Begin populating basic patient data, demographics, Past Medical History, Social History and Issues thus far known. They may go tomorrow.

6. **Constantly update**: Always update Discharges as you go if you can. Today is fresh. A month later is more than stale. Leaving blanks is fine. This will save much reverse *PowerChart* trawling. Remember, even if you have no Diagnosis, just leave that blank and keep typing the Issue out, e.g. Investigations and Management. You can give a label later easy enough. You won't remember the barrage of tests. Similarly update Plans from other Teams as you go. You don't want to look again for their notes.

7. **Only update text**: You should only update the actual letter. Leave all else to the end; including Investigations, Bloods, Lab Results, Medications and Discharge Plan, all which are likely to change constantly (though the final Plan from Consulted Teams (especially if they're no longer involved) should be inserted).

8. **Do on the fly**: You'll be busy. Between WR +/− repeats, doing random jobs, answering pages about the same thing ten times, mandatory teaching, going to Theatres, running Clinics and running down to Radiology, there isn't much time to pee, let alone do this paperwork.

    You'll have to make time. As a luxury, you can sit down and do these. But on busy Terms, do these *on the fly*, i.e. as you push the WOW and literally every moment you aren't doing something else. Do them on slow WRs when the discussion takes much longer than the Documenting or during infinite other delays which you'll soon find useful instead of frustrating.

9. **Constantly improve**: The method of your first Discharge will feel clunky and you may feel it's easier to type. Trust me, it isn't. You're just not used to it. Persist and constantly optimise to what suits you. Very soon, you'll find a way which works. That'll be the best and fastest way. And very soon, you can Discharge even with a GCS of 10.

10. **Enjoy**: Once you've established such a system, hopefully Discharges will be as rapid as printing a form. Now start tolerating instantaneous Discharges, from the Boss's end to yours.

So now we know how to do, let's consider what to do. The Template.

KEY POINTS

- Create a Master Template – from which to derive Term-specific Templates.
- Derive a Specialty flavour/Term-specific Template before each Term starts.
- Implant as many Term-specific details as possible.
- Create Term-specific auto-text including common phrases, Issues, Medication regimes and Plans.
- Start Discharges on Admission.
- Update throughout the Admission (only text).
- Do on the go.
- Persist with the method until it's a habit.
- Resist the feeling it's easier to type. It isn't.
- Consider the Template below.

THE TEMPLATE

Make it. Know it. Use it.

All Discharges, whatever the Term, generally follow a standard format. Included is a common one, but feel free to adjust/use whatever is most suitable for you.

The idea behind the Templates is to avoid typing everything that is the same all the time, and merely inputting customised data points, e.g. Name, Age, Gender, Medical condition, Admitting date (changes monthly), Admitting Doctor, Length of Stay and Disposition while the actual prose is already there.

Your Template should also include the major headings, including Past Medical History, Social History, Allergies, Medications (+/– On Admission and On Discharge), Issues During Admission +/– History Presenting Complaint, and Discharge Plan. Many elements of the Plan are often the same, and these should be Templated.

Finally, there are Boss names which you must include. These are usually many, long and hazardous to get wrong. So get it right once (titles inclusive), for each Term, and include all of them in your standard Template. When you're actually Discharging, just delete the rest except the one in question. This will save much difficult typing.

And, of course, at the end, there's your own beautiful sign off saying you're the XXX JMO on behalf of [some] Boss. However much you like your name, you don't want to be typing it some thousands of times, especially if it's long and it's 8 p.m. Nor do you really need reminding of what Term you're doing. Hence, build it into the Template and adjust based on Term (the Term, not your name, unless you want that too.)

Try to use _ (underscore) for blanks/adjustable terms, as in eMR, pressing F3 skips between underscores so you can input data quickly only at given points without needing to find and click on them. This is particularly useful when you have poor hand–eye coordination. And you'll be surprised how quickly hand–eye coordination deteriorates, especially after a 14-hour shift. As a final check, when about to print, click F3 to make sure there are no blanks left. If there aren't, the document will auto-scroll to the end. If there are, fill them out.

Now the best way is to show, especially if one has never done a Discharge. So see the potential Template below:

NB:

- **[Bold]** are mere comments, not to be included in the real thing.
- XXX should be built into your format *each* Term.
- _ is to be updated *each* Discharge.
- [ ] = explanation of what's in the _.
- /= one or the other, e.g. male/female.

Dear Doctor,

Thank you for your ongoing management of _ [name], a _-year-old **_male/female** who was admitted to XXX Hospital on the _/XX[update monthly]/20XX[yearly] for _ [insert medical condition] under Dr _ [AMO name] (**XXX** [AMO's Specialty]). There were no significant complications [or if there were, say 'complicated by … [most likely each Issue listed]']. S/He was managed … [general/major details]. [Insert other details here as required]. S/He was discharged to _ [discharge disposition, e.g. home] day _ post-admission in a medically stable condition [if they were, or state other condition]. Please find a summary of their admission below.

[Naturally you can add more in the introduction as required, and if it's a complex admission, sweeping details.]

Presentation
[Synthesised ED presentation/HPC]

Examination (in ED)
[Relevant Exam findings]

Background
[As named, but try to chase multiple prior Discharges to include all conditions. Extra fancy is to arrange them according to organ System and divide Medical and Surgical, details of multi-organ diseases, e.g. diabetes, and their complications. If relevant and major, try to include major Procedures/tests done regarding condition, their results, clinical course of major illnesses and Bosses/Hospitals they're known to, e.g. Ischaemic Heart Disease, known to Dr XXX, PCI to LAD in 20XX, etc.]

Social History
Lives with _ [include who, e.g. family/alone/etc.]

_EtOH [drinks or not, amount if significant]

_Smoking [active, ex- or non-smoker, +/- number of pack years]

_ADLs [independent or not]

Mobilises _ [independent or how if not]

Works as _ [employment]

Has had _ recent travel [Y/N and to where]

Issues during Admission
1. _ [the medical condition/issue]
– Patient presented with _ [the issue] diagnosed clinically and on _ [salient Investigation findings/diagnostic tests]

– [+/– include here salient/diagnostic elements of history, exam and Investigations]

– Patient managed conservatively/operatively with _ [include treatment here]

– _ resolved [or describe other progress]

– Patient improved clinically [hopefully]

2. [Repeat above, n times over]

Medications on Discharge
New Medications
[as stated]

Changed Medications
[changed doses of regular Medications]

Ceased Medications
[as stated]

Regular Medications (unchanged)
[as stated]

Discharge Plan
1. Please follow up with Dr _ [whoever] in _ [when] at _ [where].

2. Please follow up with GP within _ days.

3. Please have the following outpatient investigations: [details]

4. Please continue with the following treatment: [details, especially for antibiotics and duration]

[Keep adding more Plans here; ED re-presentation is always last]

XXX. If condition worsens, including _ [include important symptoms] or any concerns, please present to ED.

Kind regards

Dr XXX [Your name]

XXX [Your Term] Intern/Resident/SRMO/Registrar

On behalf of Dr XXX/XXX/XXX [the long names of the infinite number of bosses which you won't need to type again]

Evidently, any of the bits above that are too hard and/or you didn't get can be deleted.

Further details of each major section are included below.

MAJOR COMPONENTS

Background

Essential.

You really must include this as the first thing ED reads is the latest Discharge and it's very helpful if the Discharge is up to date. You too will be in ED so pay yourself back in karma with good Discharges starting with yourself. Consider the following to help:

- **Keep adding**: Always keep adding to the Background. While you may've taken the time to document trawl, others may not have that time so save them it when you can.

- **The patient**: Can be an excellent source of information about themselves, though often neglected. Ask them first or if you're having trouble finding things out, especially if they're Medically savvy. They're usually the easiest to reach, won't make you wait, and will give instantaneous responses.

- **Use several past Discharges**: Many people copy/paste the ED history but, as ED is often time pressed, it's of value to read +/– copy/paste a few Discharges before this present Admission and combine them. A relatively relaxed JMO in daylight hours doing a Discharge is less likely to miss important Background than an ED Reg who has just finished a priority patient (BAT) call to send this patient home at 2 a.m. Also, try finding Medical history from Medical Admissions. The Surgical ones may be brief. Very brief.

- **Use Med Reg/Medical Consults notes/GP summaries**: These reviews often have excellent, comprehensive, summarised Backgrounds (especially in their Specialty) for you to plagiarise so make use of them and let not their talent waste in the electronic ether.

- **Use Allied Health Discharges**: These have excellent summaries of the patient's progress in each Allied Health domain, which likewise can be included in the Discharge.

- **Synthesise HPC (History of Presenting Complaint)**: You can use the ED one, but it may not be as succinct as you like and you may need to synthesise a little with the benefit of hindsight.

Issues/Summary of Progress

Template each Issue.

This is the real meat of the Discharge (apart from the Plan), and where the most work is.

The main idea behind Issues is summarising and *categorising* the blow-by-blow progress of the patient's journey through the Hospital.

Think of your daily Progress notes as a sort of story, which you narrate, chronologically, every Issue all together, simultaneously. Your Discharge will tease out each Issue and show how you addressed them through the Admission. Essentially, what you're doing is re-categorising. Progress notes are categorised by time. Discharges are categorised by Medical problems.

Think of it like noodles. The Progress notes is a bowl of noodles. The Discharge is essentially pulling out each strand to dry.

First stage: General format

With each Issue, the general flow is a mini-History, Exam, Investigations, Treatment, Progress/Resolution.

Naturally, with minor Issues like Hypertension (unless it's major), it'll be more concise, and with majors, e.g. the reason for Admission, e.g. unknown cause of Acute Renal Failure, it'll be more extensive.

But, essentially, each Issue is a sort of Diagnosis. Hence, you'll include (only) salient findings and relevant negatives in the History, Exam, Investigations, supportive of that Diagnosis and what you did to manage it, and the Progress/End result. Thus, if a patient had rhabdomyolysis, you would indicate the long lie, the statin use, the urine colour, the CK, the Cr/eGFR but perhaps not the ROM (range of motion) of the right greater hallux. Here's the opportunity of using Med School knowledge. A good guide is to pretend, if you were diagnosing the patient, what information you would've wanted to make the diagnosis, then what you did about it. That information is likely what another would like to see in the Discharge. You'd also mention what Teams you've Consulted and the relevant Specialist Consultants who were involved in the patient's care.

Next stage: Further customisation

As you go along, you'll find many of the Issues are the same within a Term and, often, the same between Terms. One gets Hyperkalaemia or Hypertension under any Team, and often enough, the History/Exam/Investigations/Management/Progress is the same.

Hence, it'll be optimal to develop Templates for each Issue.

Every Issue you ever meet really deserves a Template for it's almost certain to arise again. And again.

Even the rarer ones, say an Epidermodysplasia verruciformis, may well turn up once more, for the simple reason if it's turned up at all, you're likely to meet it again, especially if you happen to be in a Dermatology Clinic.

Hence, once you encounter a new 'Issue', especially common ones, always try to render it generic first and turn it into a Template. This may feel like a pain, but you'll certainly see Exacerbation of CCF again and again, so that bit of effort initially will repay you at least a hundred-fold, a return as good as the lottery and mostly guaranteed.

For example, instead of typing out the whole Issue of urinary tract infection, by simply typing 'UTI', you could instantly get:

Urinary Tract Infection/Pyelonephritis

- Patient presented with urinary tract infection/ pyelonephritis diagnosed clinically and on urine MCS showing _, with cultures growing _, resistant/ sensitive to _.

- Patient experienced dysuria, fevers, rigors and had left/right renal angle tenderness.

- Peak WCC was _, peak CRP was _. Creatinine was _ and eGFR was _.

- Urine MCS demonstrated WCC _, RBC _, and urine cultures grew _.

- Patient managed with IV and PO antibiotics, including _trimethoprim/cefalexin/ceftriaxone/ Augmentin/ampicillin/gentamicin (etc., per your Institution guidelines) for _ days.

- Patient also managed with IV fluids and anti pyretics for _days.

- Urinary tract infection/pyelonephritis resolved.

- Patient improved clinically and symptoms resolved.

And by inputting the appropriate, and deleting the irrelevant, the Issue is complete.

As each type of Issue follows a similar logical progression, this makes it possible to generate a Template for each Issue with the expected course, and to add in the specific findings as they occur.

Make the Template

1. **Have a generic 'Issues' Template**: See above in 'Templates', for example. Useful for creating Templates of new specific Issues.

2. **Render 'Issue' generic**: Do the Issue as you would normally, but double a copy and render as general and generic as possible, i.e. standard, expected, salient History, Exam, Investigations, Management, Progress. Delete all the atypical, patient-specific findings and replace with general ones.

3. **Leave blanks appropriately**: Wherever there are numbers/variables, leave _ blanks, e.g. creatinine always needed in AKI (acute kidney injury) so have 'Creatinine is _' etc.

4. **Include multiple options of Investigations/Management**: Be more comprehensive rather than less, e.g. include more detailed Investigations/Management for each Issue, and adjust to the actual. It's easier to delete than to type. You can delete just as quickly with one hand, but certainly not type as fast. And as you'll always be one-handed, as you're on the phone, or charting Meds, or writing Outpatient forms and as you don't want to develop torticollis, try to make everything one-handable. Also serves as a reminder of what to look for.

5. **Add as needed**: However, don't worry if you don't have everything. You can always add to it. And less typing is better than more.

6. **Save**: Save your newly completed generic Issue with a simple-to-remember auto-text, e.g. 'UTI'.

7. **Enjoy**: Watch your 'Issues' bank grow and Discharge time melt.

Thus, very quickly, you'll build up a databank of 'Issues' which will be instantly accessible, and you only need to customise it with a few numbers and a few patient-specific details. Instead of typing out some dozen Issues, a few keystrokes will complete most of the 'Summary of Progress' while F3 jumps will finish it off. 'Tear off' the 'Results' screen to save toggling between screens as you input numbers. This way, even if your 200-day Admission seems to have as many 'Issues' as days of stay, you'll be able to generate them semi-automatically.

Common Issues you'll rapidly identify as the Term goes on, so it's best to start this on the first day, or the first slightly less busy day. For these Issues, Templates start paying off as soon as you make them.

Formatting considerations

Beauty is (a) pain.

Formatting is another bane of JMO life so it's best if everything is as fast and as beautified as possible straight from the start. Consider the following:

- **Pre-format**: Your standard Template should include the usual headings, already formatted. Note that sometimes Office shortcuts don't work so set up in *Word*.

- **Use *Word***: The 'Summary of Progress' section which we mostly use for the whole Discharge can be a terrible pain for often no keyboard shortcuts/spell-check/auto-correct work (test this out yourself, some places they do). Hence, use your favourite word-processing program. Also saves 'Tear[ing] Off' screens as they are different programs so you can 'Alt+Tab'.

- **Use 'Physiotherapy' notes section**: The difficulty in using *Word* is you must remember to pre-fill all expected auto-text as none work in *Word*, nor does F3. Also, you may forget to save. Hence, as you become familiar with your system or for simple Discharges, consider working completely in eMR. But use the 'Physiotherapy' or non-'Summary of Progress' notes section directly under 'Summary of Progress', in which, ironically, all shortcuts work. Then, before signing, transfer the whole thing into the right place. Also allows you to save. Don't worry about borrowing that space illegally. It's not like anyone else will be doing the Discharge for you in any part whatever, so the whole document is yours to do whatever you like until you sign.

- **Format only once at the end**: Difficult for obsessive formatters but as you're constantly adding things to the Discharge and copying/pasting from various sources, the format will always be deranged. Don't waste time. Only format when ready to sign. This will beautify everything instantaneously.

Medications (N/A for eMeds)

A critical part of the Discharge is to reconcile the Meds, i.e. make sure the Meds are correct. But this cross-checking is neither exciting nor short. Try to make life easier with the following.

- **Auto-text Medications**: eMeds users won't need to do this but for the miserable ones among us still on eMR2, or earlier, nothing is worse than typing Coloxyl and Senna 2 BD PO some hundred times. Save as auto-text with the doses, etc., using the Medication's name, e.g. generate Coloxyl and Senna 2 BD PO by simply typing COLOXYL. Adjust doses as needed. Also consider auto-texting rafts of drugs together if they're often used together, e.g. Palliative care crisis Medications are often similar, the doses only need adjusting.

- **Constantly update**: Always update Medication changes as you go. The other way is to photo the Med Chart and grab stickers so you don't need to refer to it again later (or walk back). Of course, subject to change. Usual check of Institution policies is needed re photos. Try not to include any sensitive information.

- **Pharmacist**: Obviously excellent at Meds. Ask them what method they use. They also help to reconcile Meds so if there've been many changes, ask them to help, e.g. via a Medication Reconciliation. They may also have special programs they can show you to update Meds.

- **Template Meds**: More common in Surgical Terms where many patients go on the same aperient/anti-emetic/analgesia regime. Build into Template as needed.

- **eMeds**: Usually, once you've completed the 'Discharge Reconciliation', just clicking this section in the Discharge auto-populates all the Medications. The only issue is if, after you've done so, there is a change. If this occurs, you can modify the 'Discharge Reconciliation' as appropriate, then right click this section in the Discharge and 'clear' it. When you save the document and come back to it, it should repopulate with your changes.

KEY POINTS

- Background: Use multiple sources, including multiple past Discharges, the patient, Med Reg Consults, GP letters and Allied Health notes (esp. for SHx).
- Issues: Generate standard/generic Templates for common (perhaps all) Issues each time a new Issue type is encountered with blanks for variables.
- In future, simply fill in the blanks.
- Each Issue follows usual Medical problem progression: Relevant Hx (History), O/E, Ix, Mx (Management), Progress details.
- Formatting: Aim to pre-format everything as much as possible and adjust in *Word*.
- Only formalise formatting at the end.
- Medications (N/A for eMeds): Auto-text standard Medication regimes.
- eMeds users have auto-populating function once 'Discharge Reconciliation' is complete for Meds.

THE PLAN

Illnesses have a Plan. Do you?

The most important and easiest part of the Discharge. Just write Boss's/Reg's words, verbatim, formalised.

A few useful tricks below to give your Discharge the rapid and professional finishing touch.

Standard Template

- **Follow-up**: Always have a line for follow-up, Specialist and GP. Everyone follows up with someone at some point in time.
- **Deterioration**: Always include a line regarding deterioration. Everyone comes to ED if they deteriorate. You may include elements regarding what to look out for, but this will be case dependent.
- **Disposition**: Optional, but you may want to make explicit where the patient is going, e.g. home, nursing home, respite. More for the next HCW's eyes. The patient usually knows.
- **Medications**: Optional. You can emphasise what Medications they should take, e.g. *Please take the following Medications as discussed … .*

Customised/Term Template

Everything else will be rather case and Term dependent so format your own other standards. For example, Surgical patients always tend to have similar dressing, wound care, analgesia and follow-up Plans so Template these.

It's also useful to cumulate little, short-phrase auto-texts, which allows you again to *only* input the distinctive data points.

Consider the following:

- Type 'ABX' and get: *Please take the following Medications/antibiotics as prescribed: _ .*
- Type 'FOLLOWUP' and get: *Please follow up with Dr _ on _ at _ .*
- Type 'CARE' and get: *Please continue care in _ .*
- Type 'OUTPTIX' and get: *Please have the following Investigations as an outpatient: _ (form provided).*
- Type 'GPCHASE' and get: *GP please kindly to follow up on the following: _ .*

Etc. You get the idea.

By having these one-liners at the ready, you may simply type a capitalised word and instantly your beautiful, full English, error-free prose will appear without the actual effort of typing and your rapid Discharges won't look like you failed Year 5 English, with spelling the weakest domain.

Capitals for auto-text are often best as you only trigger them when you want, and not when generally typing. Mostly you don't even need to type the whole word and the option will appear.

This skill is readily applicable to any sort of documentation. Identify which phrases you're always typing, then auto-text-ify them.

Of course, always clarify the Plan with the Team Reg before you complete it.

When you're pretty certain that other Teams have finished Consulting for you, copy and paste their Plan into your Discharge. You can beautify it later, as this too may change, especially if you re-Consult them later and their Plan changes. But this saves you hunting for their note buried in the millions.

If it's a complex Discharge, break up the Plan via Specialty and specifically what the GP Plan is. This not only categorises it well for the patient and the GP, but also is easier for you to type as, obviously, the Respiratory Team would not write a Plan for the Cardio Team and you can simply copy/paste all their Plans directly under beautiful headings and spellcheck.

Keep updating the Plan for complex Discharges as you'll forget the Issues and the countless Consulted Teams involved, which each have their own Plan. Again, this saves note trawling.

KEY POINTS

- Use standard Template.
- Generate auto-text phrases common in Plans.
- Break up the Plan according to Specialties involved in complex Discharges.
- Update constantly.

USEFUL DOCUMENTS TO ATTACH, BUT PAINFUL TO DO SO

In addition to the Discharge letter itself, there are often many additional reports you need to attach, which are highly useful for future reference and Specialist referrals but painful to attach. This will show a quick method to attach them all without going in and out of *PowerChart* some twenty times for the ten different Scopes and Sestamibis the patient has undergone.

Medical Certificates

In hot demand on Surgical Terms and ED, everyone seems to need a Med Cert. As usual, paperwork is painful and Med Certs one of the most painful. Plus, you'll be hassled for these possibly even more than for scripts, as they're immensely important to the patient. To minimise agony:

- **Check if they need one**: Generally, if they're not of school/working age (either end) *or* un/self-employed, they won't. But ask.

- **Print one with the Discharge**: Saves the trouble of writing one. Simply fill in the dates at the end of the Discharge letter and it'll auto-print one for you. If it failed to print, simply print as a 'Report' and choose Med Cert. Now, instead of writing a million things, your one beautiful signature will do. A similar method can be potentially adopted for family. But you'll need to addit the family/carer's name in addition to the beautiful signature. Or you'll have to write the whole thing.

- **Plan your route**: You have to *go* to the printer and sign the thing. Make sure you print first and remember to sign when you make your Ward tours.

Investigations

Some patients appear to have gone through every investigatory department in the Hospital, from Endoscopy to Nuclear Med, and had every test in between. And these are all important, expensive, hard-to-get tests. So you should certainly include their reports in your Discharge. But trawling through all the entries in eMR and copying/pasting them one by one is, again, painful. However, there's a way to do it in one go.

1. **Go to Lab Results section in the Discharge Summary**→Brings up a new window with many Results.

2. **Right click the grey bar at the top**→Click 'Change Search Criteria'→Adjust to 'Admission date to Current' or other date restriction you prefer→Relevant Results will appear.

3. **Scroll to the absolute bottom**: Ignore all else for most of it is Nursing stuff, and while it's useful to know the patient's glucometer reading on day 26 of Admission, it was probably on day 26 only, and not day 100, when the patient is going home.

   But the absolute bottom is where the money is. Here are all the key Imaging reports, major Investigations, e.g. Endoscopy, and even Operation reports.

4. **Select all relevant cells and Ctrl+C**: Instead of copying each, one by one, opening and closing windows as on the Results tab, and finding each, and getting lost, then becoming paranoid about not including some, then starting again, and generally raising your systolic into calling criteria, simply highlight all you need, and hold 'Ctrl' to select non-contiguous cells. When everything you need is highlighted, just 'Ctrl+C'. Done. All the reports are now *copied*. Remember to go right instead of left for the most recent.

5. **Select Bloods**: Now choose all the Bloods you want included and hit 'Include Selected'.

6. **Paste reports**: Go to any text box (mostly 'Non-Theatre Procedures'), hit 'Ctrl+V' and voila, every report you want is pasted (i.e. if you've selected it, and not accidentally clicked something and only included CRP = 50 on day 3 Admission).

7. **Done**: You've now saved yourself going in and out of Results and reports (×20), copying some two dozen reports into *Word* then copying them back into eMR.

If you love trees, go and delete some of the useless things like the introduction of each report, e.g. which Hospital the scan was done at (you should have a good idea) and include only 'Report text'. If you hate trees, include everything (you should all love trees).

The main bane is actually to remember to paste all that data directly after you've selected the Blood Results.

However, if you've unfortunately forgotten, and already chosen a bunch of special autoimmune Bloods stretching over 2 months, don't despair. You won't need to select them all over again. Simply click the 'Lab Results' section again, and hit the 'Refresh 'button. This will again bring up the original list of all the Results. Do the steps above again but don't press 'OK'. Just click 'Cancel' and your selected Bloods will be intact while, this time, you should remember to paste the copied Investigations.

For Operations/Theatre Procedures, this method can also be used or generate a Filter for 'Operations' then copy it directly across. There's an auto-populating function; however, it unfortunately generates more trouble for it often only auto-populates an abbreviated Operation report (generally only includes post-op Orders) and isn't very informative regarding the operation itself.

KEY POINTS

- Medical Certificates: Aim to print with the Discharge or as an eMR 'Report' then sign.
- Investigations: Go to 'Lab Result' section, select all needed Ix, Ctrl+C then paste into where you want all Ix to be attached.

NO eMR

It's likely that, even without eMR, you still need to do Discharge Summaries (and much other Documenting, though it's more likely to be paper based). Is the above system obsolete? Naturally, the attachment of various Investigations, etc. will be harder as it'll probably be done manually. But as the letter-writing process is almost identical, doing Discharges can still be as simple and rapid as above.

Still generate all your Templates as above, except this time in *Word* and save everything on your USB as a master file. Now, instead of F3, consider using the Ctrl+H or 'Find and Replace' function in *Word*. Set the 'Find what' section as '_'. Then simply sequentially replace each '_' with the data you want to input. With a steady four 'tab' clicks→Input data→Two 'tab' clicks→Click 'enter'→Repeat cycle, you can rapidly populate any of your Templates with customised patient data and still generate flowing and instantaneous reports without fancy computer systems.

Similarly, auto-text in *Word* is still possible if you don't want to repeatedly copy/paste from your *Word* master file. Depending on your *Word* version, see its Help program/search online (all these questions have been answered) or use below.

Create all your auto-text as above advised via first selecting your text→Go to 'Insert' tab→Go to 'Text' section→Click 'Quick Parts' button→Go to 'Autotext' →Click 'Save selection to Autotext Gallery'→In the pop-up which appears, the 'Name' part defines the code for the block of text. When you click OK (+/− adjusting the other options as needed), that text is now auto-text. When you want to insert it next time, simply start entering the name and click F3, and, instantly, all the saved auto-text will manifest.

To transfer all your auto-text between computers is dependent on Institution regulations. You may need your own portable version of *Word* or always use one particular computer for Discharges. Some other fancier methods do exist, e.g. copy your own 'Normal.dotm' file (which stores all your auto-texts and is located in the C:>Users>[User]>AppData>Roaming>Microsoft>Templates) to a USB and load any *Word* files from that file; however, Hospital computers sometimes restrict various programming methodology so you'll need to trial and error.

Done. You now have a *Word* version of the eMR.

BENEFITS

Infinite.

Benefits abound if you prepare Discharges as above, but chiefly consider three:

1. **Instantaneous Discharges**: If they're always prepped, you can attain the state of bliss known as 'Instantaneous Discharges'. That is, even if the Boss clears for Discharge at 4.45 p.m., the patient can go at 5 p.m. (from your end at least) and you'll avoid the state of perdition known as 'Staying Back' or the worse state of 'Coming in on Weekends to do Discharges'.

2. **Instantaneous Patient Knowledge**: Patients are complex. Discharges help dispel the fog and clarify what's going on with the patient. They also provide you with a reference for all the patient's information. Especially helpful on Boss Rounds, who generally expect eidetic memory from JMOs regarding all patient info, at least instantaneous responses to their questions. This will do for now if you haven't got eidetic memory. Also helps your learning and identifies unclear points which you can check with the Reg.

3. **Consults Reference Sheet**: Another person who expects you to know everything about your patients is the Consulted Reg, who will habitually ask an infinite number of questions, which, however obscure, you should know. Your Discharge will be your main answer book, as you hopefully have all you need right before you, without needing to trawl. This also saves much time in preparing for Consults. Ideally, if you haven't prepped a Discharge yet, prep one as you make the first Consult. The effort of gathering patient data hence won't be spent twice and you'll be ready for most future Consults.

Effectively, your Discharge becomes the most updated patient data bank for the Admission, and while it usually helps the HCW in the next Admission, if prepped, it can assist tremendously with this Admission (the one you specially care about). Besides, the Discharge needs doing sooner or later. Better sooner, so it can help you out now.

KEY POINTS

- Instantaneous Discharges.
- Instantaneous Patient Knowledge.
- Consults Reference Sheet.
- You have to do it anyway.

THE INTRANET

This is the second most common system you'll be looking at, after eMR, and you should be very familiar with it. Its importance stretches across Rostering, contacts, resources, forms and virtually any aspect of Hospital life. It's critical for organising your life in the long term so be familiar with it ASAP.

Unfortunately, many Hospitals will have different systems so you'll need to learn this from scratch each time you change jobs. However, the effort is again well worth it. We'll detail what you need to look for. You'll go look for them. Everyone knows these things. You will too.

ROSTERS

Highly essential if you want to plan your life at all, both at work and out of it. Often, Rosters are stuck somewhere on the wall and you'll just have to photo it. Biggest issue with this is it obviously can't be updated in live time. And there are frequent changes (Bosses, like JMOs, swap/give/take shifts or On Calls). So, be diligent and find it online. Often found under a 'Clinical' tab or 'Rosters' (as expected). Be sure to choose the right Hospital.

Rosters you'll need to know include:

- **JMO After Hours Roster**: To see when you're on After Hours and not get the On-Call person called in because you forgot. Often you'll be emailed these anyway. Plan your life accordingly, and if there doesn't seem much of it left, start swapping/giving away early, or start taking if you want extra experience/money.

- **JMO Roster (others)**: Any JMO Roster which you're involved in, you should know. Many Specialties have an After Hours JMO, e.g. ICU, Paeds, Cardio. If you're doing those Terms, you should also know when you're on and which type of shift.

- **Team Roster**: Mostly for pagers to call for Consults. Every Team should be on there, Boss to Reg to JMO, so this is an essential document. Follow closely the instructions. There'll be random things on it about who is on, e.g. which days of the week, and sometimes even what times, e.g. before midday. Don't be the person who spends half an hour paging one Reg only to be told to page the other one. Knowing the exact Reg also helps as the Regs rotate, so you may well know them. Also, you may know which friendly JMO can help you get in contact with the sought Reg.

- **Med/Surg Reg Roster**: Helpful for After Hours so you know who you'll be working with that night and who to report to. They're often happy to share numbers with you, especially at Handover, so you can call them if there's anything urgent or update them as needed rather than using the clunky pager system.

- **Specific Team Reg Roster**: Important especially in terms of Consults and who is holding the pager. There's often a separate Roster for ICU, Anaesthetics, Obstetrics and Gynaecology (O&G), Paediatrics and various Surgical sub-specialties, including General and Orthopaedics, and others still depending on size and services a Hospital offers.

- **ED Roster**: Chiefly useful when you're in ED. ED doesn't usually follow a regular working week so you should pay close attention to its details so you don't randomly come to work when not on.

- **Specialist On-Call Roster**: Critical in all Specialties. This is when the floodgates open for your Team. This is essentially when patients *will* be coming. This isn't an issue for some Teams who are always On Call (as there's only one) and hence constantly 'on take', i.e. will take any patients relating to their Specialty any day, in which case every day is variable and unknown. But for Specialties with multiple Teams, the 'On-Call' state constantly rotates so you must be aware when your Team is in the firing line. Usually, you'll be most busy, the day after take, or 'post take', when all the patients have descended on you. You'll then work colossally hard and try to get them all off you (i.e. fix them so they can go home), until the next 'on-take' day.

  Hence, it's essential to know when your Team is on and be prepared. Usually, the Roster will just have a surname on it, so you'll need to know all your Bosses' names, see when your Boss is on and plan accordingly. Similarly, the post-take Boss will often come in on that day (roughly), so expect them. Otherwise, if you don't know, you'll be perpetually perplexed about why suddenly you have fifty patients, why now you have none, why sometimes this Boss is coming, and why that one.

  On the flip side, this Roster is useful when you do ED. Then, it becomes the Consult Roster, and you'll know which Boss you're trying to sell your story to.

RESOURCES

Everything is generally under your own State's Information Portal. In NSW it's CIAP. In Vic, it's Clinicians Health Channel. In Qld, it's Clinicians Knowledge Network. In SA, it's SALUS. In Tas, it's searched for as EPOCH. In WA, it's WA Health Libraries Network. In NT, it's eLibrary. You'll be told which, depending where you work. Usually found under a 'Clinical' tab, or you can go straight from the *PowerChart* tab.

These are very helpful and will guide your practice so know how to use them. Consider the following.

- **Meds**: AMH (*Australian Medicines Handbook*), eTG (*Therapeutic Guidelines*), MIMS (*Monthly Index of Medical Specialties*), AIDH (*Australian Injectable Drugs Handbook*) are probably the most common. AMH is simple and easy to use, just hit the right tabs, especially 'Dosage', as is eTG. MIMS is more in depth. AIDH is great for infused Medications.

- **Clinical resources**: Very variable, but can include UpToDate, eTG, BMJ Best Practice and many others. Very personal preference and availability based.

- **Forms**: Usually under a tab called 'Forms'. Mostly you can just search it, and the most common is 'MRI Safety Form', though this will be case dependent as there are many others.

- **Protocols**: More for Seniors. Regs will usually make treatment decisions, but they often reference the various clinical protocols. You should know where the various policies/local guidelines are as you'll be a Reg soon enough, and will need to use them. They hide in various places on the Intranet, often Specialty dependent and often in Clinical as well. Also searchable. Check with your Institution.

KEY POINTS

- Rosters: Know the following:
  - o JMO After Hours (when you work and who you're working with)
  - o Any JMO Roster you're on
  - o Specialty Teams (for Consults)
  - o ED Roster (when you're working)
  - o Specialist On Call (especially when your Team is On Call or who to call for Admissions in ED).
- Resources (often on Health Info Portal):
  - o Medications: AMH, MIMS, AIDH
  - o Clinical guides: eTG, UTD, BMJ
  - o Forms: All sorts
  - o Hospital protocols.

MISCELLANEOUS

There'll be many other things you need to know and do, scattered about. You'll just have to find on a PRN basis. A few common ones include the following.

eMR PACS

Very useful when eMR *PowerChart* is not installed on your computer. You'll need to login like you do to your HR system, but you'll get access to the eMR software at least. Usually under 'eMR Advanced Users (credentials required)'.

Mandatory training

Each Hospital/Health District will request you do certain education modules. Check with your local policy and do them.

HR system

Very important for sorting out admin, if there's time (see *Chapter 10*, section *IT matters*). Know how to access early, i.e. check with your admin. Usually there's a big link to it on the Staff Intranet.

AMS (antimicrobial stewardship)

For antibiotic approvals if your Hospital has this. You'll be paged much for this. The best way is just to do them, when you can.

Simply login via your AMS section: Guidance App, then select your service and go through the approval process. The login is usually given to you, else it's often your HR system login. Check with your Hospital.

Unsigned documents

Sometimes you forget to sign docs. Which is not surprising if you're speeding with a WOW at a rate faster than most bicycles through a Ward which is harder to cross than a motorway at peak hour, on foot; with beds, other staff, trolleys, cleaning apparatus, pans with various matter in them and patients, hurtling out at you from all directions.

You won't remember. But Clinical Information Systems will and they'll also let you know about it. Once again, do when you can.

It's a waste of time to trawl the notes. Simply go to 'Quality Informatics'→Then Click 'Unsigned documents'→Choose 'Your patients' or your Hospital's→Find your name alphabetically then sign everything.

MedCalc

For calculating all sorts of stuff, especially actual Creatinine Clearance. Under Charts→'Med Calc 3000'. Has every formula you want under the Hospital fluorescence.

Sticker printing

Extremely useful when you don't want to write and there's no Ward Clerk.

Go to 'Documents' (same bar as Change User)→Hit 'Eye' symbol (top left)→Enter Patient Record Number/details→Choose which encounter you're considering (usually the current inpatient Admission)→Hit OK→Choose 'Inpatient Label' →Print (choose the right printer and number of copies)→Collect Labels somewhere.

Report printing

If you need to re-print any official document, e.g. Discharge Summary or Medical Certificate, simply go to Top left→Task→Report, then choose the report you want and select a printer.

Theatre Lists

Often needed when chasing Surgical Teams, to find where the Surg Reg is at. Go to 'Explorer Menu'→Choose 'Theatre Lists'→Choose the Location→Execute.

However, variable between Institutions, occasionally also on the Intranet. Know where it is.

KEY POINTS

- eMR PACS: For alternative login method when eMR not on desktop.
- Mandatory training: For accreditation.
- HR system: For pay/HR matters.
- MedCalc: For various calculations, e.g. Creatinine Clearance.
- Theatre Lists.
- Report printing, e.g. Discharges/Medical Certificates.
- How to print patient stickers.

DOCTOR VIEW

This is an application being increasingly rolled out across various Health Districts. Those who use it will have orientation for it. Overall, its system is similarly intuitive to the rest of the Cerner eMR system with a slightly different look. Most functions are the same and located on the side tab.

The look of the Patient List is also a little different. At the end of the day, you'll use what you're comfortable with. You can switch easily between the two views or you can contact IT (depending on Health District) to permanently switch if you favour one or the other.

A chief difference is that there are Documenting Templates which can be activated in the 'Documenting' section at the base. This can be quite useful as it auto-populates Documenting Templates based on the type of note you wish to write, e.g. Admissions, WR notes, Procedures. The headings within each Template are mostly appropriate and can be removed if not useful. It also auto-populates some data, e.g. the latest observations and your name at the end of the note. The main issue with it is each heading is in a distinct text box and there can be difficulties in switching between headings or text flowing between them. Formatting according to your wishes may be complicated.

Additionally, the Orders and Referral section is similar to ScratchPad with similar search and sign functions. The Favourites section requires more clicks overall. 'Patient Summary' is also moved to near the bottom of the usual tabs.

Overall, 'Doctor View' offers an alternative viewing experience with largely similar functionalities and is really up to user preference.

FIRSTNET

Some EDs use this system. In truth, the meat of the system is the same as eMR *PowerChart*. You'll also get training. Only be aware of some differences and use all prior principles.

- **Tracking List**: The main page of ED. Shows all the patients in table format similar to Excel with various columns of information about them. You'll get teaching for the details, key ones including the 'Doctor responsible' (especially important when it's you) and 'Team responsible', 'Patient location', 'Patient data', etc. Main thing is to filter using the tabs, e.g. by Team (i.e. your Team, often Acute or Subacute), or location, e.g. Short Stay Unit. A big use of the Board is the column of free text or 'Comments' which allows you to update *everyone* regarding the patient's progress and also for Nurses to feed back/update you regarding where things are up to. Essentially, it's a key area of communication and keeps everyone on the same page.

- **Home Page:** Sometimes not much used so is near the bottom as 'Patient Summary' or 'Emergency Department Summary'. However, functions the same.

- **Bloods**: All are 'Clinician Collect' as you/Techs/Nurses will be taking blood, not scheduled collectors.

- **Symbols**: There are a whole raft of symbols which you can institute next to the patient to describe their progress, e.g. 'Admit', 'Discharge Ready', 'Consult Placed', 'Medical Clearance'. The significance of each will be Institution dependent. Just follow local policy. They'll tell you which ones you must do. If you forget, they'll call you.

- **Discharges**: See section 'ED Documenting'. Principles are the same, only you sometimes can't free text the 'Diagnosis'. Search their provided list. Ask your Seniors. Note the list is very extensive and includes symptoms or unknown, so you will find one to fit without much difficulty.

A JUSTIFICATION FOR AUTOMATION, EFFICIENCY AND MINIMISING MENIAL TASKS

TEMPLATES: VICE OR VIRTUE?

There'll be many people, particularly of the old school, who, despite in principle agreement with the methods advocated here, will still avoid them because of a nagging feeling that you're taking a shortcut, an easy way out, and thus you may become negligent, that you're not looking after the patient and recording what happens to them as you should.

Ideally, you'd do everything to perfection. However, the thing perfectionists overlook is that there's only limited energy and attention span you have each day. Whether you use it on things that do *demand* attention, or that don't, it'll be used. Now if you use it on every little thing, doubtless, all those little things will be well done.

At the beginning of the day.

But after? Since you've used your attention quota of the day, why everything after will be poorly done, and prone to error.

Now it's far smarter, more efficient and hence better for the patient if you only use the keen edge of your attention where it's actually needed, e.g. during patient Assessment, while all the menial yet necessary tasks could just take care of themselves or use as little energy as possible.

That's the aim here. For you to use brainpower and energy *only* when your abilities *as a Doctor* are needed, and save it being wasted elsewhere.

And one of the largest absorbers of time and energy is Documenting and other admin tasks. Typing about the endless things you did, which it was faster to do than to type about. Ordering and charting the same things repetitively. All the random jobs which in collective absorb more than 50% of your time (conservative estimate). So tremendous a time absorber it is that the system has created a special position to absorb them, the name of said position it seems superfluous to mention.

But you're here to think, to learn, to experience, and not be a perpetual paper-pusher.

Yet paper must be pushed.

Hence, Templates, who shall now paper-push on your behalf, who can do it faster and more accurately than you, whose sole aim is to save you time and strength and allow that precious energy to be spent on patient care.

ON PETTINESS

People often think about the pettiness of it all. Isn't it just typing? How long will it take? Why are you so protective of your fingers, that you're protecting them even from the keyboard?

That is not the point.

The nature of much JMO work is repetitive. Very repetitive. Hence, any gain in efficiency, *any gain*, is multiplied a thousand-fold, a gain that will leave you time, attention, energy, to do the thing you want to and need to do.

Look after patients.

Spelling 'pateint' wrong won't kill them. Missing a Blood result might.

But you want to spell 'patient' right too, you say. So you go back and correct it because you're so very professional. Multiply that by a hundred, and you're staying back till 8 p.m.

Effectively, every time you're doing the same paperwork, every time you type 'Hosptial' wrong or the name of that Boss who you could never get right, or 'diarrohea' (because that's how you spell it, right? Especially at 9 p.m.), you're wasting precious time.

You want to avoid this.

When there's only one Discharge to do, all this is nothing perhaps and petty enough. But when there are a few thousand of them, especially if you've got busy Terms each year, even if you save 5 minutes off each (it will be more), you'll save much time overall. In fact, at that conservative estimate, 60 hours or more of straight work.

Straight as in no rest, no lunch, no toilet breaks. That is, more than an extra week of Annual Leave.

It adds up.

And it's possible. Suppose you never spelt anything wrong. That you didn't even need to type, except a few data points of variability, and the Documenting required would manifest itself?

Templates.

Hence, Templates simply save you time, save you errors, save you effort, and yet are more accurate and reliable than you are yourself, for you're using the machine advantage, the ability to do the same things instantaneously and accurately. For a lot of things in Medicine, you know what to look for, you know what to do, exactly, precisely, it's only the effort of doing them, the practical side, of actually sitting down and sorting them out that takes time.

You're here for head work. Don't you wish there was a minion who would sort everything out once you knew exactly what to do and told them to do it? No, we don't mean the JMO. But work has to be done. Who will do it then?

You will, or, rather, the extension of yourself will, who will never tire, never grumble and do it a thousand times faster than you.

The system.

But since the system has no mind, here's where you may use your own. You spend so much brainpower looking after patients. Perhaps just a little in organising your own tools? For that system needs but a little cortical capacity before it's organised to your will. After that, let it be and reap the benefits. The savings in time, energy, sanity. The system will do the rest.

ON ERRORS

The chief objection to automation and Templates is negligence as people may auto-text things that are generic and hence not true, generating errors.

We can only say that there are two types of people in the world: the careful and the negligent.

For the negligent, whatever system you use, they'll take shortcuts. With no Template, they'll type too little and hence be wrong. With Templates, they'll 'type' too much and still be wrong. Whatever the system, they'll be inaccurate. They need help to stop being negligent.

But it's the careful who need saving, the careful, who, through sheer volumes of work, stress and exhaustion, become 'negligent' perforce and generate outcomes which aren't normal or worthy of them if they were but in their normal functional state.

Consider the usual JMO on Discharge duty, staying back till 9 p.m. to finish these important legal documents which aren't read. Would a reminder not help them in their exhausted state? Or saving them the twentieth typing of 'Dear Doctor, Thank you for your ongoing care of …', won't that save time without reducing the value of their training?

Consider a busy JMO on After Hours, with multiple, simultaneous Clinical Review calls and Protocol-Based Reviews. Several are serious, the others simpler. Is it not better for patient care as a whole if the JMO could rapidly address and document the simpler/Protocol-Based Reviews while throwing full energy behind the serious ones?

The alternative case would be the same JMO bogged down by multiple and continuous Reviews, trying to document for all of them, yet each is incomplete as they're constantly being re-called to other Reviews. As the memory of one fades, another comes and mixes with the first. Add to that fatigue and constant interruptions, is it possible for good Documenting to be maintained? Documentation written in exhaustion, in retrospect and under the influence of numerous other matters which have taken the processing capacity of the first matter?

While with Templates, the JMO, with a few keystrokes, can document the whole Review in virtually all essentials, with slight modifications for each circumstance and can go to the next Review without being swamped by continuous typing.

Now, they need only apply their clinical acumen, while, effectively, the documentation materialises itself even with the thought.

Furthermore, Templates can even act as a learning tool, by prompting JMOs to look for relevant symptoms and signs when they may not be at peak performance and hence solidify learning and Assessment technique through repetition and cross checking.

And even for the negligent, if you make it easier for them to be accurate, won't they try to comply more often, considering the lower barriers of access?

Besides, with a little forethought as shown, Templates can be built in such a way that obliges you to indicate the result of an Assessment, or else be rendered non-sensical and hence null. Consider the spaces and underscores left to input the actual finding, the final 'Find' function checks to make sure all spaces are filled or deleted, the last read of the completed document. For who can deny reading is faster than writing, and the time saved from writing the repetitive will thus make available more than enough time for reading?

What we need is Doctors, not typists. And though Doctors do need to type, the amount they type is certainly far greater than what's needed. It's that gap we're trying to shrink.

KEY POINTS

- This whole system exists to save your time and energy for higher order tasks related to patient care, intellectually and emotionally, while simple tasks are completed with peak speed and accuracy with maximal automation, so overall to maximise patient outcomes.
- You have limited time and energy. They must be used on the areas that demand them.
- Each particular method may seem to save a petty amount of time and energy, but their aggregate in repetition is far from petty by sheer economies of scale. A minute is not long. Times a thousand is.
- The risk of errors will always exist, whatever method. The aim is to minimise them with safeguards; when you have more time and energy, you will make fewer errors.

ACKNOWLEDGEMENT

We acknowledge Cerner Corporation as the proprietor of *PowerChart* and *FirstNet* electronic medical record (eMR) programs and related and subsidiary names and terms within those programs. References in this work to eMR predominantly relate to the aforementioned programs. These references and descriptions are made based on the author's experiences, discussions and observations only.

CHAPTER 5

The Term: Organisation

The daily genius.

Organisation.

Probably the single most important tactic to the JMO's (Junior Medical Officer's) survival. Everyone has 24 hours, but some achieve stratospheric results while others struggle with basics.

The difference is here.

Now, the need for organisation lies in the difference in the way work comes and the way people work.

People like to work in their way. Be it steadily or in bursts, each person has a way and they'll stick with it.

However, work won't come in that way. No, work comes in its own way. And its way usually doesn't match yours. And that mismatch is where chaos is born, and where organisation governs it.

Essentially, organisation is distributing your time and strength to match your energies to the tasks in a way such that both the tasks are performed in time and you're not exhausted.

We'll detail helpful strategies below. However, it boils down to two states. There'll be busy days and chill days.

There isn't much to be said about busy days. Strategies are helpful, but people are similar. Push on.

But it's the chill days where you determine your survival. It's here where you can make sure there are no busy days (or at least none overwhelming) for you.

Organisation comes down to only five elements and their interplay. Know these and you can accurately complete maximal tasks with minimal wastage in time and effort.

1. **Know your Jobs**: You should have all your responsibilities spread before you. They should be explicitly clear. That is your field of campaign and by knowing, i.e. being on the ball, you'll be saved most surprises while nothing is missed. Creates the foundation for point 4.

2. **Know your priorities**: Know what you should do first, then next. Doing the urgent first won't cause problems. Doing it last will. This allows you to create a plan. You can only do one thing at a time (sort of).

3. **Know yourself**: Your own limits are important. You can't push them far. Know when to recharge to ensure maximal overall efficiency. Also, know when to get help.

4. **Act at every opportunity**: Take every chance to complete your tasks. Chances won't be given to you. You'll need to scrape them out. Be ever alert to them and seize them when you see them. It's a virtue to be highly opportunistic in Job clearance. Only possible with point 1.

5. **Anticipate**: Do in advance whatever you know will need doing. This will prevent a chill day today being followed by a tsunami tomorrow, in which you'll inevitably drown.

Below, we'll discuss how to apply these principles to your day, centred about the WR (Ward Round) (one of the dominating events of JMO life). You usually exist in three main states: On the Ward Round, Other things, e.g. Clinics/Theatre, and Off the Ward Round. Other things usually engage all your attention or don't exist. Hence, there are only two areas that need organising: On the Ward Round and Off the Ward Round.

Organisation is not hard. All it takes is a little awareness, a little forethought, a little discipline and watch your Jobs dissolve while the theoretical possibility of finishing on time becomes a reality as you not only comprehensively complete your day job but also have the potential to achieve your other goals in career and life without being obliterated by exhaustion.

KEY POINTS

- Organisation is matching your effort effectively to incoming work, as the two are often mismatched.
- Well-planned 'chill days' lead to manageable 'busy days'.
- Know the following: Your Jobs, your priorities, yourself and your opportunities – and anticipate.

ON THE WARD ROUND

You can do more than just type it.

This is most of your life in Medical Terms and a good part of any other Term. So its organisation is paramount. Considering that Regs (Registrars) will nearly always do a daily Round with all the patients, then multiple Bosses (Consultants) will suddenly decide to Round, perhaps multiple times a day, it makes sense that JMO life often seems like WR after WR after WR.

Hence, if you can manage this system of endless WRs, you'll be able to optimise your day without being driven insane. Conversely, if the WR time is not optimised, then, clearly, ever leaving the Hospital before 9 p.m. will seem a luxury too dear. And still the Jobs won't be finished. As everyone else you need help from will have gone home at 5 p.m.

The main trick is to document quickly then clear as many other Jobs as you can on the WR itself, and leave all the formal, sit-down ones to afterwards (which hopefully are much fewer).

Essentially, *every* Job, *except* calling for Radiology and Consults, can be obliterated on the WR itself. Procedural things, e.g. cannulas, are also harder, but hopefully you'll have the help of a Student/Tech/Nurse.

Consider doing literally *everything* doable on eMR (electronic Medical Records) *and* physical paperwork in those spare moments, e.g.

- Discharges/updating them.
- Ordering everything, including Imaging, Bloods and the various Nurse-assisted Investigations, such as urines, swabs.
- Consult request forms (harder as they take longer and lock you from the rest of eMR for a while, but get them ready in *Word* on an aside).
- Consents.
- Medical Handover forms (as above).
- Charting Meds (e.g. the newly initiated, warfarin, prednisone, insulin).
- Charting Fluids.
- Script writing/Outpatient forms/Med Certs/other forms the Nurses want.

In truth, this does require a bit of multitasking, but, often enough, either the Reg will be super-fast and you'll have time later anyway or the Reg won't be super-fast and much of what's happening on the WR can be documented much faster than it can be done. Hence, there'll be a considerable time lag between having the matter typed than done/discussed. The lag is yours.

This is the *culminating point* of all the systematisation, automation and simplification of each JMO task previously discussed, the endpoint of all the shortcuts and strategies to minimise extraneous work. By being capable of performing most tasks *on the fly*, you'll hopefully have nothing left to do except two things (mostly): namely, *calling people* (mostly Radiology and Consults, some which could be done on the WR) and the *unforeseen* (e.g. Reviews and other difficulties, though you can only prep for what you can foresee).

And when your skills are optimal and you have sufficiently friendly relations with Regs who are agreeable, you may even text Consult on the WR and similarly text Handovers to After Hours for simple matters.

Thus, by adopting this system, however busy the day is, even supposing the WR finishes near 5 p.m., your Jobs too will end even as the WR does.

To achieve this, consider the following ... .

Document

That's your main Job on the WR. Get that right first. All the rest is secondary and can be done later. But this you need to get right, *now*, on paper or on eMR, not only for you, but for the Team too and every other HCW (Healthcare Worker) associated with this patient. These are legal documents and serve the Reg's memory as much as yours.

Hence, use all the tactics mentioned previously (see *Chapter 4*, section *Documenting/Ward Rounds*). Templates should already be at the ready. Prep your documentation (prior to the WR starting if possible), especially the opening line and Issues (the bulk of both usually carry forward). Other elements may also persist, e.g. an ongoing element of the Plan (the patient is still waiting for RACF [Residential Aged Care Facility]) or Examination (that murmur is not going away) or pertinent Investigation Results. You can copy the prior day's note then edit and save it or just transcribe elements to *Notepad/Word* and copy across to eMR. Whatever works for you. Afterwards, use all the Documenting tactics previously mentioned.

All these strive to maximise the speed of Documenting while preserving accuracy, which makes the rest of this section relevant. If you barely even have time to type, so much for doing anything else.

Know your Jobs

You *must* have a meticulous system of keeping track and prioritising all your Jobs *as* they cumulate and as they're done. We recommend the Excel List (see *Chapter 4*, section *Personalised List/Excel List*) with extra columns. Consider prioritising using colours, separating the to do/to chase/completed statuses of Jobs with an empty box/half-coloured box/full-coloured box and acronyms for Jobs, etc. Major Jobs, e.g. Consults/Radiology, should be emphasised and written on your List. Minor Jobs (the rest) you'll probably have no time to write physically, so clear them by combing your whole List sometime later and check everything is done. Whatever works for you, so long as you capture all the Jobs in one place for rapid assessment and action.

Do it *now*

Jobs are often lost because there are too many. Even if documented. Even after Paper Rounds. Sometimes you're too busy to document or Paper Round.

To prevent this, do it now. Try optimally to do the Jobs even as the Reg speaks. Consider doing all the aforementioned Jobs (save Consults/Radiology calls/other calls). Did they ask for an Add On Blood test? Add it on now. A Dictician Consult? Now. A CT Abdo Pelvis? Order it, even if you'll need to call. If the fates conjoin, the patient may have 'arrived' in CT before you've even finished Rounding.

Because this is what you've prepared all those shortcuts for. To do it right now, within, say, 20 seconds. The Reg will often wait that long. Often, they won't even need to wait as they're trying to get somewhere near the patient's lung bases without breaking multiple backs or trying to stop the patient talking about how unpleasant Hospital food is. That time is yours.

Anticipate

When you get better and are longer in a Term, you'll be able to anticipate what the Reg wants for various common scenarios. Pre-order those Investigations/ Managements in ScratchPad, get the Reg nod, then sign. This will speed you up immensely and appear impressive as you're so very proactive.

Handover

Always let the Nurses know what you did, especially Investigations and changes to Meds, because often Documenting is not enough. If the patient's Nurse is there, tell them. Else, ask another Nurse to take a message. Make it easier for them and what you want will have a higher chance of getting done. Especially the Investigations, e.g. urine/faecal/wound, etc. swabs/cultures. These are harder still as it's a three-way cooperation: you, Nurse, and patient. You have to Order it, the patient has to generate it, the Nurse has to collect it. A break anywhere on the chain means no outcome. The patient will do their thing in their own good time. The Nurses have their other Jobs too. So do your bit as well as you can. And help the Nurses as much as possible. The patient, well, they'll poo when they like, stool culture or not.

This also goes for the rest of the Teams, e.g. Allied Health. If you can opportun- istically engage them on the WR itself, that makes it easier for both and saves the two of you playing page tag. See *Chapter 6*, section *Ward staff* for more.

Bedside matters

You don't want to keep walking back to the patient's bedside. Especially when your Hospital is a skyscraper height, ranch sized, complex. And your patients are diffused throughout, uniformly. Hence always:

- **Collect stickers**: Collect as you go to save yourself writing out stacks of addresses that you never want to see again and twenty-letter surnames which you'll spell wrong, especially for scripts and Outpatient Investigations.

- **Discharge and other documentation**: Scripts, Outpatient Investigations, Med Certs for relatives and the like, you can do them as you go and hand them directly to the Pharmacist or patient, then and there, if there's time. Especially as you have stickers. And all the patient-involved forms may be doable right now, e.g. Consents, MRI forms (see *Chapter 2*, section *Things to bring/Documents/Folder*).

- **Med Charts**: Take pictures of Medication Charts as you go, especially for those who are for Discharge to save walking back (irrelevant for eMeds [electronic Medications]).

- **Charting in general**: Check and write up new started Medications, Fluids, insulins, warfarins, prednisone doses, cease/start/note days of Abx (antibiotics). Do this even as you walk. Ask the Reg if unclear. This is the best time. But you need to be looking for these things, else you won't even know what to ask.

  Here's also where keeping a stash of charts is of infinite help. There'll never be a spare Med/insulin/Fluid Chart, ever, on a foreign Ward until you've lost half the morning looking for it.

- **Replace/address electrolytes**: You should be looking at all the Bloods at the same time, but especially check the EUCs and CMPs. And if they're deranged, replace/treat, as per the Reg. Then, at least you know to address them now and not discover 3 days later that the magnesium is 'critical'. Or be told by the Reg an hour later to walk back down the ten corridors and seven levels to chart Magmin.

- **Preparation for Other Jobs**: There may be multiple Jobs arising from the WR. Some which require further preparation prior to completion, e.g. Consults. Know what Jobs are coming, what their preparation is, and, hence, what you can do now to prepare, e.g. Cardiology Consult = Cardio letters needed = ask patient now which Cardiologist they see and in which rooms. Other things include a System-specific History/Examination for the Consults Reg, gaining Consent for various matters (or prompting the Reg to do so) and completing other patient-involved documentation. This is quite case dependent so be flexible. Hence, always ask yourself 'Does this require the patient's help?' as each new Job arises. If it does, do that part now. Doing this will allow you to harvest many efficiencies, so be alive to the Plan. Think spatially, rather than linearly.

Prep documentation

Mainly Discharges (as discussed). You can commence these, from day 1 Admission (or even before then, for elective Surgical patients) and add the current WR's progress into it, as you do the WR.

Have multiple windows open, the patient at hand and the patient soonest to be Discharged and not prepped. Thus, while the patient delays in answering questions, or is tangential, or the Reg is examining (longer to do than to write, especially with the Examination Template), you can finish Documenting, finish Jobs and commence Discharges. Sometimes you can even have a third window open in *Word* just to type as switching windows is not very easy in eMR. Use the 'Tear Off' function.

If it's difficult to multi-think, consider inputting the parts of the Discharge which don't require thinking. Add in the patient's demographics, Background, Social History, tick off the yellow boxes in the Discharge form, the number of copies to print or even just insert your Template. Every moment counts.

Even for the prepped ones, keep adding new Issues even as they arise to prevent trawling through an aeon of Notes. Is the patient constipated today? Very well, a new Issue you can add in right now.

It *is* possible to Discharge someone without ever having sat down.

Another option is to prep the Notes of the next patient you'll see (if that hasn't been done already). This also keeps the WR smooth and saves the Reg time. It also allows you to look coherent, especially when the Reg/Boss suddenly starts asking questions about them, again with the assumption of JMO omniscience in patient data.

Divide and conquer

Not a matter you can usually decide as a JMO but you can as a Reg. However, something you can suitably suggest, if appropriate. Essentially, on crazy busy days, if the whole Team stays together in a pack, you'll never get anything done, especially if it involves other people. You'll never get any Imaging nor will Consults be made. And tomorrow will be worse, as tomorrow will bring new Jobs, while today's are undone.

Hence, it helps much if you and the Reg split up, with the Reg continuing the WR alone (likely taking the Student to type) as seeing patients needs clinical skills (which the Reg has) while the JMO gets the essential Jobs done, i.e. Radiology and Consults, and re-joins the Reg when able. If the day is getting very bad, the JMO will 'Job stalk' the Reg on eMR, i.e. track and complete the Jobs the Reg documents as the Reg inches forward down the Patient List. This is probably the only way that both patients can be seen and Jobs completed as early as possible without both remaining till midnight. It also ensures that patients get the care they need ASAP.

Though this method is useful, it's very Reg dependent so you'll have to adapt ad hoc.

Learn

The above may seem like a lot, but, through sheer repetition, you'll be expert at it very quickly. Then, you'll become bored. Unless you start learning something. This is where the WR can teach you much instead of being the field the Job monkey tills.

At first, you're perhaps only too happy to be said monkey and likely too flustered to learn very much, with a stubborn focus on just keeping afloat. That's fine. But when you become proficient and you're surfing the work rather than being body slammed by it, then it's a good time to be more proactive. Essentially the WR is Medical rugby, or tennis, or any sport for that matter, just much slower. Here, you get the blow-by-blow Investigations and Management of the patient and all the various vicissitudes of their progress as you're treating the whole person and not just the Medical condition. You'll see the thought processes of other clinicians in dealing with various patient scenarios and directly see their effects. You'll see the direct application of Medical knowledge and you'll see practicalities.

Observe. Experience. Remember. Reflect. Learn. And, eventually, anticipate. Then, before you know it, you'll become confident in managing more and more Medical conditions, even on your own, with the Reg there to back you up. And soon enough, you'll be a Reg yourself.

Students

Part of many WRs, as you know. As you also know, often bored as they're often not sure of what's happening and find it difficult to ask questions as everyone, except themselves, seems busy. Also, they may be intimidated as it's a foreign environment. Remember the awkwardness you felt as a Student and the preference to march in packs? That's how your Student feels now.

The best way is to both teach your Student and make them feel helpful. We know you're flooded with work, but optimally try to engage your Student. They want to do something, most of the time. If they don't, they'll disappear quickly anyway so you won't need to worry about them.

Inform them of the patient's progress. Teach them about common scenarios. Ask them questions (in a nice way).

Everyone already knows to ask Students to do Procedure-related work such as IVCs and spirometry as this gets them ready for JMO life. But, also, let them assess patients, answer pages, call GPs and do safety forms as this helps with their communication. They can essentially trial everything you can do except actually sign for anything.

But, once they're proficient, there isn't much need for them to do it further, especially if they have exams. Students need to study, more urgently than JMOs mostly.

Hence, Students can indeed become your right arm, saving you much invaluable time while they learn the ropes of the Ward and the practicalities of JMO life. For they'll be doing all of it soon enough, and it's a good idea to acclimatise them to it without throwing them suddenly in the deep end. Turn their Ward time into a sort of work experience. However, try not to make it burdensome for them, i.e. be nice to your Students and let them go early enough so they can actually study.

KEY POINTS

- Rapidly complete documenting then do all Jobs (except Radiology and Consults and sometimes even those) on the fly while the WR happens.
- Use the lag between documenting the WR and the WR actually happening.
- Calling people (Radiology/Consults) can sometimes happen, e.g. as you migrate between Wards.
- Know your Jobs by creating a system, e.g. coloured pens, checkboxes.
- Do as many Jobs as possible right now. Possible with eMR shortcuts.
- Hand over tasks to other HCWs when they're ordered, e.g. Nurses, Allied Health.
- Do all you can while at the patient's bedside, e.g. collecting stickers, providing paperwork, doing paperwork, such as Consents, charting all Medications/Fluids, preparing for future Jobs.
- Prep as much documentation as possible, e.g. for next patient/Discharges.
- Divide and conquer if too many Jobs and complete Jobs separately while re-joining the Reg on the WR once critical Jobs complete.
- Learn as much as you can.
- Let your Students help with all manner of Jobs and teach what you know.

OFF THE WARD ROUND

Liberty. Use well.

At last, it's over. The Reg has disappeared into Theatres/Consults/Clinics/Procedural suites/Boss phone calls/other Reg lands.

Now's the time to sort out everything else.

In a nutshell, prioritise as per:

1. Clinical Reviews (hopefully none and everyone is stable).
2. Radiology.
3. Consults.
4. Jobs dependent on other Teams, e.g. Allied Health or scripts to Pharmacy.
5. Jobs dependent on only yourself, i.e. remaining Jobs/Discharges.

Do as much of each level before proceeding to the level beneath. Of course, note the above is sometimes variable and always subject to clinical urgency.

Using the Surgical Day as a model (these Terms usually have longer times off the WR), below is a schedule of how you may consider organising your day for maximal outcomes.

You'll be constantly interrupted. You'll be constantly disturbed. Your schedule will collapse. But, for all that, push on. Revert to your plan when you can. For all the tossing of the waves, the wood plank floats. Use this as your wood plank.

The Surgical Day Off the WR

Consider the following order of events:

1. **Pre-WR WR**: May or may not be required pending Teams. However, the following often needs doing. If you can do it faster, you can come in later.
   a. **Set up Lists**: Set-up time is much reduced using the Rounds List. May require a custom List as detailed in *Chapter 4*, section *Lists*. Physicians are variable. If you can set up and print in around 5 minutes (not hard if you follow the procedure), you can arrive closer to 7.30 a.m. Also add to the List any new patients from overnight.
   b. **Overnight progress**: Check all Bloods/Obs (Observations)/drains/overnight reviews, and make the Boss/Reg aware if they're significantly deranged. Make a note in your little box, the first box for Investigations, the second for Jobs, single tick for Obs, double tick for Bloods, if all good. If not good, record numbers.
   c. **Prep documentation**: Pre-type some Notes as detailed in *Chapter 4*, section *Documenting/Ward Rounds*, especially Issues/context. If still using paper Documenting, it'll be harder and you may need to pre-collect and write in patient files/charts.
   d. **Start Jobs**: If the Reg is delayed or for some particularly time-dependent Jobs, you can do that now. Uncommon, but be alive to that opportunity.
2. **WR**: You *must* get the Plan and the justification for all Imaging and Consults. Optimally, you can type. Mostly, you can't. If you have a Student or two JMOs, get two WOW/COWs (Workstation/Computer on Wheels) so one person can type while the other checks Investigations or sorts out small Jobs to cut down the hordes of tasks. The Seniors will often want to look at Results/Imaging, so when one WOW/COW is occupied, the other can work. This is utopic. Mostly, only expect to scribble down the Plan and hope for the best.

   You *must* highlight Imaging and Consults, e.g. in another bright colour, preferably red or green. It's very worthwhile when you're on such a busy Term to invest in a multicolour pen (it's tax deductible; also, humans have colour vision) so, with one scan of your three-page List, you can instantly start ordering the emergency Jobs instead of eMR trawling.
3. **Radiology**: Organise and Order all Imaging (see highlighted/bright Jobs). Order the first moment you get to sit, from X-rays to MRIs, in one massive sweep, and, simultaneously, *even as you order,* get on the phone to Radiology (which shall stay online for the next hour) and get every scan you can, approved over the phone. Avoid double calling and hence double holding.
4. **Journey Board/Nursing/Allied Health Handover**: This usually happens. It's usually fast so sort it out quickly and people will thank you for taking the time. People don't always read your Notes anyway. This is one of the chief communication exchange points. An excellent opportunity to hand over Jobs to the

Team Leader that you didn't manage to hand to the Nurses on the WR. Good time to receive feedback from other HCWs to the Team.

And now do steps 5–8 all concurrently…

5. **Document**: Start writing the WR for all those people you didn't have time to write for earlier. You can do especially step 6 concurrently. This will also help comb/organise Jobs and catch any missed. It also helps coordinate and provide Medical authority/clearance to other HCWs, e.g. Nursing staff, Allied Health. Remember, you're the interface, so, if you don't work, nobody knows what's going on medically.

    Depending on how good a multitasker you are, you can make Consults simultaneously, but, remember, most Teams are still Rounding at 9 a.m.– 12 p.m. anyway so, often, there isn't much point as most people just won't pick up their pager. Or they'll tell you to call back in 3 hours.

6. **Order/start all other Jobs**: eMR Order as you document, i.e. clear the minor Job as you write about them. Call the Ward if you're not there to ask them to do the things that're urgent. Try to have done this in Journey Board but you may miss things and this is the safety net. This step should take care of all Jobs save the Big Two (Consults and Radiology), i.e. various Nursing-assisted Investigations, Allied Health Consults, Bloods/other Pathology and simpler Imaging. If on eMeds, you can also order the Meds and Fluids now and save the Ward wander.

7. **Simple calls**: Simple means not Consults. And you will make many such calls. Chasing Clinic letters, chasing other HCWs, booking appointments and updating patients, do all these now while it's early concurrently with the other simple Jobs (see steps 5, 6 and 8), especially as each call will make you wait. Give that fax the 4 hours it needs to come through. When you're typing with one hand, Ordering with another, on hold in one call and answering another, you know the Jobs are getting cleared at an adequate pace. Note that this step shouldn't delay step 9 or onwards and you can go to step 14 if needed.

8. **Chase Bloods/Investigation**: Concurrent with steps 5, 6 and 7. Optimal at >9–10 a.m., especially if you've marked your Bloods as 'Urgent'. This is your major comb of all the patients. This is your chance to make sure nothing has been missed and for you to sort them out if they have. If there are Issues on Bloods/cultures/other Investigations that are urgent and/or missed, note down in a new colour and probably go into Theatres at this point. If minor, e.g. minor electrolytes derangement, sort them out yourself, but not necessarily right now. Go in one swoop later.

    Meantime, you can 'Bookmark' or 'Mark as read' all the Results as you go. This'll save you checking patients one by one later if any Results are still pending, one glance at the whole List will tell you where the new Results are.

9. **Theatre visits**: This may happen multiple times. Once you're fully updated about all the patients and there are a reasonable number of questions/notifications, go. Early. More time is better if more Investigations are needed. You want to catch the midday Blood collection Round if you can (if your Hospital offers this). Remember to get contingent plans for each scenario to save excess return trips.

10. **Radiology trip**: If approvals are needed in person, go now. Make sure everything is prepared, e.g. MRI safety forms. Aim to sort everything in one trip.

11. **Consults**: Hopefully some of the other Regs will have finished their WR and are in sufficiently good mood to hear your presentation. While you were on the WR, if you knew you needed to Consult for a patient, take a picture of their Med Chart (obviously unneeded if on eMeds). You may need to go back and clarify some of the History and Exam. This step should start ideally around midday or per local customs but as early as possible after Radiology. Only placed so late as often only possible after midday and you can't really just wait ad interim. If earlier is possible, always aim early (right after Radiology if you can).

12. **Nourishment**: Have food/toilet breaks ad interim here somewhere. Especially while waiting.

13. **Other**: Random things will appear here like various Clinics/meetings. Find out the urgency/necessity of each at the beginning of the Term from your prior JMO and/or Seniors. Then, you'll triage and do them as needed.

14. **Discharge documents/Order Bloods**: Do these all throughout steps 1–13, e.g. write scripts etc. on the fly, especially when waiting for people (which will happen as said). Also Order Bloods for tomorrow, and do any other Jobs which need no help and are relatively subcortical. Any moment is good for these, as long as it's spare. Ideally, this isn't even much of a true step, and you'll send people home even as you complete all other Jobs. But if you have fortunately completed all the above, you may well have earned the luxury to do Discharges at leisure.

    You'll be under a lot of pressure to do these. But your chief duty is to look after the sick Inpatients. If you can, send them down to the 'Discharge Lounge/ Transit Unit' or other similar facility where patients wait for Discharge. You'll probably be called even more from there. Tell them you're coming shortly. The biggest advantage of this Discharge Unit is everyone to Discharge is in the one place and the Unit usually has every document you need, e.g. scripts, Outpatient forms. And, of course, only one NUM (Nurse Unit Manager) is after you instead of a dozen. When you go down, send them all in one go.

15. **Theatres/Team Handover**: Ideally, here, go into Theatre for Handover and let the Team know what's happening. Usually, they'll be still operating/gone home/studying. Choose the least busy Senior and hand over. Thus, you can avoid waiting for a Senior to get unscrubbed before things start happening and will also ensure you may actually leave on time and leave enough time to tie up any loose ends or perform the new instructions they may give you. Depending on your Team, this process can start at around 3–5 p.m., possibly later, again depending on Term and busy-ness. Also, if you want more Theatre experience, now is a good opportunity if your Ward Jobs are under control. You can't assist if your pager is going off every 10 seconds. However, acquiring/avoiding extra Theatre experience will be highly Team/other JMO/ Medical Student/Term dependent. Organise what you want early and coordinate with the Seniors and your other JMOs.

16. **Ward wander**: When all above is done, and everyone is sent home who needs to be sent home, start wandering through the Wards, and start sorting all those random non-urgent Ward Jobs you've accumulated, e.g. warfarins, recharting Meds, non-urgent IVC resites, you'll know soon enough. Order Bloods if you haven't yet. Now go for your electrolyte Rounds where you trick'n'treat all the patients (who need it) to the KCMPs (potassium and CMPs) and so on. In other words, simply clean the Ward of all the remaining Jobs.

You'll probably be attacked at this time, to do all sorts of things, which, by then, is fine, as all other urgent things are cooking, and hence you'll be very ready to be distracted in all directions. It's also the most efficient way as you can clear your tasks all in one go, rather than the intermittent trickle of Jobs which keeps dripping on your forehead all day. Think of it as sleep. If a whole bucket of water was emptied over your head, you'd wake up. But, once dry, you'd sleep again soon enough. But if the same suspended bucket dripped over your forehead all night, even if was just half the amount of water, you'd need quite some willpower to get drowsy.

So, let that bucket be emptied in the afternoon.

17. **After Hours Handover**: Obviously the Team can't be onsite 24/7, for, surprisingly, you too need to sleep. But for time-critical matters, someone needs to follow up, tonight/over the weekend. Hence, it's important that if you need certain things done After Hours or have unstable patients, 'AdHoc' them on Medical Handover or hand over to After Hours as comprehensive a plan as possible. Most preferably in voice and certainly on the system. After Hours can pretty much do anything you can do. Just give very explicit instructions and as complete a contingency plan as possible, addressing each scenario likely.

18. **Home time**: Hopefully it's still on time now. Go home.

Various things will disturb this optimal schedule, including Clinical Reviews, MET (Medical Emergency Team) calls, random Boss Rounds, repeat Team Rounds and MRIs. You'll be called away to do random things. Use Phone Orders when you can. If not, just do it.

These interruptions will break the pattern of your day.

It may even break your day.

However, be not perturbed, keep calm, prioritise and revert to this schedule when you can, despite the craziness around you. That way, today, you'll float, tomorrow, you'll swim, and soon, you'll surf.

The Medical Day Off the WR

Pretty much the same as above but as there's usually more time 'on the WR' than off, most of the above steps will be compressed into the WR itself and everything save Radiology and Consults will be done *as you Round*.

You can almost think of it as a fire. Surgical Rounds are flash fires. You get everywhere, but nothing is really done per se, and you'll need to come and burn through the work later. Medical Rounds are slow burns. The conflagration spreads slowly enough, but, wherever the WR has advanced to, all the Jobs should be burnt out.

There'll be much more multitasking on Medical WRs; see section 'On the Ward Round' for how many things you'll need to do simultaneously.

On the plus side, your Regs are much more contactable (one doesn't need to unscrub to answer the phone) so there'll be far fewer Procedural suite/Theatre trips (unless your only Reg is always in Scopes/the Cath Lab, etc.). Even if they're not at your side because of Clinics/Consults, etc., they're always a call/text/WhatsApp away. There's also often a BPT (Basic Physician Trainee) always available to handle most things.

In addition, days are closed not with Theatre Handovers, but Paper Rounds where your Reg and you will sit and cross-check Jobs, monitor patient progress and make sure the patients you leave behind are safe enough. You can initiate this too as above.

When busy, there may be multiple Paper Rounds during the day, mainly to check how things are going, clarify your questions and exchange live-time responses to patient progress, e.g. from other Teams. Good time to ask anything. Sometimes, the whole process is performed via text/online, especially if the List is not long.

Otherwise, a similar schema as above should streamline the Medical Day as much as the Surgical.

KEY POINTS

- Prioritisation is key but, generally, Clinical Reviews>Radiology>Consults> other people-dependent Jobs>self-dependent Jobs.
- Generally follow the Surgical Day off the WR:
  - o Pre-WR note preparations
  - o WR
  - o Radiology ordering
  - o Other HCWs Ward Handover
  - o General Jobs + Bloods/Ix checking
  - o Consults/other necessary visits
  - o Nourishment
  - o Discharges/Jobs/Blood Ordering (throughout in all spare moments)
  - o Team Handover
  - o Ward visit
  - o After Hours Handover.
- The Medical Day off the WR follows a similar schema, only mostly merged into the WR itself.
- Paper Rounds are important and frequent.

LOGISTICS OF THE UNEXPECTED

Now, if everything went to plan, there'd be no issues. You could just follow the Plan. Done.

But things don't go to plan.

If the above were a guide on how to plan, below is a plan to deal with the unplanned. And the biggest issue with the unplanned is how to integrate them into your Plan, so it seems as if it was your Plan all along. And make it really so.

Essentially, there are two simple questions you should ask when something unexpected turns up.

1. *Should I be disturbed at all?*
2. *Where shall I put this disturbance?*

That is, assess then triage the interruption, and, despite all the unexpected, it'll appear you've foreseen them all, and, more importantly, sorted them.

Distractions/interruptions

These are disturbances. And there are many ways to deal with them so you're not so. Consider the following sequence.

- **Minimise**: The best way to deal with the unexpected is to minimise them. You're subject to a barrage of distractions and interruptions daily, many of which have nothing to do with you. The main strategy is to avoid becoming a nexus of attraction. In fine, sit somewhere discrete. There are many little portals over the Ward apart from the Doctor's room and the staff station. There are even places off the Ward which don't mind an extra Doctor, e.g. JMO offices/common rooms. The trek is worth it. This will considerably minimise the frequency of distractions as it's easier to just interrupt you, than page. And though your multitasking cells will increase exponentially from the beginning of Internship, in a busy Term, it's still not enough. Don't overstretch your system.

- **Prevent**: Adopt habits to prevent unneeded interruptions. Try to pre-empt and set up everything prophylactically. Sort out Jobs in advance (appropriately) that you know need doing, e.g. warfarins, insulins, Fluids. When you go to the Ward, always announce to the world at large if anything else needs doing as you leave. That way, you won't need to be called back (mostly). Advise likely duration of exit, i.e. to page after a certain time unless urgent.

- **Settle remotely**: Use Phone Orders when you can. Remote print Order forms. Document remotely. Chart Meds/Fluids remotely if you have eMeds. If non-urgent, ask the task to be placed on Task Manager, JMO Job Book, JMO whiteboard or wherever else Jobs are put. Moving is an effort and disrupts your flow. Solving problems doesn't have to.

- **Hardware**: To continue working even through distractions, it's a good idea to have access to *either* multiple phones *or* a relatively exclusive one *and* a well-charged mobile or bring your charge cable. You can hence page *and* call numbers with long holds *and* have a spare phone to return pages, all simultaneously, without destroying your page/long hold. There's a chance of getting too many calls at once, but that's a small chance and you can always triage. But the time savings are immense and the Ward and world at large can stay under control.

- **Coalesce**: Distractions are inevitable. But their timing is malleable. Hence, to both satisfy the Ward and not be driven crazy, set a period for yourself to be distracted and thus coalesce all the distractions into one limited time frame. Have some low-attention tasks at hand, e.g. Ordering Bloods/Recharting Meds, sit in the most conspicuous area and prepare for the onslaught. If this becomes your custom, it's very possible everyone else will hold off the page and find you then. It's not like anyone likes paging any more than you do.

- **Assimilate**: More on this in section 'Prioritising'. But unavoidably, despite the above, your schedule will be disturbed by unexpected tasks. When you can, absorb them into your programme. Note them, triage them and clear them in your own time, e.g. via an urgency/location basis. People will trust you more if you do the things they ask for, in time, and hence not page obsessively. But, when you can't, you'll integrate the new tasks in a manner that doesn't destroy your day, as we shall see below.

KEY POINTS

- Minimise them – be discreet.
- Prevent them – pre-empt maximally.
- Remote solutions – Phone Orders, remote printing, etc.
- Good hardware – multiple phones available on standby.
- Coalesce them – gather all Jobs in one time point.
- Assimilate them – into your schedule.

Dangers of interruptions and justification for regulating them

Again, some may find the above excessive. But interruptions do considerably hamper any work and greatly reduce efficiency. Have you ever wondered how a simple task, e.g. one simple Discharge, could take all afternoon?

The main reason is recurrent mental reorientation.

Suppose you start something. You have to focus on it, and plan in your head how to do it, then prep the things needed to do it, then actually do it. Now if, anywhere along that chain, someone breaks in, all that effort is wasted. For you'll have to attend to this other person, answer/fix their problem, wait for them to go away, then try and remember where you got up to in your original task.

And it's even worse if that person actually wants you to do something, now. For, by the time it's done, someone else will come. And want you to do something. Now. Repeat.

The end result is you'll know and semi-start about a dozen tasks, of which none will be done, and you've probably clean forgotten about your original task, of which the Team will give you a very apparent reminder tomorrow.

You want to avoid this.

Ideally, you'll finish one task then start another. But, as that's often not possible, consider the strategies above to both maintain your own workflow and solve other issues. You can't change others (easily). But you can change yourself. Change yourself for the better.

Prioritising

Now for the tasks that *must* obtrude into your flow. The best way to sort them is by prioritising, and hence integrating them into your schedule, as if you received them on the WR. This can be confusing. However, consider the following general guide and avoid the pitfalls to prevent your pristinely planned, highly efficient and streamlined day grinding to oblivion by a few Job spanners in the works, however hard they were thrown.

Consider the following:

- **Usual rules**: You have your usual rules for prioritising Jobs as above (see section 'Off the Ward Round'). Just follow these for the interrupting task and you can't go wrong by much. Think what category this new Job falls into, and triage appropriately.

- **Ask**: The Team always knows. And if they don't, well, you can feel better not knowing either. And it precludes them from castigating you later (somewhat).

- **Assess**: If still unsure, consider two things. Is the matter:
  - Time sensitive? i.e. *must* be done by…
  - People sensitive? i.e. someone else *must* help you to … (more difficult the more people needed).

  Of course, clinical urgency takes precedence but this is usually defined by the Team, though you should ask if there are doubts. But, for most other things, follow the above. The more 'yes-es', the more urgent.

- **Speed**: The speed a Job gets done is also influential. Many things can be done quickly, even if not that urgent. It's worth it just to do them. However, have a threshold, e.g. if it takes less than 1 minute, just do it. Else, leave for later. It's like any game. You need to go where the money is, and not be bogged down by trifles. And, if there's time at the end, you can come back and collect the trifles. But if the trifles are just *there*, you may as well get them.

KEY POINTS

- Apply usual rules.
- Ask the Team.
- Assess via asking time sensitive? People sensitive?
- Speed – do if can be done rapidly.

Pitfalls

- **Chillin' when it's chill. Then getting smashed. Unnecessarily**: Work is wave form. If you follow it, your life will be too. That is, you'll have super-chill days, then be super-smashed. And more of the latter owing to the carry forward of incomplete Jobs. But despite work's nature, you can still sail smoothly. Often. The key is to work steadily, i.e. pre-empt all Jobs when chill, then reaping the benefits when crazy (see section 'During the chill'). Your life will thus no longer have as many of those crazy peaks and troughs. And, with some luck, you can even smooth out the tidal waves of work.

- **Not prioritising**: You can't defy the general priority system already defined. You also can't have no system. And you can't operate on a first-in, first-served basis. If you just do whatever, there'll be total chaos. You'll be destroyed for no reason. Hence, you *must* keep a constant and meticulous watch over your Jobs, and not only have a firm prioritisation system in place, but be continually re-assessing them as circumstances change.

    Swimming against the tide is hard. But, to avoid, you first need to know where the tide flows. Thus, organise the tide of your work, or be drowned by it.

- **Being prioritised**: You may well have a good system. You may well know what's important. But it's not enough. Because other people will know what's important too. In their opinion, at least. And they'll insist. And prioritise for you. That's nice. However, you need to stick to your guns (unless the new matter is really of higher priority). You, or rather the Team, should know what the patient needs most.

    Otherwise, instead of doing what's most important, you'll do whatever grabs your attention. You'll be attention prioritised, not urgency prioritised. And there'll always be things that grab your attention. Often, much more than the things that *need* it. And your time will be expended by the former at the latter's expense.

    Note that often attention-grabbing things aren't that urgent. Some are, but many aren't. Little will happen if your attention isn't grabbed by such. But if you do attention-grabbing things and let urgent things slide, the latter will certainly grab your attention very soon. In a way you'll regret. And in a way the patient will suffer.

    The sick, dying patient often is silent and kicks up much less of a fuss than the howling one. Yet one is dying and the other may well be far from it. The one needs saving *now*. The other after them.

    Remember that, when you wish to succumb, it's a disservice to the patient to delay the most critical elements of their care. The patient isn't here to insist, unfortunately.

- **Excessive rigidity**: On the flip side, you need to be adaptable. Medicine and patient progress is dynamic, and they all need different things, at different times. Hence, always carefully assess the new task before consigning it to the 'later' basket. There may be many synergies you can pick up if you address it now, especially if the Job is person dependent, and the person is right there. This will also prevent ridiculous scenarios like still going to Radiology when a MET call is happening.

- **Documenting**: A common trap, especially for the orderly person on crazy Terms, is to complete all their Documenting, then start everything else. But you can't. By the time you've documented properly for your forty patients, a good chunk of the morning will be gone, and you'll find the Radiology queue has looped a few laps around the Hospital. And that scan will never get done. So always do time- and people-dependent Jobs before those only dependent on yourself. The latter you can do whenever. The former you can't.

- **Excessive persistence**: You'll find some things just aren't working, however hard you try. A Consult. A scan. A booking. Though persistence is mostly a virtue, it can be a vice if it's absorbing your whole day. Avoid this. Try something, say, two or three times, then *change your method*. Try a different angle. Or stop.

  Infinite things may make something impossible. Someone is on Leave. Has an ADO (allocated day off). Is sick. The pager is at home and not diverted. Pathology is broken. Radiology is broken. A million sick patients in ED, etc.

  But, however hard you punch a brick wall, it isn't going to break. Your fist might. And many things (as seen) may well be brick walls, at least today. Know that early to preserve effort and sanity.

> **KEY PITFALLS**
>
> - Not preparing during chill times.
> - Not prioritising/being prioritised by others.
> - Not adapting to circumstance/excessive persistence.
> - Documenting everything first, rather than doing everything.

During the chill

Yes, good things too are unexpected. And need managing.

Despite the apparent impossibility, you'll have days where you've sorted out absolutely everything (for today at least). It's early, and the hours are before you, unpaged, untroubled, free.

You could just relax, indulge yourself a little, chill. Or you could know what this really is.

The calm before the storm.

As mentioned, it's during the chill when you determine your survival (or lack thereof) in the time ahead. And there's only one rule to ensure the former.

Pre-empt your Jobs.

This is the only secret. This is what allows you to calmly absorb a tripling of your List over the long weekend. This is what allows you to send some ten to fifteen patients home in a day even if half were long stays, and still get out on time. This is what allows you to surf the patient tsunami instead of being rolled by it.

There are only two categories of pre-empting: first, Job pre-empting, then personal pre-empting.

Job pre-empting

- **Prep Discharges**: Probably the single most important pre-emptive Job, and the most time consuming (see *Chapter 4*, section *Discharges*). Don't ever grudge the effort. It'll always pay you back. There's also nearly never wastage. Even in TOCs (take over cares), it's common courtesy. And there's no time too early for it. You can start these on the day of Admission. And you've only ever exhausted pre-empting this Job if *every* patient on your List has an up-to-date Discharge. So start them for those who don't have them, and update the ones that do.

- **Bloods**: If chill, Order them *now*. You never know what the afternoon may bring. But one thing won't change. Patients will need Bloods tomorrow.

- **Chasing**: Make sure all the people-dependent Jobs are chased. There are things which you can't get around to chasing when crazy. Chase them now. Make sure they're as far on the road as possible. And you'll be one step closer to getting your long stays moving and delayed/blocked Jobs going.

- **Any other Jobs**: Prep whatever you can prep. Med Charts, scripts, forms, etc. for tomorrow. But the key is to avoid wastage. Know *for sure* before acting. Preparing too much can backfire. So make sure it's needed, then do it.

- **Optimising your system**: There are many bits of maintenance you need to perform on your existing systems and refinements you can make through experience. The months need changing on your Discharge Template. A new Boss has arrived. A certain Blood test needs to be favourite-ified that you haven't got around to doing. Use the calm to maintain, then optimise your system. Always seek improvements, but now is the time to put them in place. The system is your ship. Tie up your rigging, mend your sails, grease your decks and plug your leaks, so, when the tempest comes, you'll cleave through it rather than be cleaved by it.

- **Help out**: Your peers and you are in this together. Save each other to save yourself. Also, karma exists. Make some of the good sort.

Personal pre-empting

- **Study/getting extra experience/career development stuff**: Obvious for your career and becoming a better Doctor. Study is obvious. You can also see extra patients in your desired Specialty, get involved in projects, seek out other learning opportunities, etc.

- **Life/career admin**: Takes up much time. Do it now if you can.

- **Other**: Wow. If you still have spare time, you can figure it out yourself.

KEY POINTS

- Pre-empt all Jobs, including Discharge updating, Blood Orders, chasing and system optimisation.
- Help your peers.
- Study/clinical experience/career development/admin.

ACKNOWLEDGEMENT

We acknowledge Cerner Corporation as the proprietor of *PowerChart* and *FirstNet* electronic medical record (eMR) programs and related and subsidiary names and terms within those programs. References in this work to eMR predominantly relate to the aforementioned programs. These references and descriptions are made based on the author's experiences, discussions and observations only.

CHAPTER 6

The Term: Human Relations

INTRODUCTION: HOW TO HELP OTHER PEOPLE HELP YOU

People get things done. You need to get people.

If you're from a science background, you may think that Medicine is all about treating people, relieving them of their illnesses with good evidence and a really scientific approach. Unfortunately, you're in for a very rude awakening. From a practical point of view, there's very little 'science' for you, at least, little enough for you to decide. The science and evidence for everything, developed and to be developed, is often years above your pay grade. You may learn, sure. But the decisions … well, not yet.

Rather, the true practical side of Medicine is immensely about human relations and navigating the little canoe of yourself through a tremendous sea of all sorts of other vessels, including yachts, ferries, cruisers, frigates, warships, submarines, aircraft carriers, and sharks, i.e. other seafarers generally much more potent and, importantly, much more destructive than yourself, a collision with any *one* able to turn anything from your day to your whole Term into a floundering nightmare.

You'll deal with a vast array of people. Doctors, Nurses, Allied Health, Admin, Supportive Services, Special Services, in all their ranks of seniority, on your Home Team and off it. And, of course, you'll deal with the infinite variety of patients and the more infinite variety of families and friends with them, each with their own special set of needs that need addressing.

You are only one person. There's only so much your one person can do, even if you were a Consultant Professor. And if you're reading this, you're most likely a PRINT (Pre-Internship) Student or JMO (Junior Medical Officer), which means that you're effectively able to do almost nothing (so you feel), while you request/

wait for someone who is more qualified to do the job you need done, the job you really want to do, but can't completely. That is, look after your patient.

Now, is that possible? Yes it is, for there are experts in literally everything in Medicine who can help. However, the guardians of that knowledge aren't machines who you can simply summon, anyhow, to save you. They're people, and with people come all their attitude, quirks, preferences and everything else that will make them unhappy to do whatever you need them to do. And therein lies the importance of human relations. For, let's face it, nobody likes extra work. And when you ask anyone for anything, you're essentially giving them more work. However, when well conducted, people are mildly less discontent. And that slightly less resistance (cumulative) may well make all the difference, from your day to your career.

So, make this process as painless and as strictly necessary as possible, and not only will everything that needs doing be done, but you won't murder everyone along the way with sheer annoyance, or be murdered, though likely in a different manner.

Below, we will discuss some general guides relating to all the people you'll likely encounter in Hospital and how you can win maximal cooperation from them in the areas where your paths cross. Use this as a start, follow your local policies, improve constantly and you'll find yourself gliding over your sea of work, buoyed by a thousand friendly wings, instead of drowning in an avalanche of Jobs, while a thousand hands pile on chores the more.

PHONE CONTACTS

Direct access – save your contacts.

You'll find the most time-consuming work is on the phone. There's extraordinary time waste in just finding the right person to talk to.

As said earlier, as a JMO, you're pretty powerless, i.e. you can't do most things that need doing. Hence, a lot of your job involves calling on those who *can* do, *to* do. And as people generally don't like being summoned, least of all to do more work, and less still to meet you face to face to receive more work, you'll find much of your human contact, and much of your work, is over the phone lines.

Phones are clearly superior to finding the person in person (from a purely logistics point of view), but, nevertheless, their methodology in Hospitals involves severe inefficiencies and are hence great time eaters.

One does not simply call the mobile, like in the real world. Generally, you must first go through Switch, wait for Switch to pick up, wait for Switch to find the number, wait for that number to pick up, +/– speak to a secretary, wait further and, after all that effort, be informed, very usefully, that Dr XXX is on Leave and won't be back for 3 weeks. Or worse, you go straight to voicemail. The paging system is worse, for there's no one even to speak to, yet you still have to wait for the paging line to pick up. Then, pager return times take anywhere between a few minutes to never. If the matter is urgent, you still must, out of courtesy, wait for a return call for a certain time interval, ranging some minutes to a quarter of an hour, then warily page again while wondering if someone will be annoyed at you for paging at half hour intervals. It's very easy for one Consult to eat up 1 hour of your day, possibly more. And that's just to get through.

Hence, if you had only four or five difficult Consults, that'd be enough to destroy your day, as it'd leave no time for anything else.

It's thus extremely important to obviate as many of the intervening steps as possible, for each extra motion is wasted time and energy.

You can't help it if people don't pick up. Besides, not picking up is an outcome in itself. But try to minimise all the other steps. And to skip all the other steps, there's only one way.

Direct access.

Try to obtain direct access for all the services you commonly require. For Doctors, it's often the Team Reg (Registrar) mobile +/− speed dial, and, for everyone else, it's direct extensions +/− mobiles.

The direct numbers suggested below you should have on the back of your hand, if the back of your hand were so permanent. And if you don't have a permanent dorsal aspect of hand, then your phone. Get them at the beginning of each Term, even the beginning of Hospital life. You'll need to call them, endlessly. And you don't want to use Switch unless obliged.

View Switch *not* as someone to transfer your calls, but as an identity information portal. Get names, get direct numbers and get who is on. They know best, and the person must pick up, eventually.

It will be a bit of effort finding and saving all those extensions and mobiles. But, like many other things that need a little effort, it'll pay off marvellously. Don't spare it. At least you won't need to wait half an hour to know that Radiology is not available at the moment, a matter which will be very common.

Many Hospitals give a lanyard with common numbers, so use that if comprehensive. But, often, it's not quite complete, it's very long and one must squint. Your phone is much more user friendly. Therefore, consider saving the following contacts.

NUMBERS

The bold are saved.

- **Essential services**: Namely Switch, Hospital external extension (add this prefix to the in-Hospital extension so you can call back when there are no phones about), paging line and Code Blue/MET (Medical Emergency Team) call number. Few need to be saved as you'll use them extremely often, or someone else knows them and will do it for you (e.g. MET calls). However, if you're jumping between multiple Hospitals e.g. locuming, you may well need to. It's slightly embarrassing for the Senior Resident Medical Officer (SRMO) not to know how to page.

- **Radiology**: Every number possible. But basics include Reception, X-ray, CT, Ultrasound, MRI, Nuclear Medicine, IR (Interventional Radiology) and the Registrar for each of the previous (if there's one callable). Depending on the Institution, you may need to call different people for scans, e.g. Radiographer versus Reception versus Radiology Nurses. Get all their numbers and save them all under Hospital Radiology.

  When you're next level in the Radiology game, you'll know there are multiple phones in Radiology, but only one is published, and that's the chronically busy one so you'll never get through. Know the numbers to the other phones as well and you may hear the ringing instead of busy tone, one step closer to being picked up. Switch is an excellent resource for these.

  When you start saving multiple numbers just for 'CT Radiographer', you know you're on the right track. These methods will maximise chance of contact even at the busiest times and obviate the strenuous walk.

  The Radiology Reg number is likewise essential, especially to approve scans or to seek advice. Ideally, you could call the Boss (Consultant) too, but usually Bosses are Consulted in person. Once one of the Radiology Doctors gives approval, you can count your scan as done (but still check with their bookings person).

- **Team Reg numbers**: Not pagers as mentioned, but mobiles and speed dials. This will be detailed later, but assiduously collect these. Don't even consider if you'll Consult them again, for you will. You won't call them so liberally, but the hours you'll save through updating them via texts and receiving instructions will be a blessing (this is the digital age). Same for speed dials, which you can call unhesitatingly (as they're speed dials, not slow ones). Frequently give away your own number so they can return the favour and text you to facilitate communication. Regs don't enjoy paging JMOs and being left response-less.

- **Pathology**: Essential as everyone has Pathology of some kind, even if just Blood. You'll need to call them to expedite certain Bloods ('Please do CMPs first' or certain Bloods have become 'Life threatening' rather than just 'Urgent') and some 'Add On' Blood tests. Pathology is usually extremely reliable and tests will always be done unless they can't be. It's mainly calling to confirm they're getting done (and not find out the test you're desperately waiting for is cancelled 2 hours later), timing, technical matters like special tubes for special tests (usually printed on the Order form anyway) and if certain Blood tests can be added on and so forth.

  Have the Blood Bank's number as you'll be giving Blood, and not just taking it. However, the Nurses may often arrange this.

  Depending on the Term, it's sometimes worthwhile to have various departmental numbers in Pathology like Biochem (everyone), Haematology (everyone ×2), Cytology (if you asked), Anatomical Pathology for specimens (common in

Oncology) and Microbiology (always common) so you can chase them rapidly instead of being ping-ponged around the department.

- **Pharmacy**: Same as Radiology in multiple respects; like them, a high-demand service (including from Nursing staff) and, like them, has multiple numbers. You'll need their guidance for all sorts of drugs, infusions, approvals, scripts and the like. If confused at all, just call. There's always someone there (in business hours). There's often a Ward Pharmacist onsite, but it's easier to call directly than page if they're away.

- **Special Services**: Whatever other Special Service you frequently require, be it EEGs (electroencephalograms), NCSs (nerve conduction studies), Neuropsychology, Echocardiography, Dialysis or anything else, if you require it more than twice, it warrants a contact saved. The decision to save contacts is also proportional to effort. The harder it was to find the right person, the more it warrants saving. You don't want to spend that effort, times greater than one, even if it's every 6 months.

    There are also often Special Services associated with each Term, e.g. Dialysis with Renal, Cardiac Care and Echo for Cardio, Endoscopy Suites for Gastro, Theatres for Surgery, Diabetes Educator for Endocrine, EEG/NCS for Neuro and the like. Whenever you have much to do with them (you'll know within the first week or so) or believe that you will, just save their contacts. Often, they're very sub-specialised and there'll be a world of pain in going through Switch, so make life easier for yourself by saving and calling directly.

- **Clinics**: Whatever Clinic is associated with your Term, their number is also a must. You'll be making a lot of appointments, follow-ups and who knows what else, always 'in Clinic', hence continue with Switch avoidance.

- **Boss rooms**: If Bosses are in the habit of asking you to book appointments for them in private rooms, these too should be in your contacts. You could Google, or you could Google once. Take care, however, that you save and provide the right contacts as, often, Bosses will have multiple rooms and you don't want to send the patient half-way across your city only to find the Boss has a clinic next to their house.

- **Ward phones**: Almost unnecessary as you'll remember the extensions from sheer recall as you stare at your pager for the tenth time in 20 minutes. However, some Wards do page less, and when you do need to call them often, it's worthwhile to know multiple phones there as the Ward Clerk's always busy. Take note that, mostly, the phone will ring on deaf ears so you'll have to be patient. Think how often when you're in a Ward and the ringing phone becomes background noise. Put on speaker if you can.

    Always get the fax number, however. Hospitals often lag a good few decades behind the rest of the world in terms of technology (as it's a virtue to be conservative) and all sorts of documents will be faxed. And the inevitable question of the fax number will come. So save it and you won't be frantically calling the Ward for it while on the phone to an external clinic, hoping someone will pick up.

- **Faxes in general**: Faxes are generally pervasive so, in addition to saving the Ward fax, you need destination faxes saved. Usually less required as if someone wants something from you, they'll do the frantic search for their fax number. However, some services are so rare or high demand or require pre-faxed referrals so you must be even more on the ball than usual.

Faxes worth saving include:

- MRI (for MRI safety forms, though you usually must go down anyway).

- Pathology (for special Blood tests and other Pathology tests that may require approval).

- Other Imaging (including PET [positron emission tomography] scan, which, likewise, need special approvals).

- Various Clinics you often refer to (which won't book the patient unless they receive a referral).

- Inter-Hospital services: Any of the above and others which you may commonly refer to, e.g. IR. Their faxes will be even harder to get so save these.

Often, if you need to re-Consult these services, you can pre-emptively fax referrals over and hence obtain appointments and bookings easier. By later calling, this also rapidly identifies any documents lost in the fax void ('Have you received our referral?' the reply to which invariably is 'No') so it can be re-faxed and hopefully escape devouring.

Always remember to retain copies of documents faxed. It'll be ten chances to one that the fax won't be received. You don't want to write out the document again. Also, call to confirm fax numbers and faxes transmitted. Often the one on file is wrong, and even if right, won't transmit until fifteen tries later.

- **Allied Health**: A tricky one, for there's usually one Allied Health Team member you look for in particular and they carry a pager. So the same issues with pagers. The offices are often unattended, or unattended by the person you want. Besides, your patients will be spread between Wards and they often each have their own in-house Allied Health. But if you have one main Ward/ Allied Health Team, save the number, especially speed dials, mobiles and pagers occasionally. Allied Health often give their pager at the end of their notes, else it'll have to be via Switch. You can also transfer to mobile if the pager isn't answered.

- **Other Hospitals**: If you frequently refer to other Hospitals, especially a higher referral centre, you should save their numbers as per rules above, especially department numbers, e.g. IR, Surgical Sub-specialties, Pathology. You don't want to wait for two Switches, and multiple inter-departmental transfers before getting the right place's voicemail.

- **Pagers**: Optional and less worthwhile as they're pretty much on every Intranet. And if you need to call a Reg, you'll need both phone and computer. Besides, the effort of looking up your phone and looking up online is almost equal.

- **Door codes**: Not really a contact but very useful to save for direct access to resources. Especially of store rooms, equipment rooms, kitchens, toilets, other utilities. Save PRN into your phone. Especially helpful in After Hours.

- **Phone directory**: The ultimate contacts book. Usually only Switch has these, but if your Hospital has made public the whole Hospital's phone directory, know how to use it and save even the first call to Switch.

AD INTERIM

Golden rule 1: Work as you wait

So now you have direct access, but, inevitably, you'll need to wait. And, unfortunately, you won't have that luxury. If you want to finish at any tolerable hour, you'll have to optimise every minute.

Hence, prior to any sort of phone contact, it's always best to have something to do.

Always remember that you'll need to wait for *everyone*, from patients, to Nurses, to Admin, to other Doctors to even non-living objects, like computers, the paging line itself and lifts. Everyone, and thing, will make you wait. Hence, instead of hanging out your neck till you get a C2 spondylolisthesis for them at last to grace you with their attention, have something to do. And there's always plenty to do, electronically and personally. But …

Golden rule 2: To wait on hold is better than to wait in person

If you must wait, try to wait on phones. Because there, at least, you can sit, be comfortable, relax, eat and do the host of things you need to do on eMR (electronic Medical Records). Consider Discharges, Ordering Jobs, e.g. Investigations and Consult forms, Documenting your morning wave at the patient, checking Results, text communication to anyone needing communication. Try to do something using relatively low cortical capacity. A top favourite is Ordering Bloods for those fifty Surgical patients. Also, use speaker. And when there isn't that option, invest in an unlimited mobile plan +/– headphones and bring a charger. Save your own neck *and* have access to two hands, instead of one.

It's nerve-racking sometimes, especially when you're making a Consult, to wait for the phone to ring and have your purportedly pristine presentation constantly at the ready. Ten minutes may seem an age. And just when you thought you had everything ready, and they've made you wait sufficiently, and at last the phone is ringing, your own phone pings to announce a flash Boss Round, now. It seems hard, at such moments, to spare your attention for anything else, apart from keeping the presentation ready in your mind. Unfortunately, even so, you still can't just wait for this, especially when there are multiple Consults to be made. You'll have to choose the most brainless task and commence it. See section 'Consults (Other Medical Teams)' for more on this. But the point is, you simply don't have time to just sit and wait for the phone to ring. Otherwise, think 9 p.m. finishes.

Golden rule 3: You can still work if you must wait in person

Now sometimes, despite all above tactics, you still have to go in person. Yet there are still things you can do to defeat what seems the universal conspiracy of everyone to make you wait.

Everyone is excellent at procrastinating on their phones. However, consider doing work-related, paper-related procrastination. As you wait, you can write up scripts, Outpatient Imaging and Pathology referrals, organise/cross out Jobs, fill in the infinite number of forms you need to do and even your own Term assessment, which can take quite a lot of time (note that all these can also be done while waiting on the phone).

Remember, all the above will help get stuff done, but, most importantly, pass the time quicker and prevent you from simply trying to wring the person to your attention, social convention the only thing stopping you. And a weak stop it is when you're hungry, thirsty and it's 4.30 p.m. and you have still ten Discharges to do.

Everything *will* make you wait. But, unfortunately, you can't. So use each moment. It may seem hard at first. But with a little mindset, a little organisation and a little discipline, watch the work and frustration melt.

KEY POINTS

- Contacting anyone in Hospitals is often very inefficient: Consider multiple holds and pagers.
- To minimise inefficiency get direct access where possible and save it.
- Phone number classes to save include:
  - Essential services, e.g. Switch, page line, emergency line
  - Radiology (every department within it)
  - Team Reg mobiles/speed dials
  - Pathology (each department)
  - Pharmacy
  - Clinics (those you frequent)
  - Boss rooms
  - Term-specific Special Services
  - Ward phones
  - Faxes (where you commonly fax to and receive; keep the original document for the inevitable re-faxing)
  - Allied Health
  - Other Hospitals you refer to.
- As you wait, on hold or in person, do work.
- Much waiting = much work done.
- Prepare work in advance, especially easy Jobs.
- eMR Jobs when on hold, paper tasks when in person.

HOME TEAM

Your Boss(es).

This is the most important interaction of each Term.

This is the Team you'll be dealing with for a Term at least, and for who knows how long if you end up on the same career path.

These people will also know you best as they'll be working with you constantly, day in, day out.

So, it's almost critical to make sure you forge a good working relationship with them, for one Term at least.

Most will be pretty familiar with the Team structure since Med Student days. However, as a JMO, it's a significantly different dynamic and you need to be familiar with the new cues and keywords in interaction, usually as the Team always wants you to do something. So be familiar with the Team structure and interplay so that you can do everything they require with minimal pain and frustration while you can also get out of the Team the most you can, i.e. learn something and form positive relationships.

WHO?

The Team's members are variable. Mostly, it'll consist at least of a Reg and a JMO (you). However, it could be expanded to several Fellows, ATs (Advanced Trainees), Regs, SRMOs and JMOs. And, of course, your Team will consist of the Consultant(s).

ROLES

Consultants

- Give orders: They're the Big Boss. You do what they say (within reason). However, mostly, Consultants don't contact you directly. Their orders will be filtered down through the Reg.
- Look after only their patients: Don't discuss with them patients who aren't under their name. They won't know and can give only general advice (sometimes not that either).
- +/– Teach, +/– grill: Personality dependent. You may learn much or little. Be proactive and just do your part, ask questions when appropriate and show interest. You do what you can do.
- Term assessments/references: One of them will do these. Know early who. Similarly, usually referees need to be Consultants. Again, you'll need to be proactive to get these. Unless you're absolutely amazing or very much loved, people don't usually just offer themselves to be referees.

- Help: Usually Regs are the first point of call. Bosses should be happy to be contacted if the Reg isn't available. At times, it may just be you two.

Fellows, ATs, Regs

- Give day-to-day orders: They're your direct Boss and will be your chief contact. They'll lead the Team on a daily basis. If there are multiple Seniors, the most senior will generally lead. They'll work it out. They're all more senior than you. If any of their instructions fall foul of each other, inform both and let them figure it out.
- Look after *all* patients on your Team.
- +/– Teach, +/– grill: As above. But as you generally have much more contact with them, there are more opportunities.
- Help point: First point of call. Call them whenever in trouble. Start with whoever is available and generally the most junior. They'll escalate as needed. You may feel some decisions are Consultant decisions. You may also be wrong. They know these things better than you mostly.

SRMOs/other JMOs

- Split up Jobs with you.
- Work alongside you.
- The more senior members are semi-JMO, semi-Reg.

Medical Students

- You know who they are.

MINDSET

Someone once said that the JMO is the glue or cement of the Team, i.e. the one who holds everyone together.

That's a nice way to think about it.

It's also true, however, that whenever, wherever there's a hole, the JMO, like cement and glue, is applied to plug it.

Is there a problem? Step 1. Apply JMO liberally.

You may well feel this way, pretty soon into a Term, especially a busy one. But, remember, you're never truly alone. JMOs, after all, can only plug holes of a certain size. Any further, like glue, they stretch, crack then disintegrate. So always call in something heftier when you feel out of your depth. Namely, what you've been gluing together in the first place, i.e. the Team.

For you're effectively the Team's peripheral nerve.

If the Team was a nervous system, the Boss would be the brain, the Reg the spinal cord and you the effector sensory and motor neurons.

Hence, your job is mainly to detect things and effect things.* That is, let the Team know about Issues, and make their instructions happen. Note you're not an actual effector most of the time, you just make things happen. This accounts for your uncomfortable position, as you're reliant on others, for both orders and execution. And people don't command as clearly as neurons, nor execute as reliably as muscles, say.

We'll discuss the execution in later sections, as it's most of the work due to the plethora of effector personnel you must deal with. But, first, you must get the orders. In a way that can be executed.

Hence, you must get as much info from the Team as possible regarding their requests. This is true for most matters, more so for anything you anticipate resistance and *especially* true for Consults and Imaging. Thus, you *must* get the reasons behind Imaging (what we're looking for/ruling out) and Consults (what's our question). If possible, get even more info, like tips and tricks in getting the above, relevant preparation, compromises, contingency plans and the Team's bottom line, but, at the least, the reason must be clear. Then, even if there's no answer, at least you can say this is the Team's request and you'll look marginally less stupid than if you had just misunderstood the Team.

Note that your Seniors aren't being mean in not telling you these things first, it's just because everyone in Medicine is so preoccupied thinking about whatever it is they're thinking about, and orders are almost subconscious, that they've forgotten that it's possible that someone may not know what they know. But since everyone is mostly, and should all be, nice, then if you ask, they'll tell. Besides, it'll help them get the Job done so, even if they're not so, they should still be happy if they want to help themselves. Everyone would rather tell people to do something than do it themselves, so they shouldn't grudge you a little more telling. Also, it's a great learning opportunity to know the thought processes behind the actions.

ORGANISATION/PRIORITISATION

You must get stuff done. Hence, you need clear access, clear instructions, clear priorities and clear feedback. To get these, you need to be proactive.

Access

As you're usually the most dependent and the chief sorter out of stuff, you need to smooth access to those you depend on. Don't make contacting your Home Team as hard as getting a Consult. Know everyone's names, get everyone's numbers, do a WhatsApp group (especially if there are many Team members), piggyback onto existing communication systems, whatever it is to keep you guys connected. Unfettered communication is the first step to sorting out stuff, especially when you make nearly no decisions.

---

* Of course, everyone is encouraged to think and you should always raise any concerns and ideas you have with your seniors. We flag this as a simplified analogy and not to be interpreted as construing any medical officer as a nerve.

Instructions

Clear instructions is quite obvious, but where people are tripped is contingency plans. The idea is to sort out everything in one call as back-and-forth-ing wastes time. Hence, get the bottom line, for every scenario, for everyone. Always imagine it's the last call you'll ever make to them before you go interstellar, including to your own Team. This will sort out most Issues. Anticipating is the key. Get everything ready so that you don't need to call again, i.e. a Plan for each likely scenario. Some things are dependent on unpredictable clinical courses; in which case, you'll ask if you should call them with the patient's condition (the answer will be yes), and, hence, you'll preclude them from getting annoyed when said call comes.

The hardest to prepare for is for what you don't know. Obviously, you don't know what you don't know. Hence, the best way then is ask directly if anything else is needed to *complete* the involvement of the person currently involved. If you can't logically deduce it. The Reg's knowledge, being broader, and being so prompted, may awaken and save you both grief.

Priorities

Prioritising is hardest. Follow what's been said previously in *Chapter 5*, but get the Team to prioritise when it's getting complex. The Team knows what it really wants done first and most, even if you don't. So ask, and you will too. Plus, if the Team changes its mind, why, then they have no one to blame.

If the Team doesn't organise very well for you your whole raft of tasks, or if you're split between multiple Teams, don't despair. Prioritise yourself by gauging how urgently the Team wants something. You'll be told everything is urgent; however, you still have to do things one at a time, so ask them what's the most urgent. You may need to ask for each task. Then you'll find many things can happen in a magical land called 'Outpatients'. Similarly, many other things also don't need to happen right now (often, the Team will be more than happy if something happens at all during the Admission). And all those things will be more matters you can throw off your 'today' plate. If you don't, you may be a little stressed as you try to sort out a week's worth of work in 24 hours.

Feedback/update

Medicine is dynamic. Patients are dynamic. People are dynamic. Hence, what may be the best Plan in the world at one moment may be the worst in the next. Hence, always remember to frequently feed back to your Team regarding progress and especially about difficulties encountered. Live time.

You are the Team's livestream. Here's the benefit of the group chats and trigger-happy texting. Regs may say they're happy for you to sort things out. But, really, they want to know too. And even if they don't respond, know that they're patrolling their phone.

The best thing for you is that this feedback ensures things are sorted out in a timely manner. Regs can step in or escalate as needed. It hence ensures delays aren't caused by you. The Team should be happy to help. But you need to ask for it early.

LEARNING

The Team is a well of knowledge in their field. So, this is of course your best opportunity to learn about the Specialty on a day-to-day basis and investigate your career pathways. Be keen, show your interest, and the Team will be happy to engage you. Ask for things within reason such as teaching sessions, procedural opportunities and the like and you'll get the most out of your Term. And, naturally, if this Specialty Term is your career goal, prepare for your future job in knowledge and connections.

ADMIN

Get a good Handover from your previous JMO (see *Chapter 7*, section *Getting Handover*). This will make the transition much smoother. The main thing to ask for is what they wished they knew before they started the Term, then drill to specifics.

Communication is key. Most people are reasonable, and, if you have circumstances, they'll accommodate, so long as you tell them about it.

Find out who does your Term assessments. The Fellows/ATs/Regs can often do them, but, sometimes, it must be a Boss so it's critical to track them down early. You don't want to miss them if their only day in is in week 8 and then they're flying out for a 6-month conference. Check with your Institution.

Find out also who signs Overtime. Whether you claim or not is another matter, but you should know who at least.

If there are disputes, they're often best resolved privately face to face if you're pretty sure it's a misunderstanding. Anything further, your best friend is the JMO office, where the Director of Training/JMO manager lives, or potentially discussing with a more senior colleague. They've been around much longer than you and have seen pretty much everything or at least know someone who has seen everything and can help you out. Else consider other support networks but check what your local policies are.

WORKING HOURS

It's always hard to leave work, because, even at 4.59 p.m., somebody will want you to do something. No, they don't want you; they just want the hands to do the thing they need done. And it so happens those hands are, for now, grown on you.

But really, save in emergencies, you only answer to your Team, and only till 5 p.m. (technically). And many Teams are reasonable in terms of working hours; they know them better than you do. But, it's best, safe and courteous always to hand over before you leave. Depending on the busy-ness of the Term try to do this before 5 p.m., say 4 p.m., so once you've gone through your thirty-patient List, if there's still anything that needs doing, you still have a chance to do it without costing the taxpayer so much extra money and your own life outside of the Hospital. Essentially, the end-of-day Handover constitutes your dismissal, as it's the end-of-day wrap up. Initiate it as needed.

KEY POINTS

- Your Home Team consists of:
  o Consultant: Big Boss
  o Registrars (up to Fellows): Day-to-day Boss
  o JMOs: Compatriots
  o Medical Students: You've been there.
- Mindset: You must extract explicit instructions from the Team and their reasoning behind their requests, especially for Imaging and Consults.
- Organisation: You must have good access to the Team, including contacts, group chats, clear instructions from the Team including contingencies for each scenario and understand their prioritisation.
- Updates: Constantly update the Team regarding patient progress.
- Learning: Especially regarding the Specialty and Doctor life in general.

WARD STAFF

Know your Team. What they do, and what they want you to do.

This is the group of your colleagues who, after your Team, you interact with the most for you'll work with them, day in, day out. They can make your life very simple or very difficult, a matter chiefly dependent on yourself.

The main principle is just be amiable. Be nice.

Consider the following in assisting:

- **Names**: Learn everyone's names. It's most likely their favourite word in any language. It may be awkward at first, but it gets progressively more awkward the longer you leave it. It's fine if you don't know anyone's name in the first week. It becomes a touch weird after 10 weeks.
- **Simplify**: Try to make things easy for the other staff. Put the request form in the folders. Hand over to someone. Explain complex/out-of-the-ordinary things when needed. Apart from courtesy, the easier something is, the more likely it'll get done.
- **Courteous**: Just be generally nice and polite. Things get done quicker when people are happy.
- **Professional**: Hospitals are high-stress workplaces. It can't be overlooked that people can be *dying*, something not common in other workplaces. Hence, it's common for people to be grumpy and have their tempers frayed. Including yourself. But, when it happens, when someone is having a go at you or when

you start becoming frustrated, just keep calm (easier said) and don't engage (in conflict). Just focus on the patient's care, then move on. Remember, keep professional. Mostly, it's not personal. And if it is, it isn't for you. Of course, repeated offensive behaviour is not tolerable, but you'll get a feel for if it's the situation or the person.

- **Organised**: People are depending on you for certain things. The sooner they get them, the sooner they'll be happy, and if they're happy, you'll be happy. Hence, being organised will immensely lighten your day, by avoiding the tenth call about the same Discharge. Keep yourself on the ball and no one can roll you.

Now for specifics. Everyone has their own special abilities and their needs from you, so as long as you satisfy the latter and get their help for the former, your life will be much easier while patients will get the best of care.

Disclaimer: The powers and requirements are those that predominantly directly relate to you as the JMO. We're sure all the staff listed in Table 6.1 are even more talented than shown. But this is, after all, not a job description manual.

KEY POINTS

- Be courteous and amiable.
- Be professional and organised.
- Learn names and keep it simple.
- Know everyone's role and their expectations.

Table 6.1   Summary of Ward staff powers and expectations

Role	Powers	Expectations
Ward Clerk	All administrative matters and contacting families, interpreters	D/C (Discharge) papers, booking/appointment times
Nurse	All things, e.g. performs Ix (Investigations), gives Meds, other patient care. Special departmental expertise	Ix Order forms, IVCs/Bloods, patient reviews, most other Jobs, handover (verbal, written, meetings)
Nurse Unit Manager	All things difficult + sorting D/C-related Issues + Ward Issues	D/C patients, cooperation in sorting out Issues
Nurse Specialist	Expert in their area, takes Consults on Reg's behalf	Referrals (Online and/or phone)
Pharmacist	All Meds/Infusions, e.g. reconcile, dispense, education	Charting per their recommendation, approvals
Allied Health	See section 'Ward staff/Allied Health'. D/C clearance and assist patient function	Medical D/C clearance, early referrals, meetings attendance
Physiotherapist	Mobility, chest PT, rehab	Clearance for mobility

(Continued)

Table 6.1 *(Continued)*   Summary of Ward staff powers and expectations

Role	Powers	Expectations
Occupational Therapist	Function, cognition, ADLs (activities of daily living) Ax (Assessment)/Mx (management)	Medical clearance, likely goals
Social Worker	All complex social situations, RACF (Residential Aged Care Facility), services	Medical perspective at MDT (multi-disciplinary team) meetings, MMSEs (mini-mental state examinations), Geris referrals
Dietician	Nutrition + special feeds, e.g. NG (nasogastric)	CMPs (calcium–magnesium–phosphate), charting supplements, interventions to support feeds
Speech Pathology	Aspiration risk + communication Ax/Mx	Medical agreement for diet level
Podiatry	Feet!	Mx of underlying disease, e.g. DM (diabetes mellitus)

WARD CLERK

- **Powers**: Contact family, book interpreters (phone and in person), book appointments, handle Discharges, mail stuff to people, find forms, fax forms/stuff, fix computers and printers, Admin supplies, access a potential Ward email for staff email matters, generally anything administrative.
- **Requirements**: Discharge papers in general (the whole bundle), timing of Discharges +/− other 'Bookings'.

They are essentially Ward fairies. Usually, there's one Ward Clerk for the Ward and they know pretty much everything, except the Medical stuff, though often a reasonable deal of that too. One of the most important things for them is when to book transport and when the Discharges are ready.

Really, Discharge readiness is almost a sort of religion with almost all the Ward staff, *except* the Medical Team, who, often enough, couldn't care less about the exact timing, so long as the Plan is enacted and the actual Discharge is done some time recent. But, to everyone else, they're almost like the boarding pass for patients to embark into the outside world. And since it's your job as the JMO to sort it, everyone will be jumping on you to do them.

So it's best to have this ready early, as naturally everyone expects it to be almost instantaneous, as if you really were printing a ticket.

Similarly, if there are certain appointments or other bookings, the Ward Clerk needs to know about, let them know (it's true Nurses mostly tell them, but check local policy).

If you can let the Ward Clerk know of Discharges, transport and bookings, they'll be very happy with you and can generally help you sort out anything difficult administratively. Which, by the by, is at least three-quarters of your work, if not more.

Have you got a family member impossible to contact? The Ward Clerk will sort it.

How about an NESB (non-English-speaking background) patient with no translator and no further treatment until they get one and, for some reason, the translator won't answer your call or you simply don't have time to sit on hold for them for the next 2 hours only to be redirected? The Ward Clerk can sort it out. (They just have some secret channel, and when the other Service sees it's the Ward Clerk calling, then all is express. And if it's a Doctor, they put them on hold.)

How about getting appointments at Clinics which never pick up? Why, they'll pick up for the Ward Clerk.

Certain forms which some Special Services must have before they'll even record your patient's identifier? Well, even if the form is frozen in an iceberg in Antarctica, the Ward Clerk will source it, or at least get a faxable copy. And if you're nice to them, they'll fax it for you too.

How about printers which don't work? Here's the printer and computer whisperer. All rebellious technology, at their step, will instantly begin to behave, at least while they're in the department.

And, of course, all the million day-to-day things, beautifying Discharges, booking transport, replenishing the many pieces of stuff the Ward needs, etc., and finding you a pen in desperate times, all this the Ward Clerk can do for you if you only help them out with their two things. Which you have to do anyway.

Hence, you should often seek the Ward Clerk's help, as they'll streamline your day and cut down tremendously all the various Admin tasks which you hate, but is easy bread and butter for them.

NURSES

- **Powers**: Do pretty much everything, including Investigations you order (and those you don't, like Obs and BSLs [Blood sugar levels]), enact most of your Plans (give Meds, infusions), provide patient updates, generally look after the patient when you're not there in multiple ways that you don't need to worry about.
- **Requirements**: IVCs, Bloods, various Order forms for the things you want them to do, various patient reviews, most of your other Jobs, e.g. recharting Meds.

They pretty much run the Hospital. They do almost everything and touch on every part of patient care, including much of the stuff you mostly don't get involved in at all, like patient feeding, cleaning, linen, toileting etc. They also inform you of what's really going on with your patients. Remember, you see a patient for only 10 minutes a day (if that) while the Nurses see them for the whole shift.

However, as they're so frontline, you'll get most of your Jobs from them. Not because they feel like giving you Jobs, but, rather, they're essentially an extension of the patient's voice telling you what they need (often what the patient doesn't even know they need).

You will work very closely with Nurses. And, mostly, very well. However, at times, there will be a clash of priorities between you.

Nurses have their own set of priorities that are often different from yours, which explains why they sometimes do things/get stressed about things in a way different from you. It's mainly because many of their tasks are protocol driven, thus the inflexibility. Things like their various checks, day 3 cannulas and the like, are due to their rule books telling them to so do. And lightning itself couldn't disturb a RN (Registered Nurse) from checking S8 drugs, let alone a mere JMO.

The main thing is to give understanding, know your own priorities and engage in effective communication to work best with them. Consider the following.

Priorities

This has been discussed. You needn't be pushed into losing your daily mojo. The main thing is to field the constant calls and pagers. It's joked that Doctors can never keep a promise and hence don't make any. But, the fact is, you may be the most reliable and promise-keeping person in the world, but suppose you promised an IVC or a Medication rechart, and a MET call occurs, do you keep your promise or try to save the dying patient?

Hence, make a note of what needs doing, and try to do it, but never promise. They'll be difficult to keep. Your most frequent response will be 'I'll get to XXX as soon as I can.' People may not be happy, but people will be somewhat more unhappy if you walk past a MET call of your patient. Besides, as you work, and when you have shown yourself reliable, people will become more contented.

Communication

The cornerstone is simply Handover.

Often, there are at least three Handovers to be effective; in person, charting it/ Documenting it and in Handover meetings. You should try to do the first two on the WR (Ward Round), the third at the meeting (obviously). You may feel the effort of multiple Handovers to get things done is excessive. But, as you want things done, don't grudge the effort.

1. **In person**: Always a lot easier. Just tell them the Plan (related to them) and you can make sure they at least know about whatever it is you want done. If the Nurse is not there, find the TL (Team Leader) Nurse and let them know or another Nurse to take a message.

   It's not that they don't read your notes, it's just that sometimes you Round at random times, or your notes are rather laconic/unclear, so if they're not able to find you, they just can't do it. In-person handover also gives Nurses a chance to clarify anything they're unsure of and you'll be spared a page.

2. **In chart/paper/eMR**: Handing over documentation provides the actual authority to do certain things. You'll frequently be asked to document, as Nurses don't want to remove that PICC (peripherally inserted central catheter) only to be told later that the Team wants it and to have to explain why they removed it. Most simply won't do certain things if it isn't written. So document early. Also, for all swabs/Nurse-involved Investigations, it's ideal, when you're not insanely busy, to leave the form in the patient folder or in their hands. That way, they actually need to hold it, and the best way to get rid of it is simply to do whatever it is, then get Pathology to hold it.

   When busy, at least tell them it's printing right now, or call them when you Order, that it's printing right now. There's no eMR patrol, nor is there a printer patrol.

3. **In meetings**: Nearly all Wards have one of some sort and this is an excellent place to hand over everything required for your patient and get any feedback so make good use of it. Usually attended by all the Allied Health, NUM (Nurse Unit Manager)/TL and many of the Nurses. Excellent opportunity to let everyone know what they need to know without paging and waiting.

Nursing sub-specialties

In addition to RNs, there are a variety of specialist Nurses (like specialist Doctors) and it's good to be familiar with their roles as they have additional abilities and different requirements of you, so know how to be helped by the former and tailor to the latter.

Department based

As always, the more senior a person is, the better they'll be. Senior Nurses are generally great. They've been around much longer and you can often rely on their expertise. Juniors are really just like you (essentially new graduates) so expect what others expect of you. Compare a CMO (Career Medical Officer) or SRMO with an Intern. There'll be a difference.

Similarly, Nurses have different levels of seniority even before they specialise, which allows or restricts them from doing things you may expect that all Nurses can do, e.g. AINs (Assistants in Nursing)/ENs (Enrolled Nurses) may not be able to give certain Medications, etc. so act accordingly.

Nurses in different departments are also likely specialised and skilled in different aspects. Surgical Nurses will know a lot about dressings and drains. Cardiac Nurses will be very conscious of fluid balance and restrictions. ICU Nurses will be skilled in all sorts of lines and critical care. Renal Nurses will be proficient in dialysis matters. ED (Emergency Department) Nurses will be very good at Bloods and IVCs and will often do these on their own initiative. And so on.

Hence, know the Ward-/department-specific skills and limitations of the Nurses and they can help you much more in managing patients with the relevant needs.

Nursing Unit Manager

Always introduce yourself to the NUM. You should really to everyone, but if you hate it and prefer life in a shell, at least try to make an exception for the NUM. They're like your Home Team, and you'll see them every day. They can be very helpful too, especially if on side.

They are essentially managers of the Ward and pretty much run everything. They're also exceedingly experienced in dealing with every aspect of the Hospital as it's essentially their job description to do so.

Whose photo do you see at the entrance to every Ward? That's right, it's the NUM's. Almost as if announcing to any passing into their domain that, if there's any trouble, you know who to find. Trouble is almost part of their job description.

Hence, as they're almost the proclaimed trouble (to be conservative) magnets, they're exceptionally experienced in sorting out, and shovelling out, all sorts of difficulties, a talent which affords a protection you should certainly place yourself under.

They, and, by extension, Patient Flow, may well drive you crazy in their relentless push for Discharges. The main reason is not that they're trying to make your life a living nightmare, so that more and faster Discharges may be milked out of you, but that they're living in a different sort of world from you. You're looking after individual patients. They're looking after the whole Ward. And all the beds in that Ward.

As such, they have significant clout in dealing with all aspects of the Hospital, so long as it helps in getting the patient Discharged.

Hence, to avoid being driven mad and, instead, to be assisted by these agencies, the best approach is to have them help you push through obstacles to Discharge (and they're much more experienced than you at doing that). This help extends to a whole range of matters from administrative issues to various Services hard to get, etc. And they'll do it with extra good will if that is the sole impediment to Discharge. Once those magic words are pronounced, vast resources will be mobilised to make sure any obstruction is quickly removed or, more likely, bulldozed.

Thus, if you're having any trouble with *any* administrative matters or general Ward matters, in short, anything that you're having trouble doing, so long as it's not a Medical decision, the NUM is the go-to person. They have dealt with virtually every scenario possible (or know someone who has) and will sort it. And they'll be extremely happy if you present them with those empty beds.

CNCs/CNEs (Clinical Nurse Consultants/Educators) and NP (Nurse Practitioner)

They're all essentially Nursing experts in their particular area. They can help you immensely regarding anything in their Specialty and can guide you step by step. They can provide special expert help in their particular field (which can be almost anything), e.g. Diabetes Educator for Diabetes, Wound CNCs for Wounds, Dialysis Nurses for all Dialysis-related Issues, e.g. education, accessing ports/fistulas. So always know the relevant CNCs/CNEs in your Term and Specialties you often deal with. They're also often happy to teach, especially if you show interest.

Also, remember that CNCs often will take Consults on behalf of the Specialty. There are very often Drug Health, Palliative Care, Wound and Aged Care CNCs, who you can Consult first instead of the Drug Health, Palliative Care, Surgical and Geriatrics Registrar. They're usually less nerve-racking to Consult and will always be happy to see your patient. They're also often easier to reach than the Reg and they'll bring the Reg around in time if needed. So always check if there's a CNC in your Consulted Specialty to reduce Consult stress and salvage self-esteem. To Consult them, lodge their Consult form on eMR +/– call them (like Allied Health). With their help, the number of Consults made will be cut down considerably, especially if they don't require a call and/or the Reg is not onsite.

PHARMACIST

- **Powers**: Reconcile Medications, dispense Medications, provide S8 scripts, Medication History from multiple sources, Medication Management Plans and their like, educate patients about new Medications and Medication changes, inform you about Medications (dosage, usage, side effects, interactions, administration, approvals, etc.) and infusions and how to chart them.
- **Requirements**: Scripts, recharting/ceasing/modifying Medication doses (most likely because of eGFR/creatinine clearance or other Issue/interaction they've identified), approvals for various special Medications.

The walking MIMS. Your expert in everything Medication or infusion related. And if they don't know (a difficult thing), they can find out. And if they can't, the world probably doesn't know yet.

If you're unclear about anything Meds related, you should check with the Team, but also with the Pharmacist, especially when your Team has vanished into Theatres or Consult land. They can help with not just ordinary Medications, but also various infusions and how to chart both.

They're also able to collect great Medication Histories, often better than the rapid Assessment in the ED where everything is happening everywhere simultaneously. This is particularly useful when dealing with certain sensitive and addictive Medications such as methadone, other opiates and benzodiazepines, where the patient may not be entirely reliable, but where you don't want to overdose and see intoxication or underdose and see withdrawal. Pharmacists are also familiar with the dispensing process of special Medications so just follow their advice to navigate the Hospital checkpoint and checklist system.

They're excellent at discussing with the patient the legion of Medication changes the Team will make and can provide education on newly started Meds, e.g. anticoagulation. They can also construct a dosette box/blister pack, e.g. a Webster pak (or prepare for it), to make life easier for everyone.

The main thing they'll ask you for is scripts. You'll have a very happy Ward Pharmacist if you can give the scripts on the day (or day before) of Discharge.

It takes longer to dispense those Medications than the minute or so you took to write them. So ASAP (when there will be no more changes) would be ideal. This is where, on Discharge day, you can receive the Reg instructions in one ear and, with the other hand, pass the scripts to the Pharmacist. Take note: Pharmacists don't deal with all scripts; many you can just give the patient. But when it's complex, or as per policy, the Pharmacist is essential.

Other matters they'll need you for include adjusting Medication doses after their calculation of the creatinine clearance (you should check with your Reg), other Medication adjustments due to interactions/contraindications and the like (check with the Reg) and other predominantly administrative matters like the requirement to fill out various approvals for special Medications (you can fill out most of it, check with your Reg otherwise).

Meds are a big part of Hospitals, so have the Meds experts on your side to deal with such Issues.

ALLIED HEALTH

- **Powers**: See each section.
- **General requirements**: Referrals, Medical clearance/agreement, clarification of goals, attendance at meetings.

Allied Health essentially makes people functional again in the world, after they're fixed medically. We focus on getting patients well and stable. But we often overlook that people need to reintegrate with their world after sickness and parts of their world may've made them sick in the first place. Allied Health tries to fix that world element.

They act everywhere, but particularly in Geriatric/Neuro Terms, or any Term that has a large chronic/rehabilitation element. They'll provide valuable input to patient care, but critically for you is they'll provide Discharge clearance, i.e. when the patient is at baseline or a manageable point below baseline (new baseline).

The key is to refer early. Many patients may not be entirely ready. However, like all other Consulted Teams, Allied Health would prefer an early heads up. Many things, like Discharge packages and Rehab, all take a lot of time and you can easily stress out your Allied Health Team if you suddenly announce that the patient is for Discharge and needs to go to a nursing home, today.

Most of the time, it'll be sufficient to put in a Consult request form on eMR (see *Chapter 4*, section *Ordering Investigations/Folders/categories/Allied Health*). They'll come and see the patient when they can. However, you may need to call if it's urgent, usually Discharge related. Most Allied Health staff carry a pager/speed dial, so page/dial.

As previously said, set up a filter for Allied Health so you can see their notes rapidly and chase up with them if required.

It's extremely helpful to know your home Ward's Allied Health Team early, so you can receive and give updates to them very opportunistically, e.g. when you bump into each other, and save each other's time by avoiding pagers. The best time to communicate with *all* of Allied Health is in the regular Ward meetings, e.g. Journey Board meetings. Have all your Allied Health Issues ready for *all* your patients and ask and receive information then.

It's particularly important to know what each of the Teams requires of you. By knowing, you can update them accordingly, and hence allow them to do their job and fix the patient. Consider the general scheme below for common Allied Health Teams.

- **Physiotherapist**: Able to make people move. Able to get equipment to make them move. Able to recommend a patient for Rehab. Chest Physio in Resp. Provides Discharge clearance for mobility. Requires Medical clearance for mobilising and to what degree (consider Ortho (orthopaedic) patients).

- **Occupational Therapist**: Able to make people function, physically and cognitively. Assesses function, ADLs (activities of daily living), cognition, etc. Generally doesn't see RACF (Residential Aged Care Facility) patients. Able to recommend a patient for Rehab. Able to do cognitive Assessments. Able to help patients with home equipment. Provides Discharge clearance for function.

- **Social Worker**: Able to fix complex social situations of all sorts, vulnerable groups and home help/RACF/guardianship experts. Provides Discharge clearance socially. Requires Team to confirm Discharge destination and to fill in various reports (usually Reg/Boss level, e.g. for guardianship). Requires a Team member to attend family meetings to give Medical perspective. Will require you to Consult Geris for RACF placement and MMSE (mini-mental state examination) for the ACAT (Aged Care Assessment Team).

- **Dietician**: Nutrition experts for all sorts of special diets for various patient groups/illnesses, experts in various other types of feeding e.g. NG, NJ, JJ, TPN. Can educate patients on various diets and assess nutritional status. Will require you to do CMPs. Will require you to chart various supplements e.g. multivitamin, thiamine, and various minerals e.g. zinc and copper. Requires Team input regarding if happy for various nutrition interventions e.g. TPN. Most afeared of Refeeding Syndrome.

- **Speech Pathology**: Knows if people will choke or not. Will tell you what level thickness diet the patient can be on or even NBM (nil by mouth). You or the Dietician will ask them when the patient's diet can be upgraded. Provides Discharge clearance for degree of PO intake. Also helps with communication/speech difficulties and Rehab, e.g. post strokes.

- **Podiatry**: Experts in anything feet. Especially diabetic feet.

Again, the above may vary with Institution, but it's good to touch base both with your prior JMO regarding what Allied Health require and with Allied Health themselves to see what they need/offer and you'll find the entire process smoother for all.

Remember also that there are more Allied Health Teams than the above so familiarise yourself with them early, especially if you will often work with them.

CONSULTS (OTHER MEDICAL TEAMS)

Why you no talk to each other?

Consults.

Likely the most dreaded JMO Job of them all. The Job that will leave you feeling stressed beforehand, stupefied during and stupid afterwards. Add to that overwhelmed, as you try to fulfil the hundred demands of the Consulted Team and you'll be wondering why your own Team wanted the Consult in the first place. And even if the patient needed it, why the patient isn't under the Consulted Team's care.

The chief reason is, essentially, a very senior person in your Team, the AMO (Attending Medical Officer), has a question for a very senior person of another Team, the Consulted Team's AMO. And it seems the best possible method is to Chinese whisper the question across the Medical ladder, as it filters first down the ranks, to the most junior person of the treating Team, and then flows back up the ranks to the Consulted Team's Consultant. Essentially, every question will go down the Specialty hierarchy mountain, into the valleys, and then up another Specialty hierarchy mountain.

You are that valley.

And, unfortunately, you'll always be at the lowest point of that information curve as it's the valley that bridges mountains, despite mobile phones, email, text and all the other communication bridges in the world. Hence, you'll always be talking to someone considerably more senior than yourself. At best, it'll be a Senior Resident discussing with a first-year Reg. At worst, it'll be an Intern stuttering to an AT or even the Consultant in person.

In addition, considering that seeing Consults are an effort, so the very act of Consulting constitutes a case of the most junior Medical Officer giving work to a more senior one. As you may imagine, even a perfect Consult may not go down very well.

Well, despite this Job's low palatability, they can be good learning opportunities and it's hoped the following tips will take the edge off the sting a little and make the whole process mildly more tolerable.

Always remember, though, however well it's done, you may still get a poor reception. Just keep in mind it isn't personal. You're probably speaking to a stressed, overworked individual who is hating life and that aura may wash over you somewhat. So just chill and move on. But, first, make a good Consult, so you're not getting a poor reception with reason.

As with all things, break it down into steps. Follow closely, make use of the tips, follow the advice of your Seniors and local Institution guidelines and your ego and reputation will ideally not suffer too much while your knowledge may even increase.

> **NB:** AGAIN, THIS IS A VERY GENERAL GUIDE. FOR SPECIALTY-SPECIFIC QUESTIONS, THEY'RE OFTEN HIGHLY VARIABLE DEPENDING ON THE QUESTION. WHAT'S OFFERED IS ONLY GENERAL POINTERS. FOLLOW LOCAL GUIDELINES. REMEMBER, IT'S A BALANCE. AS YOU GO ALONG, YOU'LL GET A FEEL FOR HOW THINGS ARE AT YOUR HOSPITAL, WHAT THE REGS WANT AND YOU'LL TAILOR YOURSELF ACCORDINGLY.

WHO ARE YOU TALKING TO: HOSPITAL HIERARCHY

You probably know this already from even pre-Medical Student days. But, just to clarify, there are different grades of seniority across Medicine. And it helps when you're Consulting to know who exactly is at the other end.

Generally, the flow is the following.

- **Medical**: Intern (JMO)→Resident (RMO)→+/– Senior Resident (SRMO)→ Medical Registrar/Basic Physician Trainee (BPT)/Unaccredited Registrar→ Advanced Trainee (AT)→Fellow→Consultant (AMO/Visiting Medical Officer (VMO)/Staff Specialist (SS)/Boss).
- **Surgical (and most others)**: Intern (JMO)→Resident (RMO)→+/– Senior Resident (SRMO)→+/– Unaccredited Registrar→Surgical Education and Training (SET) Trainee/Accredited Trainee→Fellow→Consultant (as above).

Within hours, you'll generally call a BPT or Surg Reg, sometimes an AT. After Hours, it'll mostly be a Boss or AT/first On-Call Reg, though you generally always call whoever is onsite, first, e.g. onsite Surg Reg. Just follow protocol.

So now you know who's speaking, we'll move on to what you should do before you speak.

BEFORE THE CONSULT: PREPARATION

This is most of the work in the Consult and the foundation of a successful one.

Here is where, ideally, you've prepped the Discharge, everything is up to date, you know everything possible about the patient and you have all before you, including Med Charts, letters and every Investigation since the antenatal scan, and you call the Reg with a flowing but succinct spiel and can read from your own Discharge whatever you need when the questions start bombarding.

That is not what happens.

The main thing is to balance between expending insufficient effort and hence appearing comprehensively inept versus so overpreparing that you vacillate between picking up the phone and more preparation. And, as you delay, you neglect your infinite other tasks while the rest of the day collapses around you.

First thing to know is never expect to fully prepare. If the Consulted person wants to, there'll always be something you've missed. And, if they want to, they're likewise able to make you feel the full pain of missing that detail, however insignificant it may be.

Forget about them. If you could do it perfectly, you'd be sitting the relevant College exams now, and not be a week 1 JMO.

However, you should definitely prepare to a reasonable standard. This is where you'll learn through experience, knowledge and Senior advice. And, eventually, you'll reach the sweet spot of providing just sufficient and relevant information to the Consulted Team without extraneous data.

It's always better to refer early. If the Reg doesn't need to see the patient, they won't, notified early or late. But if they do, it's better to hear a poorer presentation at 12 p.m. than a slightly better one at 3.45 p.m. At least, ad interim, they can tell you what to prepare to make it less poor. Plus they have time to put it on their plate. You'll then both have time to prepare, one for the Consult, the other to amass relevant patient data.

Again, there's limited time during a day. You'll need to triage your time, and Consults, though important, cannot absorb the whole day.

Hence, prepare adequately, but not obsessively.

Consider the following in doing so.

Know what your Team wants

This is critical and guides the whole Consult. Remember to ask:

- **What our question is?** If you know, check. If you don't, ask. But you must be very clear on this as that'll be the Consult Reg's first question. And the Team should know.

- **Phone versus in-person Consult?** Very important and often determines your reception. If prefaced as a phone Consult, you'll generally get a better hearing. And the Consulted Reg may wish to convert to an in-person. However, this is your Boss/Reg dependent so just ask.

- **Urgency?** What the Consulted Reg wants to know. The more flexibility, the less stress, the better your reception. Know, then emphasise, especially if Consulting late in the day (it will happen), if the Consult can be seen tomorrow. However, also your Boss/Reg dependent.

Find these things out when the Team asks for a Consult. You must catch this opportunity as, at times, your own Team is harder to Consult than the Consulted one. When you're new-ish to this Consulting business, it also helps to ask the Team (who is not new) what special information the Consulted Team wants to know.

Your preparation

See section 'Consults (Other Medical Teams)/Before the Consult: preparation/ External documents' for details of what to get. But, essentially, have at hand the relevant History, Examination, Investigations and Management so far instituted. Pretend it's a mini-Long Case, targeted at the Consulted Specialty. 'Relevant' is always difficult, but a good way is to pretend you were the Consulted Reg and think what you'd like to know. Obviously, it'll be limited as you're just post Med School and they're nearly a Fellow of a College. But you'll be surprised how much Med School knowledge can carry you.

Prepare in accordance with section 'Consults (Other Medical Teams)/Making the Consult', making sure you have all the sections, then do a practice run inside your head. Especially optimise the opening; mental sharpness is maximal at the start. If your opening is strong, you have a higher chance of fluffing on. If it's weak, the demolition will begin from the start.

Despite a mental rehearsal of the Consult, you'll still forget things, especially when you receive the questions bombardment. Hence, to maximise your responsiveness and minimise angst, *prep a Discharge* for the Consulted patient. If you don't have time for the whole thing, do at least the Issue relating to the Consult. This will massively streamline things as everything is instantly summarised for you, by you. You can hence avoid notes and Results trawling, avoid stumbling around looking for stuff, answer questions rapidly and reap the synergies of both having the Discharge done and being able to Consult any future Specialty with little extra preparation. The act of writing also highlights any holes in your current Assessment, e.g. History, and effectively tells you what you should clarify first, e.g. with the patient, instead of the Consulted Reg telling you in a much less comfortable way.

Ideally, your Discharge is good and you'll only need to Consult yourself.

Of particular importance is having ready all the relevant recent major Investigations, either this Admission (included in Issues) or past (included in Background) (see *Chapter 4*, section *Discharges/Major components*). If they're not on eMR, you'll need to acquire them (see section 'Consults (Other Medical Teams)/Before the Consult: preparation/External documents', e.g. Echo and ECG for Cardio, pulmonary function tests for Resp, scope reports for Gastro and the like.

Hence, in addition to good notes from this Admission, you often need to collate/ chase the following documents outside of eMR to avoid phone fury.

External documents

Essentially, every Team wants letters and past Investigations/Procedures relevant to their Specialty as well as Medication Charts. Think what these would be and you'll know what to ask for. Check with the patient. Double check with Reg if not sure.

> **NB:** PRIOR TO CHASING ANYTHING AFAR, ALWAYS CHECK eMR AND THE PAPER FILE FIRST. SOME POOR JMO MAY'VE DONE IT ALREADY DURING THE LAST ADMISSION AND WOULD SAVE YOU THE PAIN IF ONLY YOU'D LOOK.

Investigations/Procedures (in Hospital)

All the Hospital ones should be on eMR. However, there are some notorious ones which'll need a trek to get. Follow local guidelines. However, the general rule is the relevant Department should always have a copy and you can walk there or have it faxed over (walking is recommended). Else, it'll be on eMR, you just haven't found it. Call the Department for where. Examples include:

- **Echos/angiograms**: Often in the Department and may not be uploaded till post-Discharge.
- **ECGs**: Often in the paper file.
- **Insulin charts**: At the bedside.
- **Scopes**: Often in 'Clinical Notes' only under 'Endoscopy Reports'.
- **Special reports and Investigations**: For example, EEGs, Neuropsychologist reports, certain special Pathology. Often in the Department or in a special, unfrequented corner of eMR.

Investigations/Procedures (external)

You pretty much need to call for everything; see *Chapter 4*, section *Finding stuff/ Offsite data*. Remember always to get *everything*. If you don't know what you're getting, ask for what else there is. And get it. Of course, within reason. The further back, the less use/urgent. In terms of search, broadly divided into Pathology, Imaging and everything else.

- **Everything else**: Documents, Discharges and every other Investigation/ Procedure possible. These you generally can only get by calling the external Clinic/rooms/GP/Hospital and have it faxed +/– emailed over. Use prior mentioned rules in hunting for it.
- **Pathology**: As above, but the best way is calling the relevant Lab. They're usually fastest if you know who. There's sometimes also a login for each Pathology centre useful for mass checking of Results.
- **Imaging**: As above, but the best way is calling the relevant Imaging centre. Alike Pathology in advantages and they can easily send reports. Actual images are harder but still possible. Best to get the patient to bring them.

All this stuff is often quite critical so ask the patient if these have been done and ideally have it ready in the folder, or at least coming in from the electronic ether.

Letters

One of the terrible failings of eMR and one of the most time consuming, but necessary, of your tasks. But you must find out if the patient is known to a Consultant of the Consulted Specialty, and obtain their latest correspondence. Fortunately, many of the Investigations/Procedures will also be there (so kill two Jobs with one call) but as irritable a Job as it may be, involving difficult secretaries, dysfunctional faxes and frustrated JMOs, it's needed to guide an accurate clinical picture.

Again, get everything. You don't want to call back, nor does the other person want to fax again. The last two or three letters are usually fine. GPs have a GP Health Summary, which helps.

The best way is simply to commence the process, but if the asked for correspondence doesn't get back in a reasonable time, make the Consult anyway and await the correspondence. People need decisions made, and, sometimes, if we can't get the information, delay is more harmful to the patient than not knowing. So try (it sounds particularly smooth when they ask for it, that it's 'on the way' – only excelled in smoothness when you say it's 'in the folder') but it's certainly not a terminal roadblock to getting the Consult.

Med Chart (N/A for eMeds)

Always have the Med Chart there. However, always a hassle as the Nurses will often guard Med Charts like treasure, so just take a picture of it and leave the treasure. You could do this even if they were counting S8s. Photo used ones if the treatment course is extended, e.g. for antibiotics.

Practicalities

In the ideal world, you'll have all the above ready, crowned with a perfectly specific and concise question, backed by a flowing presentation to give to the Reg.

What will happen is that the question is extremely vague, or there's no question at all, the information is missing and haphazard, and no one will give you anything, from letters to Investigations until you have faxed over at least thirteen requests and been told that none were received.

Just make do with what you have, and proceed. Time takes priority. You've tried your best. But this Consult needs to move forward.

Each Consult's ideal preparation will be Specialty, Question and even Reg specific. But the principles are the same. Use them as needed.

> **KEY POINTS**
>
> - Know yourself/your Team: Your question(s), in-person versus phone, urgency.
> - Preparation: Have a prepped Discharge with the Consult Issue, and all relevant Hx, O/E, Ix, Mx. Prepare a strong opening.
> - Get external documents: All Specialty-specific Ix/Mx in and out of Hospital, Specialist letters, Med Charts (if on paper).
> - Avoid paralysis: Consult must continue even if not everything has arrived.

GETTING TO THE TEAM

The second most difficult part of a Consult.

You'll find it's hard to get through to people.

Very hard.

It'll happen like this. You've spent all morning preparing, finding letters, chasing Investigations, rehearsed beautifully and your Reg is breathing down your back, asking for what the Consulted Team thinks. And you've picked up the phone.

Many times.

You've long abandoned nerves, you've tried every way to get through, every communication channel spanning four centuries, and now you're up to the seventeenth pager. And still, nil response.

What then?

Do not despair. It's well known that particular Teams (no names will be named) are harder to find than the North Pole, but you can still reach them without appearing to harass them, or ruining your own day in trying.

Consider the following series of tactics to locate them. By using each judiciously, and often simultaneously, you should be liberated, either by having them or so announcing to the world that you've tried that your Team will feel sorry for you and either make the decisions themselves or perhaps Consult the other Team personally, using hidden channels only available beyond Reg level.

1. **Get paperwork**: It's good for your mental health to assume that it'll be impossible to reach the Consulted Reg. Assume you'll have to page until that pager's battery dies. Assume you'll be kept waiting for hours. Assume the pager is on the Reg's dining table. And prepare for it. That is, commence the Consult process when you're about to sit down to do paperwork.

   Lots of paperwork.

   Even better if it's for the patient you're Consulting about.

   Hence, always have some subcortical work at the ready, scripts, Discharges (e.g. of this patient), Pathology Orders (though take care nothing locks you out of eMR for long else the Consult will go badly), your own Overtime sheet (which may or may not be paid in the next century) and *always* expect to wait after paging. You can even continue to optimise the Consult and read up some more while you wait (though there's a limit). That way, if you get through, you'll be ecstatic. And if not, well, you won't have waited in vain.

2. **Page**: Always start with the usual way. You aren't particularly special (to the Reg) so use the manner of all JMOs first before resorting to further tactics. Sometimes, the Reg may just answer. You might get lucky.

   The critical thing is to make sure you have the right Reg on the right pager. Useless to try a hundred times if they're off. Or worse, that they're not on for Consults today and it's the other, even harder-to-reach Reg who's on. Check with Switch if you need to.

   Always give a good 5–10 minutes before you page again. At least give people some time to walk to a phone or finish what they're doing. You don't answer pages when you're in the middle of an IVC, nor will Regs who are in the middle of an angiogram or lumbar puncture, or scope or scrubbed, etc. It's not like they're just waiting all day for your Consult.

   Probably paging three times is enough. You should be justified in using more extreme measures if there's still no response. Note that this will already take about 30 minutes.

3. **Text/WhatsApp the Reg**: As we'll see in section 'Consults (Other Medical Teams)/Follow-up and future Consults/Strategies for acquiring', you can acquire the numbers of many people if you take a little care. Including Consults Regs. Here's where a humble text asking 'if they're available for Consults' will go a long way and make the difference between 3 hours chasing Switch and the wrong Reg only to find the right Reg is off and knowing to make the Consult tomorrow as it was non-urgent anyway, the whole process taking one text and as many minutes while saving an infinity of frustration. Remember also to use other communication methods, e.g. WhatsApp. Some places have no reception but have Wi-Fi, so leave no stone unturned or signal untapped.

4. **Text/page the Team JMO**: Dependent on how friendly you are with your peers. But you guys should all be friendly. You're all in this same boat of frustration together. Obviously avoid paging the JMO if you can as they'll be harassed enough already. But a quick text asking if their Reg is available today or not and where/when is often replied to.

   Timing is exquisitely critical. If the Surg Reg is in Theatre for a massive case, they probably won't come out to hear your Consult, even if you should page a million times. Their phone and pager are probably in their locker, in a land far, far away. Similarly, if they're on an ADO (allocated day off) (yes, Regs have ADOs too), it's unlikely they'll pick up either.

   All such inside info is only available to the Team JMO and is obviously invaluable as it'll save titanic efforts best reserved for crushing many Discharges. You'll, of course, return the favour with your own Team.

   Even if you don't know the JMO, still contact them if necessary. Alternatively, post on your group chat. We all know the feeling.

   Getting a heads up from the JMO is essential. Much of effective organisation is about conservation of effort, and if something isn't going to work, it's best to know early. You'd rather know about a brick wall from twenty paces than breaking your head against it, repeatedly. Be friends with everyone obviously for many reasons (not least being for your own general sanity), but also for Consults. If your friend is on the Term, you can get that info. Never Consult the JMO obviously, but, with their help, at least you're a little closer to Consulting who you're supposed to.

5. **Follow protocol**: Always follow protocol regarding Consulting Teams if there is one. There's sometimes some sort of hierarchy or process you should follow if you can't get through to someone. Ask if there is one. Something to lean on at least if you get blasted by a gale of shouting.

6. **Switch to transfer to mobile**: If all else fails, ask Switch to transfer to their mobile. Regs don't like this, but you're a little justified in doing this when you've tried some six times and half your day is gone just looking for them. You can apologise for the intrusion once in. They can take the apology and the Consult.

7. **Geography**: As a final act of desperation, you can stake out where the Reg usually lives (not the home address). Each Specialty usually has its own hideouts, e.g. Gastro in Scopes, Surgeons in Theatres, Cardio in Cath Lab/Echo/CCU (Coronary Care Unit), Renal in Dialysis. They also usually have their own offices in Clinics or Reg rooms. These are places you'll just have to find out and visit if you really can't lay hold of them. They will, again, be displeased, for such sanctuaries, they believe, are usually free from irritants like Consulting JMOs. You'll also be at a disadvantage as you don't have eMR open before you. You'll probably have a hard time as the Reg will very likely make you feel their displeasure. However, on the overmatching positive, you'll get the Consult, to your Reg's relief and your overwhelming triumph.

8. **Document**: Document after every attempt to contact. Something simple will do, e.g. 'paged XXX Reg XXX times, will try again' would be sufficient. That way, at least when your Reg or the Boss asks, you have something to show for it, *instead* of 'I did try, but …' *angst*. However, avoid ranting on eMR on how hard it is to get hold of them. It's a Medical record, not a frustration record, though the latter would be thicker than the former. Also, you won't get hold of them any faster.

9. **Tomorrow**: There's always a tomorrow. Tomorrow never dies, as they say. But you're likely to if you Consult at 4 p.m. Reg moods worsen exponentially regarding Consults after 2–3 p.m.

10. **Consult forms/Administrative matters**: Always fill these out if they're requested by the Consulted Team. Many Teams won't see a patient unless a formal form is put in. It'd be a pity to waste your Herculean efforts in finding the Reg, then present pristinely, only to get a cancellation because a check box wasn't ticked. You can copy tracts of your Discharge into the Consult form for their viewing pleasure. The key part is to satisfy all their strange tick boxes, which are different for every Consult, but, usually, the best way is to speak with the Reg first and ask if anything further is required.

11. **Help**: As usual, don't suffer alone. Reinforce yourself with your own Reg and the NUM, etc. if you really can't get through. It's not always you.

KEY POINTS

- Get paperwork to do while you wait for the Consult to pick up.
- Page two or three times.
- Text/WhatsApp message the Reg.
- Contact Team JMO to be aware of Reg status.
- Follow Hospital protocol re Consults.
- Switch to transfer to mobile.
- Locate yourself to Reg's common haunts.
- Document every attempt.
- Comply with Consult paperwork, e.g. Consult forms.
- Try tomorrow.
- Get Senior help.

MAKING THE CONSULT

At last, you have them.

You've defied all efforts of invisibility, you've seen past all disguises, you've pierced through every barrier, defence and buffer that's been raised, and you feel almost qualified for another branch of the Emergency Services.

And, finally, you hear the phone line say, 'This is so and so [a part you didn't pay much attention to or they said it so fast you didn't hear anything vaguely resembling any language, proficient linguist though you are] …', but the next part you did hear because you've been waiting for it all this time, that's right '… the [insert Specialty] Reg'.

> **NB:** ROOKIE MISTAKE 1. ALWAYS GET THE REG'S NAME. AS YOU'LL SEE SHORTLY, WHEN DOCUMENTING, YOU NEED THIS. AND IT'LL SAVE YOU TIME FINDING OUT AFTER.

In presenting a Consult, it's rather common for JMOs to start at either extreme, to either present/prepare too much or too little, i.e. to either assume the Reg knows the patient, e.g. 'You know Mr/Mrs [XXX], right?' (probably not, but if they do it'll save you both much time) or tell the Reg absolutely everything about them. That is, everything. Including the pre-conception History. And the patient's 80 years old.

Neither is necessary, but the balance between the two is essential. The key is to be sufficient. That is what the Reg wants too. Comprehensive in their area of concern, but not much more. That is sufficient.

Mindset

There are two useful mindsets to consider when Consulting.

1. **Long Case**: A very common way to present Consults. Naturally everyone knows about ISBAR (Intro, Situation, Background, Assessment, Recommendation), and the Long Case format, i.e. History of Presenting Complaint, Past Medical History, Meds +/– Social History (if relevant), Examination, Investigations and current Management. This is excellent and very comprehensive; however, the key is to keep it relevant.

   Hence it's also useful to adopt another mindset.

2. **As the Consulted Reg**: Imagine if you were the Reg being Consulted, what sort of information you'd like ready for you to answer the Team's question. Hence, naturally, you wouldn't be overly concerned about the many minor Medical comorbidities (the patient had pneumonia – once) if it was a Surgical Consult, nor necessarily all the Surgical History (there was a lipoma excised 20 years ago) if it was a Medical Consult and so forth. That's when Med School knowledge kicks in, because once you start thinking about how you would answer said question, then naturally you'll start preparing and answering those questions in your own mind. And what you can't answer, you'll also look for. Naturally, there are probably still many things you haven't prepared for, but since the Reg can see you've tried, that's usually sufficient. Also, the main idea is to rapidly give the clinical context, preferably in one word, the shorter the better.

Sure, you'll be worried about missing things. Unfortunately, you *will* miss things. But it's better to present a clear story, albeit not absolutely complete, but with the main brushstrokes apparent, than confound your whole presentation in an attempt to avoid omissions. The Reg will fill in the details with their questions. If all the details were there already, that's great but you'd more likely be the Consulted Reg and not a day 3 Intern.

Steps

Below are a few logical steps when Consulting. The exact details from each Specialty you'll have to work out as you go. It'll be a bit different everywhere and there'll be strange quirks wherever you go. We don't know them, but you will, shortly enough. However, in general, follow this schema to streamline your Consults and minimise mortality from exasperation.

1. **Correct Reg**: 'Are you on for Consults?' This is the absolute first question, before even the Consult itself. You don't want to be raving on for some 10 minutes only to find it's the wrong person and you'll need to repeat the rave to someone else. Regs are usually very good at screening for this, for both your benefits.

2. **Question – Specialty specific**: Always start with the Question. As mentioned, this isn't always clear, but your opening line, before anything patient specific, should be something that would vaguely interest the Consulted Team, at least somewhat involving their Specialty's chief organ system.

   Consider these key points:

- **It should be short**: Usually one sentence, even better, one phrase. Something like 'This is a Consult regarding XXX, are you able to help me with this?'
  - Note that 'XXX' can be anything, e.g. 'optimal antibiotic regime for XXX infection' or 'optimisation of CCF management' or 'drainage of pleural effusion for XXX'.
  - One of the first rules of Medicine is everyone wants things fast. Optimally instantaneously. And if it seems many people have the attention span of a ferret, it's chiefly due to insane amounts of busy-ness and not due to any genetic relation to another Order of Mammalia. Keep that in mind before giving the 15-minute talk.

- **It should be clear**: Know exactly what you want from the Consulted Team, i.e. what you want them to do ('see the patient' isn't quite enough). Often you don't, so ask your Reg. As mentioned, they have much more experience fluffing their way through these things. If they too are confused, they won't complain if you get a bad reception.

- **It should be relevant**: The hardest of all and will be discussed in section 'On Relevance'. But, essentially, the question should bear some direct relation to something the Consulted Team offers.

Essentially, ask straight up for whatever you want. Suppose you wanted to buy socks. You would not start talking about all the clothes you've worn, your style, tastes, likes and dislikes, what you look good and bad in and end by asking for a pair of socks.

You'd start by asking for socks.

And if the shop doesn't sell socks, then they can at least point you to a place that does sell socks.

But if you launch into an essay of your fashion sense, that'd take an awfully long time for both of you and end up not achieving much.

So always go straight to the point. And if your Team has no question in particular, just ask for the optimisation of the Management of [said Medical condition] or diagnostic dilemma of [something related to the Consulted Team's system].

Clinical context is important, but subsidiary to the question. Ask for what you want. Give what context you can. The other side will ask for what further context they really need.

Consulting thus is helpful as it provides a compass to listening. To absorb the useful data and filter out the fluff. Remember, the Consulted Reg knows nothing about the patient. And they only really want to know what they need to know to solve your problem and then the two of you can go back to your normal, un-Consulted/Consulting lives. By quickly asking for what you want, the listener can begin to use their long experience to filter what they *do* want from all that you're saying, and ask for what you've missed.

Another key question is always ask if the Reg's Specialty solves your question, unless you're sure. Often, it's mildly confusing which Specialty is optimal at the Management of which condition (if you don't believe this, see ED Admission Matrix). Though not everyone carries the Matrix in their head, it's likely the Specialty's Reg will have their part of it quite well memorised *and* the borderline conditions which they don't manage.

3. **Patient Name/Patient Record Number/Patient Identifier**: The Reg will usually need this, but ask anyway. If they're interested enough, they'll ask for it. If they don't care, they won't care about the identifier.

   Whether they want the identifier, etc. or not really depends on where the Reg physically is when you Consult and if they're a Med Reg or a Surg Reg. Med Regs tend to want everything so they can look through the notes alongside you and effectively Consult themselves before you finally fluff to the point. Surg Regs tend to want the story because they're usually in Theatres, and they mainly want to know if they need to operate or not.

4. **Spiel**: A bit of an art, which you'll get better at. It's helpful to follow the Long Case format; however, tailor it to chiefly involve what's relevant to the Consulted Specialty. Say you had a 50-day Admission, for sepsis, exacerbation CCF, AKI, shock and severe electrolyte derangement, but has now developed an earache, ENT will mainly be interested in the earache (and perhaps not even that but oh well…). They do *not* want to hear a blow-by-blow analysis of sepsis, exacerbation CCF, AKI, shock and severe electrolyte derangement.

   Start your spiel like you would your Discharge, only for that Specialty, e.g. 'This is a [XXX age] old female/male presenting with/who has XXX, +/− complicated by XXX, on a background of XXX [two or three major comorbidities] with XXX [any extra important info you'd like to add].'

   - **HPC (History of Presenting Complaint)**: Chiefly related to the Consulted System. One sentence on why the patient's in Hospital helps set the clinical context, but that's as much set up as is usually required.

      You'll then of course, talk in detail about the Consulted problem, from every aspect, essentially a Long Case about that one aspect, appending on all the other parts of the Assessment as an aside. Chiefly, it'll be the HPC, the Past Medical History relevant to the problem, especially if it's a recurrent one, and highly suggestive elements of the Examination and Investigations.

      At times, if the Consulted Team is heavily involved (often a possible TOC [take over care]), you'll need to talk in depth about the whole clinical course and give a more detailed sequence of events. A good way to guide you is look at the 'Issues' List in your Discharge. Naturally only involve the main and active 'Issues'. 'Constipation' for 2 days is not usually a main 'Issue' (though exceptions do exist).

      For a Consult about Management of a predominant Issue, you'll need lots of detail about said Issue (and there'll be lots to talk about) and a brief sweep of other chief Issues. For Consults regarding a less predominant Issue, a brief sentence about the predominant Issue, then at length about the less predominant Issue itself will do. Don't discuss all the Issues and how the patient developed said Issues.

      Length: Aim to be most of the presentation. You may well be cut off here and there if the Reg questions various parts. Answer, but then keep to your flow.

- **Past Medical History**: Generally include everything, but try to mention matters that are related to the Consulted System first, e.g. Cardio will want to know about CCF (congestive cardiac failure) and IHD (ischaemic heart disease), etc., but less about the patient's laparoscopic cholecystectomy 3 years ago, while it'll be the inverse for Surgery (though they'd probably also want to know about the CCF and IHD in terms of fitness for Surgery). Also remember to include the relevant Consultant if the patient is already known to someone in the Consulted Specialty.

   Length: A list, run fast over minor, irrelevant ones. But run over all of them. They may be important.

- **Medications**: Again, tailor to Specialty and mention the patient's Meds first, then the others, e.g. 'apixaban' is probably important to Surgeons and Cardio, while 'multivitamins' and its precise dose may not get the honour of the first mention.

   Length: Like Past Medical History. Group Medications if you can, e.g. 'five anti-hypertensives'. Then read them out if the Reg wants to know with doses. If they then think it's too long, well, you had clearance.

- **Other History**: Usually will be Specialty specific so tailor, e.g. Geris will want to know about Social History, especially mobility status, ADLs and home supports. Include anything majorly significant, e.g. lots of Family History for a given cancer, if the patient likely also has said cancer and the like.

   Length: A list, summarise to classes if not very relevant.

- **Examination**: Always examine, but only report relevant findings and relevant negatives. Regs don't want to hear how you looked for Janeway lesions or caput medusae (unless they're actually there, which may consequently cause great excitement in the BPT room). This is, after all, the real world, not an OSCE (Objective Structured Clinical Examination). People want to help you (and sometimes not even that), then go home and not listen to you demonstrate your prowess in memorising Talley. Generally, saying that there are no relevant findings is sufficient (if there are none).

   Length: A few sentences.

- **Investigations**: Particularly important. Include those supportive of your diagnosis and/or relevant to the Consulted Specialty. A simple summary is usually sufficient as both you and the Reg know how to read eMR. However, as you presumably know the patient, you're less likely to miss any. Also include any special tests you've already performed to investigate for the Issue you're Consulting about. Mention if you've chased letters and outpatient Investigations.

   Length: One line for each major Investigation like a scan, quick rundown of others.

- **Management**: Very helpful. You should go into very precise detail about what Management has been instituted as the Consulted Team will be highly alive to those matters. They'll very likely demolish your existing Management Plan, but that's fine. They're the experts after all. But, first, they need to know what to demolish. A common example would include exact antibiotic course, duration, types and the like for ID (infectious diseases) Consults.

Length: As needed, usually most of it.

- **Anything further**: It'd be highly bizarre if the Reg hasn't said anything by this time. But, as in Med School, you can use the strategy of presenting till exhaustion. The Reg is unlikely to have time to bear with it. And you may always end by asking them the next section's question.

Whole length: Often less than 5–10 minutes.

5. **'When will you see the Patient?'**: Essential question which you must get a firm answer to, however uncomfortable and pressuring it feels. After all, if formally requested, the Consulted Reg is obliged to see the patient and it's doing a disservice to the patient if their care is delayed. On the flip side, if only phone advice is required, at least make that clear.

6. **Plan/advice currently: Investigations, Management, follow-up**: The Reg will usually start their spiel now. This will usually include the various things they want you to do now, including additional Investigation and Treatment. Document these as they speak.

   If they aren't seeing the patient, ask if any follow-up is required (document either yes or no) and what the final Plan is, especially how Medications are stepped down/ceased. This will go into the Discharge.

   If they see, they should document.

   If you're not calling again, ask for a comprehensive Plan all the way down to the GP's Handover (i.e. up to when the Consulted Team is no longer involved), e.g. when lines can come out, oral stepdowns, contingency plans. This will save much future chasing.

   You may not know when the Consulted Team will cease involvement, but, once you do, get this extended follow-up info on that final call.

On relevance

People are always confused about what's relevant.

The ideal way is to have a list of differentials in your own head. Here's the bridge people don't blatantly ask you, but is palpable between a person who is reporting well and one who is listening well. And, hence, with that list, you begin firing off findings relevant to each differential, to rule it either in or out. And if the other side is listening well, they can hear your thought processes ticking off and ruling out progressively each possible differential until it's mostly in favour of one or a few differentials which requires their expertise to tease out. And, hence, the Reg, with their specialist knowledge, will finally differentiate the true diagnosis, often using the minutiae, which can be pivotal.

The real way is to think of all the things vaguely related to the system you're Consulting about, report everything related to it, hope the Reg pieces it together and nod and agree appreciatively as they do.

You'll aim for the former. You'll do well to start with the latter. The interim is called learning.

A good way to learn is ask directly what the Reg is thinking about and looking for so you can mimic and expand on it in similar cases.

To conclude

Despite everything, you may still feel your presentation was bad. However, remember, people understand if you did badly. The main thing they want to see is you tried. Because everyone did badly at first. But only with trying do people get out of the state of bad and into the state of skilled.

KEY POINTS

- Correct mindset: Long Case (Specialty specific) or 'be the Consulted Reg'.
- Correct Reg.
- Question: Specialty specific, short, clear, relevant.
- Patient Name/Patient Record Number.
- Spiel: Long Case like – Specialty Hx→General Hx→PMHx, Meds, SHx, O/E, Ix, Mx.
- Relevant is details tailored against differentials, to include or to exclude. All details are tailored/flavoured towards the Specialty in question.
- 'When will you see the Patient?'
- Plan/advice currently: Ix, Mx, follow-up (up to Discharge and GP Handover).

AFTER THE CONSULT

Phew. So that's done and you weren't shouted at, nor made to feel comprehensively incompetent. And the person over the phone ideally was mostly silent, only gave a few instructions and ended with the magic words 'We'll see the patient today'.

Is it over?

Not quite. There are a few loose ends you should always tie up and opportunities to seize to make the follow-up of this Consult, and even future Consults, faster, smoother and less agonising than this one's been.

Document: Always write stuff

You should always document once you've spoken to the Reg, especially if they're coming, or their phone advice plus their Plan (the Reg doesn't always document).

Something simple will do. Use a Template if needed, e.g.:

[Your Specialty] **JMO** [Your Name]

Discussed with [Consulted Specialty] **Registrar Dr**
[Reg Name]

Happy to review pt. today [or another time]

Recommendations:

— [the details]

A case of identity: Get names

Always get the Reg's name. This is actually quite hard.

Everyone always introduces themselves at the start, which is certainly ISBAR, but it doesn't help at the end of the Consult. Besides, everyone says their name super-fast. Which is fine because we know they know their name. Only the rest of us don't, and may be hearing it for the first and last time. Fix this by:

- **Getting it from the start**: What you should've done before the phone was taken by the queue of other HCWs (Healthcare Workers) waiting for it. It may not sound smooth asking for it at the end when you remember, but it's smoother than the next point. It also strongly suggests to them you're Documenting. Try to remember at the start next time. However, most understand. They've been through it.

- **Call them back**: You could, and it'll likely warrant severe irritation or, more likely, you won't be able to call back. Anyhow, it'll be awkward. Try other methods.

- **Switch**: Usually knows everything identity related. Ask who was On Call and they'll usually help out. Unless multiple Regs carry the one pager (especially in Ortho, Surg, O&G, Anaesthetics, etc.), which makes it difficult.

- **Roster stalking**: There's usually a 'Team Roster' that shows the names of all the Regs who aren't frequently rotating, with surname and initial. Fine to use as you can say you spoke with 'Dr XXX', which no one can be offended with. For rapidly rotating Regs who all carry the same pager, e.g. Ortho, Surg, etc. as above, there's often a separate Roster for each of those Specialties. Just read the Roster and it'll tell you who's on.

- **Forget it**: If you don't have time, just write the Reg's Specialty. This isn't a legal proceeding and you're not stalking criminals. Still, it's better to note who it is.

Activate the Plan

Run by your Team first, especially for major things like actual Management and major Investigations like scans. However, start activating the minor things like various Add On Bloods, etc. Nothing worse than going to the trouble of a Consult then ignoring it. It'll also promote difficulties for future Consults.

KEY POINTS

- Document the interaction. Use a standard Template.
- Obtain the Reg's name.
- Commence their Plan (after confirmation from the Team).

FOLLOW-UP AND FUTURE CONSULTS: SMOOTHING ACCESS

Get mobile numbers.

Ideally, the Consulted Team will now start consistently seeing your patient until all their Issues are addressed or even TOC.

Again, this is not what always happens.

Remember, the Consulted Team have their own set of problems and you've just added one more to them that may not be their highest priority. Hence, you'll need to be more proactive and chase after them (*your* patient, after all). Which is fine, as that's perhaps the one thing all JMOs are, or very quickly will be, very proficient at.

The actual follow-up and Plan is variable case by case. Do as instructed. Remember, the key principle is to get a Plan extending to the point that the Consulted Team no longer needs to be Consulted. Then you won't need to call them again. If in doubt, think what's stopping the patient from going home, from the Consulted Team's view. You'll know what to ask then.

Another key thing for you (for follow-up and the future) is access. And its barriers.

Pagers, as mentioned, are an immense barrier to access and, hence, an excellent buffer, but against you. You have to wait, the phone waits, you may not have a phone, your phone may be taken, people call back just when someone has taken your phone, the paged person doesn't have a phone, the paged person is not available, the wrong person is paged, the pager's battery has died, the pager is at home/on the office table/in your locker or the paged person simply doesn't answer the page.

In short, there are infinite difficulties.

All of which difficulties are obviated with one piece of slightly more advanced technology.

Mobiles.

And most of all, texting.

There's much you can do over text. In fact, almost everything, short of the actual Consult itself (and sometimes even that). After all, the aim is just communication, and virtually all of it can wait for a text reply.

Perhaps only the discussion part of communication really needs voice or face to face. The logistical/practical side is more than well served by text. And that side is probably more than 90% of communication.

The main advantage is, of course, speed, easy triaging and pure peace. People can live very well with getting a million texts. People will die with a mere thousand pages. The first, one can flick through in a moment, while the latter is able to exhaust battery and sanity in one go.

So keep both of you sane and save the patient at the same time.

Mobiles: Uses

There are a million things that can be solved by text. Yes/no answers shouldn't cost an hour. Examples of the usefulness of texts abound and include, but aren't limited to, those shown in Table 6.2.

Table 6.2   Examples of the usefulness of texts

You to the Reg	Reg to you
• Clarifying instructions • Updates on the patient's progress • Updates on the Team's decisions • Timing coordination for Procedures/Assessments • Reporting on Investigation Results (via text, images, videos) and special Examination findings • Updating on current patient status and their current location • Updates on the presence of important facilitators of communication, e.g. interpreter/family	• Updating your Team on the Consulted Team's decisions/arrivals • Requesting updates • Getting Investigations rolling/requesting new ones • Treatment recommendations • Coordinating logistics for Procedures/Assessments • Checking certain critical things are done • Instructions/requirements pre- and post-Procedures

The sheer usefulness will become far more apparent as you count the number of times you reach for the phone to page and ask something, then remember you can just text.

Sure, people should document, you and the other Team. But, for practicality's sake, a quick text is much easier and faster and it'll all be enshrined in eMR soon enough. For, in practice, things take time, and who *continuously* refreshes eMR? The text, on the other hand, will make things happen, as people *are* always checking their phone.

Many Regs are too busy to even eat, let alone take your non-urgent Consult, or even less urgent update. But there's always a quick moment for a text, and, many times, that's all you need.

And, eventually, if the Reg is agreeable, you may do the whole Consult via text. Sometimes they even prefer it.

Mobiles: Strategies for acquiring

- **Ask for it**: Works at times. Offer to update them via a text. Some are very open to giving their numbers out. Will also help when they've worked a little with you. If they feel you're not the annoying type and you have good rapport with them, they'll be happy to give it. Try not to become the annoying type after you have it.

- **Send Investigation Results to them**: Many Specialties will want to see certain Investigation results prior to arrival as a rough gauge of seriousness. Cardio wants ECGs, Ortho wants X-rays, Ophthalmology wants eyes, Surgeons want Wounds and areas requiring Surgical intervention, etc. Hence, you'll send a picture to their mobile (get patient consent first, of course). Done. Remember, of course, to save their number.

- **Give out your number**: Then you'll have theirs. No one is looking for you, hence you should have little enough to fear. It's easier, after all, for both of you. Often, the other Team would like you to do things and this method is likewise more direct for them.

- **Ask your Reg**: The Med Regs all know each other, as do the Surg Regs. Enough said. Though, again, this may or may not work, depending on how chummy they all are with each other and you.

- **Ask the Consulted Team's JMO**: Rather improbable at times, but if the Reg has declared they don't care who has their number, the Team JMO may be able to help.

- **Look at the phone**: Regs often call landlines with their mobiles as they often can't find a phone when paged. The landline sometimes has a screen. The screen has numbers on it. Enough said.

Mobiles: On Calling

There is, however, a great temptation, once you have the said number, to call for everything. It's so much easier and quicker, isn't it, than the boring old paging method.

Don't.

It's important to observe mobile etiquette. The Reg may be On Call, but not On Call for you.

The last thing they want is you to call, out of hours, regarding something that can wait a week, which they've just told you about, and make them generally regret the fact that communication advanced ever beyond pigeons and the cupped hand. Don't be that interesting person.

Hence, either send a text and wait patiently, or just page. Unless your Reg wants to call (it's their call then) or it's an absolute emergency, in which case still send a text (it may not actually be one), then call. Or perhaps call your Reg and the MET first.

It's almost guaranteed the text will reach them faster than the pager.

Conclusion

Hence, you should assiduously acquire mobiles, especially if you're likely to Consult a lot during the Term. The mobiles of the Regs in any closely related or interacting Specialties, e.g. Gastro and UGI (upper gastrointestinal surgery)/ Colorectal, Renal and Urology, Geris and Rehab, are almost essential to an efficient Term.

A note on the text Consult

Controversial to say the least. Some Regs love it, some hate it. You need to tailor.

- **Definition**: A preparatory document (aka a text) where the Reg is introduced to the Consult matter, to be followed by a formal call requesting the Consult. Call can be obviated if Reg deems it unnecessary.
- **Critical rule**: No Reg is formally Consulted until you actually speak to them, unless they consider themselves to be Consulted. They'll inform you if so.
- **Usefulness**: Extreme, on busy Terms when gluteus rarely meets seat. Less on chill Terms when it's easier to Consult normally as saves the need to text.
- **How to make one**: Essentially similar to a real one only shorter and snappier:
  - **Intro**: Be sufficiently apologetic, and increase its degree with the lateness of the day. Emphasise if the patient can be seen tomorrow (if they can) or if phone (or text) advice will do.
  - **Question**: One phrase will do. Prefix with 'The question is ...' to catch attention.
  - **Identification**: Name and Patient Record Number and age is a must.
  - **The Consult**: Consult as usual but in dot points. Mainly pertinent details here. Write no essays (your thumbs will prevent you).
  - **Include**: Key relevant positives in History of the Presenting Complaint, Past Medical History, Meds, Social History, Examination, Investigations, Management so far. Dependent on what the Specialty wants. Take photos if needed.
  - **Attachments**: Send as much info as possible, especially letters, key Investigations and anything else they usually want in a Consult, e.g. Imaging reports, Radiology images, other major Investigations, Pathology, Bloods. Also pictures of the patient's affected area are very helpful, especially in visual pathologies, e.g. wounds. There isn't always a computer so, if all the info is there, the Reg can decide now, and much more can happen much faster.
  - **Conclude**: Enquire for a good time to call. It may well be never, but they must say so.
  - **Call**: Call some time after, enough time for them at least to read (unless they've declined).

Advantages

Benefits accrue to both you and the Reg. These include:

- **Time saving**: Both you and the Reg save time, you from constant preparation, constant waiting and the straining expectation of a call that may never come while the Reg has a massive drop in paging load, can look at things at their ease instead of being constantly hassled. They now get fewer calls and have a rapid and constant return number for the Consulting Team, instead of paging.

- **Triaging**: Pagers are blind. Texts are not. With the text, the Reg with multiple Consults can easily triage and can thus judge the urgency of your Consult much easier and faster than taking the call.

  With the page, it can be anything, from something trivial that could wait a week to an emergency for which it's extraordinary that a MET call hasn't happened. There's much less doubt with the text.

- **Focused phone Consult**: Instead of scrabbling through all the data you vomit at the Reg with a normal phone Consult, the Reg has time to synthesise at ease and can hence clarify anything by calling with focused questions instead of losing you forever after the dial tone.

- **Preparation**: As the two of you aren't directly talking, this gives more preparation time for both (though you probably need it more). You can prepare what you want to present (once) and add on things dependent on what the Reg requires. The Reg can prepare additional questions or data they need or recommend Treatment or Investigations they want the Team to start. Neither of you is put on the spot. Also, both of you can act at your leisure rather than responding to another person's leisure. Leisures never seem to coincide, and, when they don't, there'll always be one stressed party, who will soon make two.

- **Ease of communication**: Few things need an immediate answer. A text, as mentioned, solves most problems. Hence, the Reg can text you to find out more and deliver recommendations. You can ask questions and deliver targeted responses. Each at their own time.

- **Speed of anything happening**: Much time is wasted in waiting for someone to nod or give their blessing. A nod or blessing, however, doesn't depreciate in value with a text. There are never phones, but there are always mobiles. Hence, by smoothing these barriers, much more can happen instantaneously. For example, giving Discharge clearance. Via the paging system, one can give Discharge clearance probably at a rate of one every 10 minutes even if you do nothing else, allowing for the Team to page, then the Consulted Team to call back. You can perhaps give twenty text clearances in the same time.

So now the life cycle of a Consult is before you, go forth and Consult, to the benefit of your patient and the addition to your learning, with the satisfaction of your Team, and without the mortality of the other Teams, nor with the annihilation of your own self-esteem.

KEY POINTS

- Obtain mobile numbers: Saves infinite trouble for you and the Reg, especially for many simple communications and for future Consults.
- Obtain via:
  o Asking.
  o Sending Ix Results to them.
  o Giving out your number.
  o Looking at the landline.
  o Ask your Reg/JMO friends.
- Observe calling etiquette: Reserved only for emergencies usually, else text or page.
- Consider text Consults:
  o Only when the Reg is agreeable.
  o Similar process but condensed into a message.
  o Many advantages but highly Reg dependent.

RADIOLOGY

Always first.

An extremely important part of your day, though, unfortunately, it's also different everywhere. You've probably heard many things about Radiology, but they boil down to two:

1. Most Radiology work primarily 9 a.m. to 5 p.m., with limited services available afterwards. You can assume that Radiology doesn't work Overtime.
2. The whole Hospital wants Radiology.

Hence, Radiology is a very finite resource that is highly sought after; indeed, competed for. And, unless it's urgent, they operate on a first-in, first-served basis.

So how can you get this precious resource? The key is again in organising.

GENERAL RULES

Generally, a three-step process.

Preliminary organisation

Get the numbers.

Always get the phone numbers of every Radiology service department, as previously mentioned.

Switch is always busy, and so is Radiology, and you don't want to wait 10 minutes for Switch only to be told the CT number is busy, could you try again in 20 minutes. You could've known that instantaneously if you just had the CT number. Also, Switch often drops out, so there goes your third attempt at trying to get through to Ultrasound.

Even if you get through, don't rely on them transferring you to each other. Though it makes sense, it likely didn't occur to the engineer doing the wiring, as they usually can't.

Remember (if you can't be bothered) that the investment is more than worth it. If you're at a Hospital, you'll call Radiology. Many times. Think about how much effort you'd save if you could get through to them directly rather than via Switch each time. It'd be enough to tilt the world backwards, even without a special point.

Also, take heed of the point regarding faxes and multiple numbers. You'll thank yourself very shortly.

Order the scan

ASAP and well.

Put this in ASAP. As in, as soon as you can link gluteus muscles with seat. Or, even better, while standing and pushing the WOW (Workstation on Wheels), if you have time. As mentioned, you should've noted (and highlighted) Imaging needed on your List during the WR.

This is very important as Radiology will never do anything without an eMR order, however well you may sell it to all the Radiologists in the world. Hence, once the Order is in, at least time is working for you and it may well be protocoled before you even talk to the department about it. The later you leave it, the more uphill the battle becomes, as, however urgent your scan is, it's always easier to occupy empty slots than oust full ones.

You *must* order wisely. Consider the History, Pathology and modality.

- **History**: Always include as good a 'Clinical History' as you can. Imaging is first dispensed on clinical urgency, then first-in, first-served basis, so if you do a good enough job of selling your case, then your Imaging will get done sooner.
- **Pathology**: Know what you're looking for (ask the Reg if you have no idea) and correlate it clinically with pertinent History, Exam or Lab Results. The more correlation there is, the higher probability of imaging actually getting done. Include all those findings pertinent to the differential, e.g. 'patient is guarding, tachy, febrile, CRP of 300, WCC of 30, RLQ (right lower quadrant) pain shifted from periumbilical, psoas sign positive' will be more convincing for appendicitis than if you just wrote 'Looking for appendicitis'.

  Radiology prioritises more serious and more acute pathologies, especially life-threatening and time sensitive ones. Similarly, if the patient is very sick, they'll also be prioritised, even if the exact Pathology isn't completely clear.

Hence, the more serious the differentials, the more acute an Issue is, the higher the chance of your Imaging getting done. You should, obviously, actually be trying to rule out these pathologies. People will notice if you put 'trying to rule out AAA' (abdominal aortic aneurysm) when getting a CT brain.

- **Modality**: Always try to choose the correct Imaging modality to rule in/out the Pathology. Ask Radiology if unsure, or your Reg. Try not to get Abdo CTs for gallstones alone (you'll be referred to Ultrasound), or PET scans to rule out SBO (small bowel obstruction) (the chance of being yelled at is high). However urgent your matter is, if the correct modality isn't chosen, it won't be approved.

So, if you Order well, with specific Pathology and a clinical correlate, not only will your scan be done, but you may even save the next step altogether (the satisfaction of calling for a scan and being told the patient is in Radiology already, is considerable).

It may seem you're diagnosing before Radiology, but, in truth, Radiology is confirming or ruling out your clinical suspicion. So the more specific you are, the better.

Call/go in person to Radiology

Well prepared and all together.

Once you Order everything, in accordance with your local protocols, call or physically enter Radiology. A general guide is included below but it'll be Institution dependent and you'll need to figure it out, preferably during the first week of Internship. It'll be the same system, probably for the next 2 years.

Calling is usually simpler (hence, the numbers), as it saves travel time and you have eMR open to answer unexpected questions. However, Radiologists are sometimes absent from the phone. There are also phone queues (permanent busy tones, where your call is not placed in a queue). Being present guarantees an eventual hearing (unless it's lunchtime).

Have everything prepared beforehand like a Consult. If organising multiple scans, call all in one go for each department, e.g. approve every CT in one call. In a busy term, especially a Surgical Term, you'll probably not allow Radiology to go offline for the next half hour.

Even more preparation is needed if you're going down to Radiology as you won't have eMR. Get everything ready, especially for MRIs, like safety forms and Consents if needed (often required in Nuclear Medicine, try to get it done on the WR if possible) and go down prepared like an in-person Consult, including the renal function if asking for contrast, coags (coagulation studies) and platelets if asking for Interventional Radiology, and with results of other relevant scans (they should've failed in excluding whatever Pathology you're looking for and hence the requested scan is clearly the optimal modality).

If you anticipate difficulties, prep a printed sheet (with patient sticker) with the relevant information. They'll very likely ask a question that you have no idea of, but, with that bit of paper, you may know a little more.

Tell them what you've already emphasised in the Order form, focus on the Pathology you're trying to prove/exclude, ask what time it can be done and, if not today, when.

Radiology will never promise anything, so if you get a 'will try for today', unless it's life-threatening, that's about as much as you'll ever get, so push no more. Perhaps aim for a morning/afternoon dichotomy. It's a good sign if they give you a time, but that's usually in Outpatient settings (the patient generally won't be content with 'sometime this afternoon').

You can check in throughout the day (if you have time) but the balance between friendly reminders and harassment is an art you'll have to practise in person.

Follow up

> *Check and chase.*

Not really a step, but you *will* need to chase things up. Assume that, and everything that happens without chasing will be a bonus to your day.

A good way to check how your scan is going is via the actual Order in eMR. If the status converts to 'Scheduled/Exam Registered/Arrived (optimal)' instead of just 'Orders', that's a good sign. Also by double clicking the actual order and going to 'Order Information', you have a suggestion of what time it's scheduled (i.e. the time next to the status changes).

Otherwise, you'll have to call or go in person if your scan just won't progress.

Occasionally, if there are major issues, your Reg will have to personally talk to Radiology. Report any difficulties early to the Reg and they'll decide. You are, after all, the JMO, and, however good a salesperson you may be, you won't be as good as the Regs who've been in the game much longer and know what to say. Leave them a field to demonstrate their prowess.

As usual, document all interactions, especially when anticipating difficulties. You tried, and that's sufficient as a JMO.

IMAGING TYPES

The difficulty for approving Imaging is often proportional to the resource scarcity and difficulty doing the scan. If it needs to be done, it'll be done. But the scarcer/harder it is to get done, the harder it'll be for you to convince people to get it done. There are generally three graduations.

Tier 1: X-rays

Often done if Ordered.

Can usually be done without calling anyone except in some places, and unless you want it done urgently. In those cases, you only need to call the Reception or radiographer, and then it'll usually be done within the day (unless the day is crazy). Hence, you need the X-ray Reception/Radiographer's number.

Tier 2: CTs, Ultrasounds, some Nuclear Medicine

Often done if called +/– go there.

The next level up and usually needs approvals. For these, you almost definitely have to call someone. Depending on the Institution, it may just be the Radiographer/Reception or the Reg. You'll then have to sell it to them by word of mouth. Document your approvals and the times.

Remember to get Consents filled out for Nuclear Med scans.

Tier 3: MRIs and everything beyond (including IR and complex Nuclear Medicine, PETs, etc.)

Go there, may still not be done.

Final and hardest level. Very Institution dependent and often requires Boss approval. So, you'll have to walk to Radiology, be prepared like a Consult and sell your story to the Boss in person. Remember always for MRIs to fax the safety form first and Order it on the system before speaking to the Boss.

Try to find the exact clinical correlation that requires MRI, rather than another imaging modality. Often it's because another modality has already been done and failed.

Remember to keep a copy of the MRI safety form. They tend to get lost, even after three faxes and walking it in person to Radiology. You don't want to do it again. A general rule in Medicine is if any document is hard to get and/or important, take multiple copies. The MRI safety form is hard. Be prepared to send it down multiple times, multiple ways.

Everything else will be case/scan/Institution dependent. Aggressively comply with their paperwork for optimal results. As usual, document.

Radiology may be hard to get. But it needn't be so for you. Use these tactics and watch your Imaging frustrations melt away.

KEY POINTS

- Radiology is scarce. Prioritise it. Consider:
  - Getting/saving *all* Radiology departmental numbers (multiple phones and faxes).
  - Order the scan ASAP: Include relevant Clinical details, Pathology (to confirm/exclude) and correct modality.
  - Call/go in person to Radiology: Have details prepared as for a Consult but mostly tailored for Radiology. Also have scan contraindication data available, e.g. eGFR.
  - Follow up: Call them re progress or check eMR Radiology Order itself.
- Tier 1 scans (X-rays) generally will be done if Ordered +/– call to Reception/Radiographer.
- Tier 2 scans (CT, USS [ultrasound scan] +/– Nuclear Med) generally need Order + Call (often to Reg).
- Tier 3 scans (MRI, IR, PET, etc.) generally need Order + preparation/extra paperwork + Consult to Boss.

SPECIAL SERVICES

Ask and save.

GETTING THEM

These include things like EEGs, EMGs (electromyography), Neuropsychologist Assessments, Sleep Studies and other special Assessments, etc. With these, there isn't much to say except use general principles. There aren't any fixed rules because each department is different and will require different methods. Why, sometimes even different people in the same department do it differently so you'll need to figure it out.

To expedite, consider:

- **Someone who has organised these things before**: Especially other JMOs as they've suffered as you have and don't usually want anyone else to suffer.
- **Post on the JMO group chat**: A wealth of experience available, as you often won't know everyone, especially not the person who knows what you need to know.
- **Ward staff**: Especially Ward Clerk and NUM, who know everything that you need to (and don't).
- **Switch**: Ask to be directly transferred to the relevant Department and their administrative person usually can help you. Also, the relevant Specialty's CNC or Technician is also helpful. Sometimes you may be put through to the relevant person directly, e.g. EEG Technician for EEGs and Neuropsychologist for

Capacity Assessments. This is easier as they'll tell you exactly what you need. Just ask Switch if you can reach them directly. Same process can be mimicked when calling other Hospitals.

- **Google**: Useful for things not in the Hospital (and life in general).

THE PROCESS: FOR NOW AND EVER AFTER

Ordering these Special Services is often painful. Hence, follow the maxims below and you'll at least cap the suffering at once. Never think it won't happen again. Because it will. And you don't want to go through it, times *n*.

- **Save**: The more painful the process is, the more effort you put in, the more the process is worth saving. Remember your pain and save yourself from it next time by recording key contacts, especially emails and faxes so it'll be an easy Job in future. Also remember to save the exact Procedure and logistics. It's certainly a flowchart easier than the various hypothalamic–pituitary axes and you'll likely use it more frequently in every Term (except Endocrine) so don't grudge the effort.

- **Stock forms**: With rather critical forms that had to be faxed over, emailed or sent via pigeon, always leave a copy with the Ward Clerk first to keep in store so that you don't have to look for it the next time and save yourself faxing, emailing or pigeoning.

- **Your own contacts**: Remember, as mentioned, to keep the Ward fax number and your State Health email at hand. Often, there'll be referrals and forms you need to email/fax. Hence, the fax number and the State Health email as either every other type of email will be blocked or the other party will have every other non-State Health email blocked. So, figure out how to use these early.

- **Follow red tape**: Don't cut it. You'll be strangled by it. So meticulously follow their rules and paperwork requirements. Things simply won't get done unless you abide by their administrative laws. Don't think about changing them, regardless of how ridiculous you think them. You'll be a retired Consultant before they change. So don't waste your effort and simply comply rapidly. Think, the faster you do it, the less time you'll be associated with ridiculousness.

- **Document**: If it's getting hard, or you anticipate it will be, document what you've done so you don't need to backtrack. It'll also win much needed sympathy from your Bosses and bring assistance from other authorities, e.g. Reg and NUM, if anything can be done. It's like an IVC. You need to try a few times before you call Anaesthetics. Whether they come or not is another matter. But to call, you need to try first.

KEY POINTS

- Process can be complicated.
- Get these via advice from other JMOs, Ward staff, e.g. NUM, the Department directly.
- Save future headaches via saving all contacts, processes and forms related to getting the service.
- Document and comply with their processes rapidly.

FAMILY

Treat not only the body. Treat the mind too. And the many minds which follow this one.

Much of your job is keeping the patient and their family updated, informed and happy or, at least, agreeable. You may enjoy doing this more or less depending on your character and tastes. However, on a busy Term, this can occupy much time, and some may feel that this doesn't actually help the patient medically, especially when multiple family members want multiple updates, multiple times of the day. This is understandable, given the family's concern for their loved one, but understandable too for the Doctor to be rather unimpressed, not only because of the latter's over-familiarity with the actual events, but, as usually you're so time pressed, you can't afford being a radio.

But how can we achieve both (as being a Doctor naturally means you wish to achieve everything)? How can we be both diplomatic and yet still have some time left to actually look after patients? Well, fortunately, diplomacy may not be so time consuming and you may consider the following common dilemmas and some ways to help solve them, to keep everyone happy and you sane.

There are often a few practical difficulties in communicating with the family (and the patient). We'll leave the finer techniques and subtle minutiae to the communications experts/tutors/texts/experience. This is the logistics. These include getting in touch at all, the NESB patient/family and general practicalities in patient/family interaction.

Disclaimer: We're sure you all have great rapport and we don't presume to lecture you about being a human. You all have 20+ years of experience at that. And as to general communication as a health professional, well, you'll need to find your own style or adopt one that works for you.

GETTING IN TOUCH: CONTACTING THE FAMILY

First, you must get into contact with the family.

This isn't always a problem. Sometimes family are apparent.

Very apparent.

So much so it seems they're doing the WR or mounting guard over the patient. So constant is their presence that you can't enter the Ward before you bump into them, where they'll most likely ask for a comprehensive update, that will turn into a day-by-day commentary of a 50-day Admission.

But, other times, it seems near impossible to get hold of any family at all, let alone the NOK (next of kin), or EG (Enduring Guardian). Especially when the patient can barely keep their own airway open and the family are needed to make a decision. Alternatively, you'll find the patient needs an urgent Procedure and they're not only NESB with a language not offered by the interpreting service but also unconscious.

You need the family. But you only have one number. And they're not picking up. What do you do now, without destroying your day? Because, remember, to provide the best care, you need to look after all your patients, and yourself too. Anything that absorbs time indefinitely threatens this significantly. Here are a few ways.

- **The patient**: The first most obvious way. If the patient can provide you with contacts, that's best. But the below assumes the patient is incapable of doing so.

- **Try again**: Obviously. Often it's the reception or something, and they may just pick up, from the second to the twentieth try. Or they may pick up from sheer annoyance. No need to wait though ad interim. Do a Discharge or something.

- **Leave a message**: Most importantly, tell them the call-back number or the Switch detour. Let them know it's super-urgent. Leave your pager if necessary. This method is variably useful, as many people don't check their voicemail, so we wouldn't rely on it.

- **Ask the Ward Clerk/Nurses**: They both deal with the family much more and are more adept at it. They also often have cunning ways that you know not of. Admin is the Ward Clerk's domain after all. But when they do page you to tell you the family is on the line, remember to pick up. Nurses also often know who's better to contact.

- **Alternative family numbers**: Pretty obvious too. Ask everyone to leave their phone numbers with the Ward Clerk, especially those who often visit. The main issue is when the NOK/EG doesn't pick up (only they can make decisions, etc.). However, remember that a chief reason people don't pick up is they don't pick up private numbers owing to scammers/stalkers/other such respectable denizens.
    Hospital numbers are nearly always private.
    It's obviously a bad idea to dial from your mobile (boundaries, boundaries). However, call another family member who does pick up private numbers. They

can hence either inform the NOK to pick up, already, or they'll call back very urgently.

- **Alternative numbers of the family**: Often, the number you have is wrong. Rather than waiting, call other sources for the right number. Use common sense. If it's a RACF patient, the RACF probably has the most up-to-date details. The GP sometimes has good details too. Trawl eMR if there are details there from the past. Other Hospitals/Clinics may have them if they're frequent flyers there. If it's an ED patient, the unconscious patient often has contacts somewhere about them, and their ID. With their ID, government or other organisations they're affiliated with can provide you with their contact numbers (especially in an emergency). Most often, their contacts will be in their phone and that may also assist you. It's been heard (this is not an endorsement) that one unconscious patient, whose phone was locked by fingerprint recognition, lent their finger to ED staff. The NOK arrived soon after. Hence, creativity is of utility (always operate within legal frameworks, though usually to save a patient's life, many things can be done).

KEY POINTS

- Repeat calls +/– leave a message.
- Ask Ward Clerk/Nurses for help.
- Try all numbers of family: Other family members who pick up to contact NOK.
- Try alternative sources (within legal framework): Government organisations, RACF, other frequently visited Clinics/Hospitals.

NESB: CONTACTING THE PATIENT

Now, supposing you have contact, the next hardest thing is if the patient/family speaks no English whatever (NESB). Evidently, their Investigations and Treatment need to proceed. Your steps will include the following.

- **Interpreter**: The best solution, both patient care wise and medico-legally. Optimally you have an in-person interpreter, mostly organised with the help of the Ward Clerk/Nurses/yourself, dependent on the Institution. The next best (but usually sufficient) is a phone interpreter, usually transferrable to the bedside, or portable phone, also organised by the above people.

  The first is primarily for major conversations about treatment/invasive Investigations and the like, but it's much more scheduled and less ad hoc, though can be if your facility has an in-house interpreter.

  The latter is more ad hoc and convenient out of hours and for more immediate matters that cannot be planned.

  Either will do. Just remember as usual to document the whole interaction, as well as the interpreter's name and ID number. Information provided and informed consent is particularly important, as the probability of miscommunication is higher and hence you'll need to make sure the patient actually understands everything said. Repeat confirmation if necessary, as sometimes it's etiquette in some cultures to agree with people in authority (which is yourself). But you definitely want to make sure they understand before proceeding with anything.

Hence, plan in advance what you want to ask to avoid the pain of acquiring an interpreter again and consider each of the different scenarios you'll likely run into.

But supposing you can't get an interpreter or for day-to-day things …

- **Other HCWs/family**: This is certainly not sufficient for important decisions like Consent and major information regarding their illness, but for minor things and elements of the History, this can help very much and save much time. There's often another HCW that speaks the language and, as interpreters can sometimes take hours to arrange, getting a simple answer to 'Are you in pain' may be solvable without that effort. You can also get the family on the phone if nobody is there; they are usually very helpful.

- **Be multilingual**: Obviously, if you know another language, that's great, but you don't have to be a linguist to be a good communicator. We don't exactly recommend you take up Ancient High Gothic, because you have a patient who speaks that only.

  However, it always pays to know some basic words in the predominant non-English languages in your local area. Consider 'yes', 'no', 'sick', 'home' and 'pain'. Especially pain. You can get through very much with just 'pain' and pointing. Then it'll be more specific depending on Specialty, e.g. nausea in Gastro, but, generally, it helps to know the words for various discomforts in several locally common languages. Also consider simple instructions like 'deep breath' or 'push against me' for Examinations.

- **Technology**: If learning languages is becoming too intense, consider miming (more or less successful but always amusing, especially for the patient) and Google Translate on speaker or better programs if you can find them. Sometimes you can get away with it by asking it to translate and speak for you. But the accent is not great so this is rather hit and miss and you'll often make the patient more confused than if you had just used pseudo-sign language.

  Always aim for words or simple sentences to avoid errors and being culturally insensitive. The longer it is, the more liable the translator is to make some ridiculous remark.

KEY POINTS

- Use an interpreter – in person or phone.
- Help from family/other HCWs.
- Learn a new language (or some keywords).
- Use technology – Google Translate on speaker, etc.

INTERACTING WITH/REASSURING THE FAMILY

Now for the other extreme. Here, we have extremely anxious patients, who need much reassurance and who, despite a stubbed toe, would like minutely updates regarding said stubbed toe.

Again, we're not going to discuss how you should interact. You'll do what's comfortable and in your own style. This is more as a snorkel when drowning.

However, you can only do so much yourself. To cope with thirty such cases, you'll need help from friends and help from yourself. You may be the ultimate diplomatist, but you won't have more time than the worst. This again is about achieving maximal results in your limited time. So, to begin…

- **Nurses**: Your best friends in this. They often know the family better, especially as their patient interaction stretches beyond your 10-minute WR. Though they often prefer you to update the family, when you're smashed, you can tell the Nurses all you know, and they can relay it to the family. Also, ask what the family's specific question to you is. This is more helpful than just 'updates'.

- **Ward Clerk**: They can help you with necessary administrative tasks in patient liaison. Things like times to pick up the patient, appointments and telling the patient's family members to be here at certain times, etc. All logistics issues they're expert at. However, try to minimise Medical matters. Nurses can help you better there.

- **Yourself**: You are the JMO, after all, and you'll often be the one who relays day-to-day matters. However, to keep it pleasant for yourself, inform the family early that only one member will be updated and the rest of the family is to get their updates from that person. That person can be the patient, but if they're quite unwell, they'll be relatively clueless to what's going on, so best choose the NOK or someone with the best health literacy and best contactability. No use getting a Professor of Medicine if you can never get through to them.

   Be patient and understanding, and know that people get stressed. This all may be familiar to you, but not so to the patient and their families. Sometimes, you're treating the latter as much as the former, the emotional effort not necessarily less than the Medical.

   Agree early on how you'll communicate. You're responsible for communication, not a running commentary. You also have many patients to look after who all deserve the same standard of care. All wheels get the needed oil, not just the squeaky ones.

   However, if you've done your best and things are still not pleasant, remember you don't need to bear with it. Enlist the help of your Seniors (as mentioned below) or the following good friend.

- **Nurse Unit Manager**: Your best friend in dealing with difficulties. Believe me, the NUM has pretty much seen it all, or knows another NUM who has. Hence, if you're running into diplomatic difficulties, seek the aid of this seasoned diplomatist. If it escalates further, they'll bring the even more seasoned diplomatists, the Patient Relations, or the Executive, or whoever else runs the Hospital, and you can be sure you won't be responsible for this matter. Don't shoulder an Executive-level burden alone. Of course, this assumes you've done your part and not merely spoken to the family once during a hundred-day Admission.

- **The phone**: Many pagers will ask you to talk to the family. If you're free right then, tell them to put the family on. The thing you want to avoid is waiting around, which saps much time to no purpose. If someone has taken the trouble to page, the family are likely there and they'll be happy to have a quick phone chat, rather than you trying to find them, then call them, then leave voice messages, repeatedly, and still not speaking to anyone alive. Even if you tell them to be there, there's a big chance they won't. People have lives outside of Hospital. So just ask the Nurses to put the family on and they'll either come to the phone or be transferred to a bedside one.

  Also, as you're usually all over the Hospital, covering multiple Wards, it'll save you doing excessive walking, to the bedside, then away, then to it again. JMOs mostly lose weight (which may or may not be desirable) in their first year or two anyway, so you need less unnecessary motion, not more.

- **Document**: Document every family interaction. This is particularly useful for you and all other staff. Family forget if they've talked to you, mostly because there are so many and some may not have chatted with you personally. Also, if you're not a HCW, you have no idea who anyone is. We're all guilty of charging to the bedside with our spiel and not introducing ourselves. And many people just bear with it.

  Obviously, you should introduce yourself. But you should also document, as, that way, at least everyone knows someone in the family is updated and will disseminate the information to everyone in the family. You are, after all, the Doctor, and not the chief patriarch/matriarch of the clan, so don't take up that role.

- **Allied Health**: Particularly helpful when there are more social/functional Issues. Social Workers are particularly amazing at this, so if there does need to be a family meeting, etc., leave this to the Social Worker to sort out. Your main task there is merely to provide a Medical update/perspective, then continue with your day if you have no more input. Similarly, enlist the other Allied Health experts to talk about their particular domain if that's the main issue or barrier to Discharge.

- **Regs and Bosses**: Once matters become complex or highly sensitive, you should leave the conversation to your Seniors. They not only understand, but don't expect you to lead such conversations but merely to learn from them, and document.

Things like NFR (not for resuscitation), breaking of various bad news, the results of complex Procedures, Surgeries and Investigations, you should generally leave to Seniors as these are highly sensitive matters, and, if bungled, are hard to un-bungle, leaving more trouble to fix than to just do it right first.

First, do no harm, sayeth Hippocrates and that applies to patient and family feelings too.

Besides, you with your grand official Medical experience of some 1 day to a few years may not do it in the best way possible. Then it becomes doubly hard to change the patient's/family's mind because 'that Doctor said …'.

You may be familiar with the Medical hierarchy, but, to the patients, you're all Doctors and, therefore, pretty much the same, from Consultant Professor to first-day Intern, sometimes even to Medical Student. Hence, avoid planting wrong impressions and provide a united front. Because, logically, as concluded by the patient, if you Doctors don't agree, how will they get the best care? Besides, the patient is in an unfamiliar environment and hungry for information, so they'll cling to anything they get. Don't make them cling to false wood.

Hence, if you see some scan result, or Pathology report or Blood result that is concerning, always discuss with your Seniors first. If they're happy for you to report it, they'll tell you the right thing to say or they'll do it themselves while you observe (good learning opportunity for when you're a Senior).

Communication is key. But none now is better than bad. At least the next person can work from a blank sheet, and not one with a paint bucket upended over it.

- **The patient**: The patient not only needs your reassurance and updates, but they can also assist you to assist them. They are a goldmine of information about themselves unsurprisingly, but, surprisingly, mostly untapped. Bits of the History, names of specialists the patient sees, various safety forms, etc. can all be sorted by asking them direct. Again, calling directly is great, especially to save travel time, instead of going there and finding they've just gone to the bathroom. Besides, a good deal of the time, patients know much more about themselves (medically too) than you. Make use of this information. It's often easier than trying to call their specialist, the Professor of XXX Specialty.

- **The family**: The family can help you very much instead of only being a source of more work. Utilise the family as much as you can. Often, they'll want to be helpful, as it helps the patient. They can bring in reports, scans and anything else Medical if they're medically aware/very organised and can save you a world of trouble in chasing these things from some distant Clinic in distant times, using an even more distant fax machine. Instead, the family can bring in a CD, a chip or even upload the scan results to the Cloud. Just make sure the Hospital can cope with these.

KEY POINTS

- Get assistance from Nurses: Can relay medical information.
- Get assistance from the Ward Clerk: Can relay administrative details and appointments.
- Get assistance from yourself: Establish one family member as the main contact who will update everyone else.
- Phone contact: Put family on the line now.
- NUM: Helps with many difficulties.
- Registrar/Boss: Helps with or performs difficult and complex medical conversations.
- Allied Health: Helps with discussing their particular Specialty. Also often helps with family meetings.
- Document all patient/family interactions.
- The patient and family are here to help also, especially with medical information about the patient.

CHAPTER 7

End of the Term

Made it. Now start again.

So, finally, you've made it to the end of a Term. You finally feel like you know what you're doing. You feel competent.

Aaaand... it's week 10. The new Term. When they'll throw you back again to that day 1 when you regretted life in general. Well not so bad, but pretty bad. You'll start all over again. And again. Five times each year, perhaps more. Why? Professional development of course.

Anyhow, before you feel too down, there are ways you can improve that transition experience. Of course, all your clinical knowledge will always carry forward and increase, but that iffy thing called your day job probably will have a whole new lot of quirks to sort out. Below are some pointers to help sort it, without feeling like a day 1 Intern, every Term.

It's all about Handover. Getting a good Handover, and giving one. The first will help survive the next Term, the latter, returning the favour to your next JMO (Junior Medical Officer).

And, of course, don't forget the healthy dose of Admin for the final weeks of Term. You don't want to come back as an inter-State Reg (Registrar) to hand in your RMO (Resident Medical Officer) paperwork.

GETTING HANDOVER

What you wish you knew now, instead of in 10 weeks.

As new JMOs, you'll nearly always get Handover first (unless starting on the ED [Emergency Department] and maybe Relief).

Often, at Handover, JMOs aren't sure of what to say or only talk about patients. This isn't because they don't want to help; rather, so many things are now instinctual that they can't think of much that isn't obvious. But to an outsider, nothing is obvious. Hence, you need to be proactive and pick their brains. Only when you start probing with the right questions will they start having 'Ohhh yes …' moments.

There are questions like 'What did you wish you knew at the beginning of the rotation?' but these are very person dependent and may not always give you very useful information.

Consider the following questions/matters to ask the prior JMO. If they can answer, you can hit the floor running, or even sprinting, day 1. If not, well, you can hit the floor sprinting day 2. But, in all seriousness, they've been here for more than 10 weeks, they know how all things work and they can pass on a wealth of tactics for you to survive, if you'd only ask. For example:

- **Inpatients**: There'll be clinical context and the like but you must focus on outstanding Jobs to do/to chase and their urgency as well as key Issues for patients, including common Reviews. Everything else is important but you'll pick that up along the way, while these things will start you off. You can also find out if a Discharge has been prepped by simply filtering for it.

- **Lists**: Essential to get this proxied, seeing it's the backbone of the Team's function. If there isn't one, make one. Especially important if you're covering multiple Teams to get all of them.

- **Team/contacts**: Get for all Team Bosses (Consultants), other Team members, e.g. Fellows, Regs, SRMOs (Senior Resident Medical Officers), RMOs, their general roles and schedules, and other key departments often involved with your Team, e.g. the Home Team Clinic or frequently associated Teams' Clinics, their Admin details, Private room details plus associated CNCs (Clinical Nurse Consultants) and other HCWs (Healthcare Workers) you'll work closely with.

- **Daily schedule**: Very important to find out how the Team works. Will often be the same between Medical and Surgical Terms, but always check. Things like WR (Ward Round) start times/location, Consultant WR times, Clinics, meetings, afternoon Handover time and general order of the day, beginning to end. Also, know what to get ready at each of these events, e.g. on arrival, on the WR, at afternoon Handover.

- **Jobs**: Will be the same usually throughout the Terms but worth checking. Good time to check if there are any Templates you can inherit, forms you need to keep, Bloods customarily ordered and frequency, special Investigations/Medications (standard doses) usually ordered and any other painful matters that can be eased by foreknowledge. Consider all the previously mentioned JMO Jobs and ask accordingly.

- **Meetings/Clinics/other duties**: Often, you'll be required to attend/do things that aren't part of the usual JMO repertoire. Ask about these and how/when these are usually done/urgency. Also try to obtain associated Templates, e.g. for Pre-admission Clinic.

- **Peri-procedure Procedures**: Many Teams do procedures of various sorts, e.g. Surgical Specialties, Gastro, Cardio, i.e. anything that needs to go to a special Procedural Suite, e.g. Endoscopy/Interventional Radiology or Theatres. There are often a variety of Jobs that need organising before and after these procedures that the Team will automatically expect to be right, e.g. G+H (Group and Holds), coags (coagulation studies), bowel preps charted, and certain Reviews afterwards. Make sure you know which of these Jobs are yours and make sure you get them right. Theatre/Procedural Suite bookings are precious and you don't want everything delayed because one coag wasn't ordered.

- **Preferences/special characteristics**: Will exist for every Team and Consultant. Useful to know these things to ensure a smooth transition, and allow you to get on easier with the Team and the Consultants, e.g. in Medications, Investigations, Treatment. Know what parameters the Team is interested in and ask if unsure. You can also start building these into the Template. In addition, be informed of the standard Investigations/Management of common presentations in the Specialty, e.g. routine screens or rafts of Treatment/Medications commonly ordered. You should still check each time, for assume no time is routine. But, since most times are routine, things flow quicker if you know and are prepped.

- **IT quirks**: Mostly, everyone will be on the same system but, occasionally, there are special, independent IT systems you need to use/maintain. Plus each Institution will do your usual Jobs in slightly different ways. Get extensive Handover from the JMO regarding this as there'll probably be no one else who knows once that JMO leaves while everyone will expect everything just to keep working. Sometimes, there are printouts/guides available. Search for these assiduously and know them religiously.

- **Wards**: Particularly invaluable if the JMO can show you around the Home Ward and how it works. Consider IV access/Procedural Stores locations and passcodes, NUM (Nurse Unit Manager) office and how Allied Health works, e.g. daily Journey Board meetings, etc. +/– introductions to the Ward staff. However, this may not be feasible considering busy-ness of both on the last day.

- **Life Rounds**: Especially important if you're new to the Hospital. Consider all the Life Round questions you presumably have already sorted out in your Home Hospital and figure these out early here. The outgoing JMO will be very versed in these.

- **Help**: Hopefully we've discussed the most common issues you'll run into but there'll be many Institution-dependent problems and Institution-dependent solutions. You just need to know where to look for them. And the previous JMO is likely to know. Ask them about common difficulties/issues they've had and who fixes them. Consider difficult IVCs (Vascular CNC/Technician), difficult patient/family interaction (NUM), difficult Radiology (NUM/Reg), difficult Consults (Reg +/– Consultant) and the like. This will save you looking for help in unlikely/wrong places and preserve your day from destruction.

- **Tips and tricks**: Always ask for these to close. Ideally, you would've got everything from the above; however, there'll always be something easier to ask and harder to find out. If nothing comes to the JMO's mind, ask what was hard to do/organise. Pain is a great memory stimulant and, if they remember, they can save you the memory. These miscellaneous things will help ease every non-usual day, which also happens commonly. Take detailed notes here. You will refer to them.

- **Pager**: Get it. Or know where it'll be.

KEY POINTS

- Mindset: Be proactive and question fruitfully.
- Inpatients: Key issues + Plan/outstanding Jobs.
- Lists: Be proxied.
- Team + frequently associated HCWs: Obtain Contacts!
- Team/Boss preferences.
- Pager.
- Daily schedule.
- Jobs: Any special quirks/differences from usual?
- Other duties, e.g. Clinics, meetings?
- Peri-procedure/peri-operative tasks.
- IT quirks: Any special additional systems?
- Ward tour (+/– virtually), including door codes, Procedural stores, offices, intro to all people.
- Life Rounds/sources of help/tips and tricks.

GIVING HANDOVER

What you wish you knew 10 weeks ago, and you hope they know now. Well, don't just hope.

The thing is to assume the next JMO has no idea of any of the above things, and tell them anyway. You'll be doing them and the Team a great favour, if neither feels like they have a new JMO or a new Term (assuming both were good).

Handover takes place in many formats, including written (email/text), phone, face to face or a combination. It's very dependent on how crazy the last few days of the Term for both parties are and their weekend.

Usually, it'll take place at the end of the last week of Term.

It would be best to tell the incoming JMO and prepare a written document about the patients.

In terms of written patient Handover, each one shouldn't be more than a few lines long, especially if you have some thirty to hand over. Things to hand over include reason for Admission, major comorbidities/clinical contexts if relevant, e.g. Transplant patient/palliative, something about progress if extended Admission, main current Issues and Plan/outstanding Jobs/barriers to Discharge. Prioritise for the next JMO if you can, especially if there are many pending Jobs.

An oral one can obviously be longer, but it's likely they won't remember, so main details especially relating to JMO Jobs should be handed over.

As to all the other stuff, it'll be dependent on how experienced the incoming JMO is. A new Intern will likely be appreciative of all the info. A final Term RMO may roll eyes. Act in whichever way is helpful.

To further assist a smooth transition, consider:

- **Handover sheets**: Usefully provided by some Hospitals, utility is variable depending on how much is filled out. Try to fill them out as you can, but you'll need to check the accuracy of what's given to you, especially the older it is.
- **Final Jobs**: Obviously, tie up loose ends as you can, order Bloods for that last weekend, and at least order newly sprung-up Investigations if you don't have time to chase them anymore.
- **Discharges**: Preferably prep to the extent of your time in the Term. This is, of course, not always possible, but try as much as you can. A 100-day admission with no prepped Discharge is no great 'Welcome to the Team' present.
- **Handover**: Talked about above, but also let the Team know what Jobs are still pending and will be chased up. The written Handover can be emailed to the Team also. This keeps everyone on the same page.

With this combination of effective Handover, given and received, hopefully you'll feel less thrown with every Term transition and, of course, patients can be best looked after.

KEY POINTS

- Give verbal + written Handover where possible.
- Do as in section 'Getting Handover' but tailored to the recipient.
- Notify Team of where all is up to.
- Fill in and pass down Handover sheets.
- Final Jobs: Do as many as possible, including prep Discharges.

CLOSING THE TERM

Goodbye. And speak well of me. Please.

We won't dictate how Terms should end. It's a very personal matter and depends mainly on the Team's rapport, busy-ness and personalities. Some members you may never see again. Some may become lifelong friends. Circumstances will decide.

However, consider the following important matters to sort out prior to the final goodbyes.

- **End of Term assessments**: You *must* fill out that red form. This assures your Postgraduate Medical Council that you've generally done your job. The hardest part is booking an interview with the Consultant who is the supervisor. Make sure you notify them early, e.g. week 7–8, earlier still if they're very busy, and book a definite time. Get everything ready, fill your part out and attend punctually. The Consultant may be late. You can't be. Also a good time to get valuable feedback, especially if there hasn't been much opportunity during the Term. There may also be a meeting with your Director of Training, where you can give feedback or raise your concerns about the Term. Book these in early too.

- **References**: You may wish to ask for these earlier, depending on the timing of job applications and suitable chances. But end of Term is often a rather fitting opportunity. Something to consider before you leave.

- **Overtime**: The final call. After this, probably no one will remember, not even yourself. If you're going to claim it, claim it now, while you still know where the Department Head or their delegate is. Else your forms, memory and money will be lost forever to the ether.

- **Hospital Admin**: More relevant if you're leaving a Hospital. Usually many loose ends to sort out, e.g. returning accommodation/locker keys, swipe cards, library items, etc. Some may give you a checklist. But, if in doubt, ask Med Admin. And get all your stuff ready to go.

- **Pager**: Remember to give that howler away (if it's attached to the Term). Either direct to the next JMO or somewhere they can find it. Worst case, leave it with Switch or the Team.

 KEY POINTS

- Do end of Term assessments + exit interviews as needed.
- Obtain References where possible.
- Final chance for Overtime approval.
- Complete exit Admin if needed, e.g. lockers, keys, swipes, subscription, parking.
- Get rid of pager.

CHAPTER 8

After Hours

The Hospital never sleeps.

You'll work After Hours.

Often.

This includes evenings (usually from around 5 p.m. to around 10 p.m.), nights (from around 10 p.m. to around 8.30 a.m. the next morning) and weekends (around 8 a.m. to 10 p.m.)

That is, you can be effectively *on* for up to 14 hours continuously.

And during those 14 hours, several Wards, or perhaps the whole Hospital, is yours to cover, the patients of which you know nearly none. The next shift is still some 5–14 hours away and there's just one Med (Medical) and one Surg (Surgical) Reg (Registrar) (perhaps a little more, the bigger the place). Both, however, will be harder to get through to than the usual Med and Surg Reg.

You must hold the fort until the break of day. How can you manage it, yourself alone?

Deep breaths

Actually, it isn't so bad and there's mostly plenty of support, After Hours Nurses, the evening and night Regs, ICU, which is never closed, ED (Emergency Department) if desperate and all the Bosses (Consultants) are (supposed to be) a phone call away. But, at times, it feels just that daunting, that it really is just you. And, in some more remote places, perhaps it really is just you.

Fortunately, most patients tend to just sleep during the night (hopefully) and there are whole legions of Nurses (relative to you, that is; actually, there aren't that many) looking after their section, or several sections, constantly patrolling, who'll let you know if there are any major issues. Besides, a good many of them will be a good many times more experienced than you are and can help you greatly.

However, you still need a new gameplan as After Hours is entirely different from regular Ward life, and hence needs an entirely different set of strategies to deal with it well, not only in keeping everyone alive in the Hospital (till the Day Team comes), but also keeping yourself alive enough to drive home.

There are three main tasks in After Hours: Staying Alive, Jobs and Reviews.

STAYING ALIVE: AFTER HOURS LIFE ROUNDS

Hold the fort till day. Yourself too.

You're actually pretty autonomous in After Hours. There are no Consultants Rounding with you (usually), no Regs chasing you to chase Jobs and no NUMs (Nurse Unit Managers) pushing for Discharges (unless you're a JMO (Junior Medical Officer) recruited specially to do Discharges).

The only real things in which you must drop everything, including food, to attend to right now are MET (Medical Emergency Team) calls and Clinical Reviews/YZs (Yellow Zones) (which you have half an hour to drop).

Hence, you do have more leeway to look after yourself so long as you take the initiative. And a healthy JMO is an efficient one.

Of course, After Hours can be insanely busy, so it's important to pace yourself as you trundle through Jobs and Reviews. You'll do as you feel best, but you should always set time aside for eating, drinking and peeing.

All the prior Life Round rules apply. In addition, you should:

- **Find relief**: At will (it doesn't take half an hour to find a toilet).
- **Hydrate well and often**: Avoid brain fog and general stupefaction. Set an alarm if necessary to drink (when you're concentrating, you don't feel thirsty until you enter hypovolaemic shock).
- **Eat normal number of meals**: Like a normal person, except during the shift period.
- **Sit everywhere**: Nobody is making you stand now.
- **Bring food**: Eat as you walk to Reviews. Doesn't look glamourous, but a grumbling stomach while you assess a distended abdomen for SBO (small bowel obstruction) is less glamorous and more painful. It also saves you walking to food, in which time, a Review will come. The time you spend walking back and forth between attempts (multiple) to acquire food and Reviews (multiple) precisely when you try is more than enough to get a three-course meal. Hence, just have something with you. Even a mouthful is better than none. Don't depend on Wards having food. By evening, it'll mostly be devoured anyway.
- **High-energy foods**: More helpful. Now is not the time to diet and JMOs are often seen diaphoretic from hypoglycaemia on shift.

- **Time-outs**: Especially if you're getting overwhelmed. Don't push on. Mistakes are far worse than the patient seeing you 10 minutes later. Find a quiet place (pretty much the whole Hospital except where a MET call is happening) and just compose yourself.

- **Triage**: Multiple Clinical Reviews will come. Multiple MET calls may come. If so, don't try to body split. You'll break. Take the details and start as many simple things as possible over the phone, e.g. ECG, Fluids, repeat Obs. Many Investigations take time, as do the effect of simple Treatments. It's possible that your simple things will have solved the problem before you get there. Always go to whoever sounds the sickest first.

- **Eyeballing**: You may not have time to see everyone formally. But you can stroll past. The phone and Obs sometimes don't encapsulate the degree of sickness. Seeing them gives you a better idea. Also good time to sign the Phone Orders you've given.

- **Phone Orders:** See section 'Medication Reviews/Medication Charts'. Main idea is to start Treatments before physically getting there. Two Nurses will take your Order, and you simply chart as if dictating a STAT Order. Good especially when overwhelmed/time sensitive.

- **Help**: You have more time to play with in normal Reviews. However, if the number of Clinical Reviews/Yellow Zones is becoming physically impossible (contrary to popular belief, there's only a limited number of people JMOs can see in 30 minutes), triage as above and notify a Senior. Very Institution dependent who to, but usually there'll be a Navigator or After Hours NUM. If in doubt, call Switch and tell them you're in trouble. They'll direct you to the right people. The Med Reg will also help, but the Med Reg covers the whole Hospital and you don't know what state of stress they're in, while the Navigator or After Hours NUM sees the Reviews happening across the whole Hospital, so they'll be better able to allocate resources and deploy staff. Worst case, it'll be a MET call due to >30 minutes. Well, you tried. Patient safety first.

- **Help each other**: Work is not always equally distributed. Though all the JMOs usually have specific cover, you should help each other out when possible. See who is slammed and, if you're not, un-slam them, as you'd like to be. Sometimes, all After Hours JMOs simply band together and sweep the Hospital. Whatever works. Remember your fellows will be one of your strongest supports.

Rhythms

Each shift type has subtle differences and rhythms that you can utilise to look after patients, clear Jobs and not get killed in the process. There's not much structure to the work as it's so sporadic, so your mealtime is one of the chief time landmarks. Consider the following:

- **Evenings**: Generally best to eat at the beginning of the shift, unless there are urgent Reviews. You won't have a chance to eat afterwards. Usually evenings are Overtime shifts from the day, so if you didn't even have lunch, you're not likely to cope well at 10 p.m.

Don't get into the mentality that you can clear all the Jobs, then eat and have a calm shift. You won't be able to clear the Jobs. Jobs will build up again, likely in less than half an hour. Then the truly urgent Reviews will come and, before you realise it, it's 10 p.m. and you haven't eaten since breakfast. And a hungry JMO makes poor Reviews, except of fridges.

The reason for this is plain. At 5 p.m., the Day Team is either still there and is sorting things out or their Treatments/patches are still working. Hence, there'll be a calm in the early evening. But by 7 p.m., unsorted Issues will begin declaring themselves through the patches, all through the Hospital. And they won't stop doing so until either your shift ends or it's after midnight, when everyone at last falls asleep.

Hence, it's important to replenish before the crazy evening rush hour comes. Remember, you've had a long day too, you've probably not eaten lunch and will have as much water in you as the Sahara. So, revitalise yourself before preparing for the next onslaught of work. You can get through more of it that way.

- **Nights**: Presumably you've eaten 'breakfast' before coming, so your next meal will likely be at around 3–4 a.m. with snacks before and after.

  The main Jobs rush hour comes at about 10 p.m. to 1 a.m., then again at about 6.30–8 a.m. Main reason is the Nurses have just changed shift. And being fresh and full of energy, they'll identify a fresh round of things you need to do. Hence, expect a Job piling/paging at those times. Unless urgent things occur elsewhere, sometimes it's most efficient just to clear the most out-of-control Ward first and while you 'wait' for all the Jobs in other Wards to declare themselves. By about 11.30 p.m., Jobs should've stopped piling and you can clean sweep the rest of the Wards. This will save repetitive walking across the Hospital for one insulin. And another one.

  The Reviews are much more sporadic here so it's impossible to plan for. Try to triage as usual.

  Try to maintain a schedule that works for you, e.g. snack/hydrate at around 1 a.m., meal at 4 a.m., snack/hydrate at 7 a.m., etc., and flex it around the urgent Reviews that come. If you have a Plan, at least you won't go too far from it and you won't forget that you, too, are of *Homo sapiens* with *Homo sapiens* needs.

  On good nights, sleep is not impossible. Usually the best time is from about 2 a.m. to about 6 a.m. Often, not much happens then and you won't be paged. Unless it's bad. Or an APTT.

- **Weekends**: Pretty much normal life and meal schedule, only in Hospital. You'll need to plan for two meals here. Again, keep to a schedule and pace yourself. There's no one really driving you here (except urgent Reviews) so don't whip yourself.

  Sundays are usually more hectic than Saturdays as it's now been 2 days the Team hasn't seen their patient, and unaddressed Issues will raise heads. There are weekend Specialty Rounds but evidently less extensive than the usual Team. Plan accordingly.

  Jobs and Reviews are also more random, though they tend to increase in the afternoon (consider shift changes again), so try to be physically ready before the rush.

ORGANISING AFTER HOURS: JOBS

It's the number left standing, not the number of Med Charts you do, that counts. But you still need to do the Med Charts.

In your day job, organisation is centred around the WR (Ward Round), and everything flexes around that. In After Hours, there's no WR, and it can be organised any way you like, with critical Reviews sprinkled about to pepper your plan.

But, if anything, After Hours is centred around Job completion. A large amount of Jobs. There's probably fewer Radiology calls, Consults and information chasing to do, and almost no Discharges or WRs, but there are exponentially more IVCs, Med Charts, Bloods and Reviews to do.

Hence, with this different nature of work, consider the following plan for Job clearance that is both efficient and not comprehensively draining.

Principles

Criticality > quantity.

First thing you should know is there's an infinity of Jobs in After Hours. You're doing the leftover work of maybe ten JMOs. You won't always get through them. Fortunately, as it's shift work, the infinity will stop for you when the time is up.

Hence, work steadily but don't stress too much if not everything is complete.

Like your day job, try to accomplish as many *important* tasks as possible in the given time. First, criticality, then quantity.

Always remember the main aim of After Hours is to keep everyone alive till Day Team review. Always aim for this first before everything else. Only start Jobs after you've attended to the urgent Reviews (see section 'Clinical Reviews').

But Jobs are important too as they act to pre-empt Reviews, by giving the patients the simple Management they need to prevent deterioration. So below are a few steps to help save both yourself and the patients.

Getting ready

There's a different preparation regime and equipment set for After Hours compared with your Day job. Leave your Day kit behind and get the following.

Responsibilities

The first thing you should know, before even starting, is your cover, i.e. what Wards you're responsible for and any other duties, e.g. first On Call for Theatres.

Usually, multiple JMOs divide up the whole Hospital. Know clearly what your domains are. Sure, you'll all cross cover. But your own Wards are your first duty, unless otherwise directed.

As said, JMOs do buddy up and clear the whole Hospital of Jobs, but that's done ad hoc and by choice. It's good to help out, but you'll be surprised how many times you're called to do the Jobs on other Wards when the actual JMO wasn't smashed or even paged. Just like, in the day, you're called about patients you know nothing about, in After Hours, you're called about Wards you don't cover, though the knowledge vacuum is the norm.

Hence, know clearly your responsibilities to do your job properly.

Know also what other duties you have and who takes your job when you attend to them, e.g. first call for Theatres means you help Theatres and obviously need to give your pager to someone. If unsure, ask Switch, who knows all things. Sometimes, multiple JMOs cover the same Ward for different things, e.g. Surgical JMO covers Surgical Paediatric patients, while the Paediatric JMO covers the rest. In those cases, ask Switch again or After Hours NUM for precise clarification. Again, remember your first duty is to your cover.

Electronic Medical Records

Your life changes, hence your eMR (electronic Medical Records) life changes too. Forget the custom, proxied Lists, the whole Hospital is now yours to look after.

Hence, make sure the following eMR modifications are in place before you start your shift to enable smooth function and minimal fumbling about.

- **Ward Lists**: Create or activate the Lists of the Wards you're covering, remembering to include 'Room' and 'Bed' as needed columns (see *Chapter 4*, section *Lists* on how). Everyone who calls you will talk about Ward X, Bed X. In the day, you merely needed to hear the last name and you knew which patient. In After Hours, you know nothing. And nobody seems to understand Patient Record Numbers. It also takes too long to search. But if you have all the Ward Lists open before you, you can check a bed number, a surname and immediately enter the file. You can then start asking pertinent questions, and initiating Investigations and/or Management, *instead* of hanging up, then reading up, then calling back and waiting. Remember there's minimal Ward staff at night and you can call all night if you like.

- **Whole of Hospital List**: You should've created this already, but, if not, make it. If you really can't find the patient, this is helpful to scan through. At least, you'll know if they're in the Hospital.

- **Multi-Patient Task List**: For Day Team Handovers. Should've been set up at Orientation, and important as Medical Handovers are often critical (though they should call you if it is). However, eMR crashes, you change Hospitals, you get seconded, etc., so best set this up prior to your first After Hours shift; see section 'Prioritising'.

- **Task Manager**: Place to view the infinity of Jobs. Set this up for each type of After Hours shift you're covering. See *Chapter 4*, section *Lists*. Know how to use it.

- **After Hours custom List**: Always set up a blank custom List for After Hours and add onto it all patients you need to chase anything for. This is essentially your 'After Hours' List and you can make eMR your massive notebook instead of the folded/scrunched A4 sheet. Use it like a day List, e.g.

  - **Reviews**: So you remember who you've seen and to chase if needed.

  - **Med/Surg Reg Reviews**: Useful as you can present the patient without trying to decipher your own hurried scrawl. You're essentially Consulting them, and though the knowledge threshold is lower than for a Day Team Consult, you should preferably still know something, e.g. the patient's name.

  - **Handover**: Both receiving and giving. Makes it easier to chase Jobs for patients handed over to you. Also easier to give Handover. You deteriorate throughout the shift. This helps you remain mildly coherent at its end. Especially when you can just read off the computer rather than dragging from the depths of your consciousness that 22nd Review.

- **Auto-text**: See *Chapter 4*, section *Documenting*. Make sure you have all your auto-texts ready, especially if you haven't come across many of them in your day job. Documenting takes up so much time at night, and the number of times you're typing the same thing is more than a photocopier. You don't want to be still Documenting a whole night of Reviews at midday. Get ready, especially the Protocol-based Reviews, Procedures completed documentation, e.g. IDCs (in-dwelling catheters), and simpler Clinical Reviews, e.g. mild asymptomatic hypertension. They'll chew up most of your time. Obviously not recommended to Template complex Clinical Reviews, but the simple far outweighs the complex in volume, so you can save energy for the latter while completing the former.

Props

Essentially the same as *Chapter 2*, section *Things to bring/Other tools*.

Usually the documents folder is less needed. Instead, *always carry a notebook* or some paper at least. You see the Med Regs everywhere carrying a notebook around? It's so they can take Consults at the drop of a hat. In After Hours, you're the Consults JMO for everything. How comprehensive a job you do is debatable. What's not debatable is you need somewhere to write. Remember, there's only limited space on your arm. And if you're practising the Five Moments of Hand Hygiene, that space quickly fades too.

Hence, with this notebook, whenever a call comes, you can easily note down everything the other party can tell you, know the patient's condition, start to address the Issues, remember what Investigations and Treatment you've commenced and, importantly, follow up and, eventually, hand over. Remember, on After Hours, you have no idea who, what or where anyone or anything is. You're also exhausted. You won't recall anything, ever. This is your auxiliary brain. Don't drop it.

Scrubs are again very recommended and essentially routine. Much more comfortable than your day clothes. You can also wear shoes actually designed for walking. And you'll be doing much walking. Also, well-made sets (including the official State Health ones) have an absolute wealth of pockets and subdivisions. On the latest review, there were at least three places for pens, five large pockets, twice as many subdivisions and a dedicated strap to hang your pen torch. And that's just the trousers. Think of your scrub set as almost a trade belt. All the tools you need can fit in it, ready to go. Add to this your neck (for the steth [stethoscope]) and you'll feel very much like a real Doctor.

KEY POINTS

- Know your responsibilities and coverage.
- eMR: Lists needed include:
  o Ward(s) List (that you cover)
  o Whole of Hospital
  o Multi-Patient Task List
  o Task Manager
  o After Hours custom List.
- Prep various auto-texts (see section 'Clinical Reviews').
- Props: Bring steth, pen torch, cannula equipment, pens (+++), notebook/paper, scrubs.

Prioritising

Now that you're ready, and the hours are before you, the next thing is to prioritise. As mentioned, you're very autonomous, which is good and bad. Good as you do what you want. Bad as you don't know what you want. Or, rather, you don't know what all the patients need, and who needs it most.

Apart from MET calls and Clinical Reviews, which everyone knows to do first, all the other Jobs are a big mush. And another person's prioritising may not be entirely accurate, especially as they don't know all the Jobs you have. Even Clinical Reviews sometimes need prioritising.

We'll briefly discuss Clinical Reviews (see section 'Clinical Reviews') further down. Here, we'll focus on Jobs in general.

The Jobs below are classed per general level of urgency. However, anything can be urgent or not, and you'll need to use your judgement. None of this is absolute. But, in general, one may consider the following.

Principles

Time sensitive. The key is to prioritise the essential Jobs (those that will make a difference to patient care and are time sensitive), over non-essentials (those that can be delayed without much impact). And to do as many of the former as possible.

Time sensitive means: any delays = badness.

The more badness there is, the more urgently you should attend to them. Consider this before launching into your work.

There's also more urgency in initiating active Treatments, e.g. antibiotics and time-sensitive Investigations, e.g. early morning cortisol (not much use in the afternoon).

Therefore, start doing…

1. **Arrests/MET calls:** Duh.

2. **Clinical Reviews/Reviews in general**: Duh (2). See section 'Clinical Reviews/ Yellow Zones'.

3. **Organisation**: Short of the above, it's important to organise your shift first before starting all the Jobs. You can't rely on people to prioritise for you and things will be missed if you don't catch them. Also, don't rely on people calling. That's very variable and everyone has their own definition of urgent. You may well get called to do non-urgent matters while the urgent ones … well, the patient can't tell you it's urgent. It's better usually to do one Med Chart less than miss doing an IVC for antibiotics already overdue 7 hours that will trigger a Clinical Review next shift.

    Hence, first trawl the online 'Multi-Patient Task List', then the 'Task Manager' List and assess the urgency of the Jobs (see below).

    'Multi-Patient Task List' has all the Doctor Handovers, which are usually very specific and sometimes critical (though they should call as said), while 'Task Manager' has the legion of Jobs. For Hospitals without 'Task Manager', you *could* stroll through the Wards and look through the Jobs Books, though sometimes it's easier to start organising when you spend your allocated time in each Ward.

    That way, you can avoid missing most critical issues, which you haven't been called about, identify urgent Jobs to clear first and know which Wards are least under control and sort them first. You can, thus, distribute your time appropriately through the Wards.

    Once you know your whole pie of Jobs, then you can start cutting it up.

4. **Verbal Handover**: Generally, if a Doctor calls you to Handover, they'll give you a pretty accurate picture of what's happening and what needs to be done. And, if they're calling, it's usually quite urgent and suggests an imminent

Medical Issue. Nobody calls at 5 p.m. to talk about a Med Chart. See section 'Clinical Reviews/Handover Reviews' for details.

They will mostly prioritise for you. You only need act. We imagine it's reasonable to trust the Consultant's or Registrar's prioritising.

Sometimes, they'll call giving a heads up regarding an unstable patient and not just Jobs. Keep an eye on these (add them to your After Hours List) and, as above, get a good contingency plan if the patient deteriorates.

5. **Multi-Patient Task List: Handover tasks**: Often, Doctor Handovers (less urgent tasks) will appear on this List. The actual form should give you pertinent details, e.g. ISBAR, especially R, i.e. what to do.

    Again, their urgency is variable, but you should review the List early, as urgent-ish Jobs often appear here. And there may be no verbal Handover as the Day Team is still getting smashed.

    Perform them as directed once they're on your Job radar. Again, the prioritising is fairly accurate as, usually, these are requested by Seniors who know what they want. If it isn't urgent, often no time frame will be given. If it is, they'll state it clearly. Pending emergencies, try to abide by these times. There's usually a good reason.

6. **Task Manager/JMO Job Books: the rest of the Jobs**: These will include virtually all the remaining Jobs, the usual JMO tasks you do in your day job as well as Reviews (not including formal Clinical Reviews).

    See *Chapter 4*, section *Task Manager* for details, but main thing is to filter via urgency. See section 'Types of Jobs' for a consideration of the common Jobs.

7. **Calls**: These are certainly not the least urgent, but they'll usually happen throughout the shift. Address ad hoc. They all proclaim themselves urgent usually. You will judge. Just remember to get the details and/or ask them to put it onto 'Task Manager'/JMO Jobs Book if not very urgent. Go if urgent. For Reviews, try to start what Investigations/Management you can right there and question as fruitfully as possible. You won't easily get another chance. The sparsity of phone manning has been mentioned.

8. **Timing**: As you commence your Jobs, pace yourself. Obviously do all the urgent and time-critical Jobs first across the whole covered area, then start cycling between your Wards. Spend a set time on each, doing their most urgent Jobs first, then move on

Your presence is reassuring. Otherwise, you'll be paged endlessly from the one Ward you haven't been to, and the time spent answering and waiting could've been used to clear the Jobs. Then, watch the Jobs and shift glide by.

Remember, ideally, everything should be done. However, you only have limited time and you need to triage to optimise overall patient care and prevent deterioration in as many patients as possible, and not simply for those who people have called you about.

For it's very possible that you may be called for patients with less urgent demands while neglecting the patient who needs urgent intervention, merely because no one has called. Only when you know what needs doing can you prevent this.

KEY POINTS

1. Arrests/MET calls.
2. Formal Clinical Reviews.
3. Organising all your Jobs across Wards.
4. Verbal Handover tasks.
5. Multi-Patient Task List tasks.
6. Task Manager/JMO Job List tasks (most other Jobs).
7. Calls (throughout shift, prioritise ad hoc).
8. Cycle through Wards.

Types of Jobs

Your most common Jobs include the following:

- Recharting Medications.
- Charting variable Meds: insulin, prednisone and warfarin, electrolyte replacement.
- Clarifying Medications and doses.
- Cannulas for various purposes.
- Other Procedures, e.g. IDCs, nasogastric tubes.
- Venepuncture: For common Bloods, Review related or handed over.
- Results checking/simple Plan enactings/reporting to Seniors.

Obviously, screen these and determine importance. Where you've been handed over to complete something by a certain time, try to meet it. For everything else, very case and judgement dependent. However, some general rules include the following.

Cannulas (IVCs)

Prioritising

IVAbx (IV antibiotics)/other active Treatments/severe electrolyte derangement replacement > IV Fluids/mild electrolyte replacement > protocol-driven change, e.g. day 3 IVC.

Remember, you're essentially first On Call Anaesthetics in After Hours and you need to triage your time. Ideally, everyone would get everything, but, unfortunately, in the real world, everyone cannot get everything. So, the ones who need it, need to get it, first.

Of course, everything is subject to clinical situation and IV Fluids could easily be more urgent than antibiotics. Use your judgement.

Hence, always ask what the IVC is for to gauge urgency. Essentially, know if they need it, when they need it by and if there are alternatives. If they can step down to orals, they may not need IVs. If they can eat and drink, they may not need the drip.

Consider that a stable, fit, young, well patient waiting for elective surgery who is NBM (nil by mouth) may well be able to wait for their IVC for Fluids. A deteriorating, febrile patient with multiple comorbidities, who already has an antibiotic dose or two missed, cannot. On the flip side, a recovering patient whose next dose of IV antibiotics is due tomorrow evening can wait. A bleeding/shocked patient needing Blood/Fluid resus can't.

Strategies

- **Set-up**: The easiest way is simply to pre-emptively set up some five or six on your Home Ward, depending on which type of Ward cover you are. Usually Surgical Wards need more, and Medical ones less. Thus, when you go to cannulate, you can instantly put one in without searching an unknown Ward for that one thing, say, a bung.

- **Common spares**: Carry tape/gauze/tourniquets/dressings as mentioned.

- **Have a glance**: If you're going to do many in a row, cruise by briefly (if nearby) and assess difficulty. It's always nice to do the easy ones first for a confidence boost and IVCs are more about confidence than anything else. You'll very quickly have a feel for who will be hard/easy. Some people have veins visible from another Ward. Others can't be seen with two ultrasounds. Act accordingly.

- **Aids**: If it's difficult, consider tapping, asking the patient to pump hands, tethering along the vein rather than across it, warm water in a glove, placing arm in a dependent position, warm water arm bath, another arm/feet/legs, infra-red vein finder, Ultrasound or any other vein-whispering technique you've heard of. The usefulness of any of the above is debatable apart from Ultrasound, try what works for you.

- **Help**: If it's becoming impossible, call for help. Don't spend all your time on a lost cause and don't torture the patient any further. Your chances of striking gold (or Blood) falls exponentially with the number of tries. The After Hours CNC/Vascular Access Team/another JMO will have much better luck by virtue of being someone else. Similarly, if there are simply too many, ask if the Nurses can help out. Institution dependent, but many Nurses can cannulate and may well do so if asked. Similarly, if your Hospital has the service, ask for help from the Vascular Tech, who spends most of their time clearing Wards of IVCs/Bloods and who naturally has an incredible hit rate.

Venepuncture

Prioritising

Extremely variable. Generally MET calls/Clinical Reviews/Reviews > Handover Bloods > timed Bloods, e.g. APTT.

Most of the MET calls/Clinical Reviews will require Bloods to be collected right there and you can send them as 'life threatening' (obviously very urgent).

Handover Bloods are very variable, from a patient going to Theatre now needing a Group and Hold to Bloods needed because the day JMO couldn't get to it. Ask how urgent or when it needs collection. If not specified, use your judgement.

Timed Bloods: Just collect it by the time needed, e.g. APTT.

Strategies

Similar to IVCs, though less necessary as less equipment and fewer steps. Perhaps more needed in Cardiac/Respiratory Wards as everyone needs APTTs because of heparin infusions.

Medication Reviews/Medication Charts

Prioritising

Very variable (N/A to eMeds [electronic Medications] largely).

Active Treatment, e.g. insulin, warfarin and Medication adjustments > recharting Medications.

It's apparently therapeutic to do Med Charts (you'll find out shortly yourself). Prioritising chiefly depends on when the next dose is due.

Nurses can't give Medication if it isn't charted; hence, by charting them, you'll prophylactically prevent many Issues throughout this shift and the next one, by 'treating' the patient's existing Issues. Hence, you'll pre-empt Reviews.

Otherwise, all the patient's controlled Issues will bubble up in addition to the one they're in Hospital for. If you don't chart insulin, the patient may get a BSL (blood sugar level) of 25. If you don't give warfarin, the patient may get a clot. If you don't titrate electrolytes, the patient may get an electrolyte derangement-associated complication, e.g. asystole (uncommon so don't freak out). If you don't chart Fluids, the patient will have low BP, then maybe shock. And so on.

So address these Issues, again based on judgement.

- **Warfarin**: Check INR and titrate. If in doubt, keep the same if INR is stable, or ask. Also, know the patient's clinical condition, e.g. not bleeding/not waiting for Theatres, etc.
- **Insulin**: Read their insulin chart and check any Team/Endocrine notes. Follow what the Day Team has been doing if stable. Follow the sliding scale (on the insulin chart) for hyperglycaemia. Withhold/reduce if there have been hypoglycaemic episodes. Very case dependent so use clinical judgement. Always ask if in doubt.
- **Electrolytes**: Mostly follow Team notes/Handover. Use eTG guidelines mostly otherwise. Ask if in doubt. With experience, you'll know how much X amount of replacement raises the serum electrolyte level by but there are a bunch of clinical provisos, e.g. active loss like diarrhoea, so be safe and clarify.
- **Recharting Fluids**: Again, follow the Team directives but more clinical judgement. Know why they need Fluids. You should assess Fluid status and if they can drink. At the least, check the patient doesn't have CCF or CKD (chronic kidney disease) and check their electrolytes so you're not making them more hypernatraemic, i.e. tailor their replacement Fluid (know the components) against their existing electrolyte profile and replace without giving excess of something else.

- **Symptomatic relief**: Give appropriate amounts as per your clinical judgement. Use PRNs when possible. Follow the Team's instructions (especially if they've just forgotten to formally chart their instructions).

- **Others:** Follow Team notes/Handover.

- **Medication Reviews**: This is as someone wrote 'R/V' on the Med Chart. You'll mostly have no idea. Often, it's due to reduced renal function the Pharmacist has noted, so you can dose reduce as per eTG/Med Reg if critical, though it'll depend on the Medication. Most of the time, be conservative and ask the Day Team to review mane. Consider if the patient really needs the Medication, tonight, right now. If not, it should be fine not to give. Do no harm, as said. Follow the Team notes and Handover notes for the most guidance. Else, make an appropriate Plan by looking at the Obs, Bloods, Clinical History and/or ask. Place for 'R/V' tomorrow if needed, so the Day Team knows to sort this out.

Strategies

- **Chart Round**: Med Charts aren't necessarily the most urgent of your Jobs but they're most of the job. Unless there are an infinite number, just clear out a whole Ward of these paperwork Jobs in one go. Go to the Jobs Book/'Task Manager', note every chart you need +/− code the type of Job that needs doing, e.g. M for Med Charts, I for insulins, etc., grab charts, then just slug through them. If the Nurses are very nice to you, they may have them all ready to go. Just ask what they need and they'll bring out their stash of Jobs for you to hammer through in one hit.

- **Sign off/cross off**: As they're so high volume, you can clear most of the Job Books/'Task Manager' in one sweep. Remember to do this crossing/signing off as it not only makes you feel better by completing so many tasks, it'll save the next shift's JMOs from uselessly Job trawling.

- **Medication Reviews first**: These are usually faster and simpler to do. They're also often more acute as Nurses usually pre-empt Medication recharts by a day so you have maybe 10 hours before the next regular Medication is due. It's also easier to write a number in the warfarin box, than rechart thirty Medications. Both are one Job on 'Task Manager'. You decide.

- **Date and names**: You must do the thirty Medications rechart eventually. Do repetitive things first across the charts to minimise thinking, i.e. Date, [Your Name] and Signature. These tend not to change, for now. You'll be surprised how slow your processing power is at 4 a.m. Conserve it.

- **Chart no extras**: To optimise patient Management and save writing, take care not to rechart ceased Medication. This is important. It's a great pain for yourself to write an extra ten Meds the patient doesn't need and a greater pain for the Day Team to cross them all off again, only for you to rechart them at night.

- **Phone Orders**: You'll have crazy days and nights. Times when any personal care is impossible, and deteriorating patients are raining so fast left and right that your pager can't receive them quick enough. And then you get a call about an asymptomatic hyperglycaemia of 15, while the three febrile, hypotensive and tachy patients are still unseen. It's times like these when you need Phone Orders. A Phone Order is just as if you were there charting a STAT, only someone writes for you. They're great for when you need to institute Management now, but can't physically get to it in time. They're excellent for many of the little things you'll be called about. Just dictate the Management you'd like, e.g. 'For XXX, 2 units, s/c NovoRapid, STAT', another Nurse will listen to the Order and this patient will be managed while you run to the three other febrile, hypotensive and tachy patients. Just remember to come and sign for the Order at some point.

You can give also Phone Orders prior to Reviews, though please know what you're doing before you give it. Obviously, you'll attend pretty soon afterwards. But the benefit is this'll get things rolling and if the patient is treated early, by the time you examine them, they may well be improved and help your Assessment, i.e. by gauging response to Treatment.

NB: NOT APPLICABLE TO eMEDS, YOU CAN JUST CHART WHATEVER YOU WANT REMOTELY.

Other Procedures

Prioritising

Variable. Dependent solely on indication and how the rest of the shift is. Know that you'll be locked from many calls for quite a while, i.e. you can't just drop the IDC, so try to time these for a calmer part of the shift, though, of course, subject to clinical indication. It'll also be dependent on your confidence in doing them. Don't be pressured into doing something you're not comfortable doing. Ask for help from other JMOs or After Hours CNC/NUM.

Strategies

Primarily in Documenting, the actual technique you need to perfect.

Documenting: Use auto-text for the whole procedure. They are almost all the same. Just adjust for gauge/sizes, e.g. for IDC, NGTs, IVC.

A possible example of urinary catheter insertion is appended below (naturally, as always, follow local guidelines; examples are for illustrative purposes only).

[Insert type here] Medical Officer Dr [insert name here]

Asked to insert IDC

Indication: _

Patient consented to procedure
Sterile technique applied
Hand hygiene performed
Draped

Cleaned urethral meatus with sterile normal saline
Lubricant inserted into urethra
Has had _ recent travel [Y/N and to where]
Inserted _French IDC first pass
Inflated with 10 mL sterile water
Drained clear straw-coloured urine
Procedure well tolerated by patient
Nil complaints voiced

Urine sent for MCS and urine creatinine, sodium,
   osmolality

Plan:
• Monitor urine output/colour
• Team to chase urinary investigation results
• Notify Medical Officer if any concerns

Results checking/Plan enactment

Prioritising
Defined.

For Handover tasks, see section 'Clinical Reviews/Handover Reviews'.

Sometimes, Nurses put a task in the Job Book/on 'Task Manager' for you to review a Result. For these, there isn't a follow-up plan after the Result's reviewed. It'll be dependent on what the reviewed Result is. Check the Team documentation usually. Follow instructions if there are any. If not, then if it's something you are confident in handling, handle and document. If not, notify the Med Reg or current Senior in charge of the Specialty's patient or, in absence of former, the Specialty Doctor On Call.

 KEY POINTS

- Cannulas (IVCs): Prioritise active Rx soon due. Set up early and triage.
- Venepuncture: Prioritise Review-driven Bloods.
- Medication Reviews/Medication Charts:
  o Follow Team directives/guidelines/Senior advice.
  o If paper charts, get everything physically once and do once.
  o Use Phone Orders.
- Other Procedures:
  o Aim for quieter part of shift.
  o Use/develop auto-text to document these procedures, e.g. standardised documenting for all IDCs, with adjustment for size, etc.
- Results checking/Plan enactment: See section 'Clinical Reviews/ Handover Reviews'.

Help

Remember, if you need help After Hours, there's always someone around. You need different help for different difficulties.

- **Procedural things e.g. IVC, IDC**: The After Hours CNC or NUM, who can either help directly or direct you where appropriate, e.g. Vascular Access Team. So, don't die of frustration if that one cannula isn't going in.

- **Medical things**: Med Reg or Surg Reg, or ICU +/– ED if they're not contactable and you think it's urgent. It's best to get the Med Reg's number at the beginning of the shift in Handover so you can text them semi-urgent things. They'll be able to judge if they need to see now or later. But say they're at a MET call, it may be hard to take a page.

- **Admin things**: Usually the After Hours NUM/Navigators are best. Where it be for availability of certain Medications, or special forms, or diplomacy with patients/family, NUMs as always are expert at sorting out all sorts of Issues, a skill they certainly don't lose After Hours. So seek their help instead of suffering alone.

- **General**: Try to know who you're working with. You can hence cross-cover or spread cannula magic. As mentioned, JMOs also band and do group Job sweeps.

- **Specialty things**: The On-Call AT (Advanced Trainee) or Consultant for Specialty-specific matters. Reserve this for if you really can't get hold of anyone else. Usually, the Med/Surg Reg will call, but if you think this warrants the Consultant's attention and you can't get hold of the Med Reg, you could do this. You could also call the After Hours Specialty Reg On Call for phone advice and generally people aren't too annoyed if it isn't too late and you call them like you would for a Consult.

  The advantage is they usually know the patient better (as you'll nearly always call about inpatients) and would appreciate you updating them of any changes.

- **Always call**: Of course, most critically, if you're concerned, never be afraid to call anyone, even the Consultant. It's far better to endure whatever flack they may dispense, even in liberal portions, than for a patient to deteriorate. Their behaviour doesn't reflect on you. Patient safety is always paramount and they're aiming for the same goal, if only in different roles. But, by seeking help early, you're doing the best service you can for the patient. It could even save someone's life.

KEY POINTS

- Procedural things: AHNUM (After Hours NUM)/CNC/Specialty Reg.
- Medical things: Specialty Reg on site.
- Admin things: AHNUM.
- General: Know who is on shift with you.
- Specialty things: Specialty Reg on site/On Call.
- Always call if concerned.

CLINICAL REVIEWS

Read a real textbook. See some real patients. Learn from real mentors. Then be a real Doctor.

As reiterated, this is *not* a clinical textbook. The aim of this book is to make it easier to do what you want to do, and not tell you what to do. None of the rules are engraved and you should always be using your clinical judgement, Senior instructions and/or local guidelines in precedence.

However, as Reviews are a big part of the JMO's life, it may be worthwhile considering the following very basic guide. This is by no means comprehensive, but, rather, allows you to start something until the Medical/Surgical cavalry comes, i.e. allows you to institute some basic Investigations and Management. As always, you'll be guided by your Seniors and the actual clinical scenario.

Generally, Reviews are divided into the following:

- Clinical Reviews/Yellow Zones (attend <30 minutes) or Rapid Response/MET calls (attend <10 minutes): both trump other Reviews, cardiac arrests/Code Blue (immediate attend) trumping everything.
- Patient Reviews (attend speed variable).
- Handover Reviews (attend as per Handover).
- Protocol-based Reviews (attend speed variable – when able).

Clinical Reviews/Yellow Zones

Clinical Reviews are probably one of the more terrifying JMO tasks. Here is a sick, possibly deteriorating patient before you, and you suddenly feel that Med School has seriously *not* prepared you to be a Doctor and how in the world you got into this. This section is in this chapter for it is during After Hours that these Reviews become the most terrifying.

For, in daylight hours, your Reg is always at hand in Medical Terms and will probably either see the patient with you, instead of you, or are a phone call away to give advice. In ED, there are sometimes more Seniors than Juniors. In Surgical Terms, they're not beside you, true, but at least they're all in Theatres and you know where they are. Otherwise, the Med Regs of every Specialty are only a page or phone call away.

But not so at night. Here is indeed the daily Hospital Halloween. There's only a skeleton team and you're almost completely on your own, or so you feel. The Med Reg may be at another Review and is perhaps an hour away. Even the MET may be at another MET call. While here you are, with a sick patient you know almost nothing about, whose numbers are heading towards MET territory, and suddenly all your Medical knowledge seems to have frozen in your sinuses, instead of thawing in your brain.

As mentioned, this domain is immensely clinical and not suitable for this book. It's also extremely patient, case, protocol and Senior dependent.

The best advice is, *ask* frequently.

However, it's best to start something, and commence a basic Assessment and Treatment. The following is a very basic guide. For a true clinical guide, read any of the clinical, Ward-based texts on common calls. As for this, just think of them as crutches before you fly.

Arrests/Code Blue/MET calls

These emergency calls won't be discussed here as the circumstances are too variable/acute to know what you'll be doing exactly. You could be doing anything from CPR to getting an IVC in (much more of the latter).

You'll find getting vascular access and sending Bloods, Documenting and calling various people tends to be a larger part of your role.

But, generally, follow DRS ABCD and local guidelines, and start something sensible (per guidelines and your Medical knowledge, e.g. BLS [Basic Life Support]/ ALS [Advanced Life Support]) until ICU and the Med Reg comes.

A note against anxiety

When you start out, you'll be expecting everyone to have Pathology. Everyone must have something wrong with them. But the truth is, most people won't. Many things will be very benign and it's very likely not a few people live happy lives in the community in constant Yellow Zone. The main thing is not to be too frightened or complacent and exclude everything serious you can. Minor Issues will be sorted out by the Day Team. You just have to keep the patient stable at night.

There'll be many more negatives, far outweighing the positives. The key is to look for the latter. And as soon as there are any positives, think about what to do, then wake up the Reg.

In a statistics sense, you'll find the key thing is to minimise the false negatives. True positives aren't hard, as you'll soon notice a sick patient. True negatives will be many patients who you probably won't even be called about. False positives will be what frustrates you, as it'll seem something is wrong, and hence require your Review, but often there's not. Which is a good thing, even if frustrating.

But the false negatives are the dangerous ones. These are patients who don't appear particularly unwell, except some slight matter is off, something doesn't add up and requires your Review. But, really, they're about to crash, they're literally at the edge of the Medical cliff. And those are the ones you don't want to miss for these patients will become MET calls in the next hour, and certainly within your shift. But it's difficult as you must screen many true negatives, to catch the false one.

The main idea is stay vigilant. Screen appropriately. You can't be paralysed by fear, but you can't be blasé either. Have a system, screen the mortal differentials, and when you've done so adequately and consulted your Seniors, continue with your shift. And follow up as needed.

Clinical Reviews: procedure

What will happen is this. You'll get a page indicating a Clinical Review, giving the location +/– the derangement/reason/call back number. Then, about 30 minutes begin.

Consider the following procedure:

- **Call back**: Unless it's a MET call, usually it isn't always helpful to go there directly. You need to triage and know what's going on. So call the relevant Ward.

- **Question fruitfully**: Get as much info as you can before seeing the patient. It'll be variable how much the Nurses can tell you (the more senior usually more), but they all can inform you of the patient's identifying details, Obs, basic History, e.g. of a fall, some visual data, e.g. Blood in the drain and if the patient appears sick. It's more helpful if they've looked after the patient for a period, but don't bank on it. Remember to ask for the Nurse who called the Review (they often get another Nurse who knows nothing about the Review to call Switch, while the Nurse who does know is doing something else). Now is also when it's best to give some instructions so the Investigation/Management ball starts rolling. You won't be able to reach them later. It'll sometimes be hard enough to reach them now.

- **Trawl notes**: Read the notes as you question. The note trawling sets the context and gives much info including live eMR data so you know what you're dealing with. Very often, the Team's answered your question in their notes and tells you what to do. It also precludes you from doing certain things otherwise logical but inappropriate owing to the patient's special circumstances. Hence, abide by it unless there's a major change.

- **Consider Meds**: Easier if on eMeds, but harder with paper. Something also to ask the Nurses and consider withholding/reducing some of the Meds and giving others that will help the issue, e.g. PRNs/withheld Meds. Ask the Nurses about the Med classes you're worried about, e.g. is the patient on any anti-hypertensives if the patient is hypotensive.

- **Initiate basic Investigation/Management as appropriate**: You can't start everything without a full Assessment, but you can often start something. Stuff takes time to happen so this is more efficient as you can get the Results of some Investigations and observe the effects of some Treatments even as you get there, rather than waiting and fluffing about. However, don't do too much unless you're sure that's what the patient needs, especially Treatment-wise. You can't un-give Treatment.

- **Prepare notes**: You may do this after the Review but doing it before has two benefits. You have to document later anyway and this saves forgetfulness. You also remember to add the patient to your List to follow up instead of chasing them all over the whole Hospital. Another advantage is Documenting forces you to synthesise and work out what's going on. However, obviously go first pending urgency.

- **See the patient (and document)**: Conduct an appropriate and targeted Assessment, often simultaneous History/Examination/Investigations. See your clinical texts on how to do it.
- **Generate differentials**: Your whole Assessment should be aimed at ruling in and out differentials, with Investigations and Management aimed at clarifying the diagnosis, then treating it. Hence, think and act.
- **Consider Senior advice**: If it's something out of your depth or the patient seems sick, notify the Senior early. For things you can handle, still best to run by the Senior especially when starting out. People get you're new to this (or should). As you get better, you'll be more confident to act independently but obviously stay safe.
- **Commence Management**: Once you've completed your Assessment (+/− sought Senior advice if needed), enact the further Investigation/Management plan. Remember to document if you haven't yet to authorise stuff happening.
- **Chase and hand over**: Follow up on your patient throughout your shift. Remember to add them to your After Hours List. Chase the Investigations. There isn't a Reg who does that, it's you now (+/− the Med Reg). And if needed, know to hand over appropriately, what's done and what needs doing.

What to get rolling

Consider the simple things you can initiate that are listed in Table 8.1. This is a basic armamentarium. You'll acquire more as you go along and know better how to use them. But the list in Table 8.1, JMOs from day 1 could very possibly start.

Each of the these things you can use as needed, is *generally* not harmful and often helpful. However, as we stress, use your clinical judgement and in consultation with Senior advice.

Table 8.1 Simple things *you* can do

Common Investigations *you* can order	Common Management *you* can start
- Bloods/cultures/ABGs (arterial blood gases)/VBGs (venous blood gases) - Any Nursing-assisted Investigations, e.g. swabs (of anything), UA (urinalysis), urine MCS (microscopy, sensitivity, culture) - ECG - CXR +/− other X-rays as needed - Obs/Neuro Obs/Limb Obs/other Obs of all types/postural BPs - BSLs	- IV Fluids - Oxygen - Symptomatic relief you're comfortable prescribing, e.g. analgesia, anti-emetics, aperients - Electrolyte replacement you're comfortable with - Bronchodilators - PPIs (proton pump inhibitors)

Common Plans
- Continue as per Team (unless not doing so) - Continue monitoring - +/− Senior Review (or d/w Senior ...) - Notify MO if any concerns

Vitals derangements

Similarly, each of the actions listed in Table 8.2 you can *consider* doing, pending clinical context. These are certainly *non-exhaustive* and only some, or even none, may be applicable in each case. As emphasised, *always* follow clinical judgement, Senior advice and local guidelines.

> **NB:** THE ACTIONS LISTED IN TABLE 8.2 ASSUME ISOLATED DERANGE-MENT. FREQUENTLY, THERE WILL BE A COMBINATION MORE SUGGESTIVE OF A CERTAIN PATHOLOGY. CAUSES ARE BROAD FOR EACH. ALWAYS CONDUCT CLINICALLY TARGETED HISTORY AND EXAM FIRST AND CONSIDER CAUSE AND DIFFERENTIALS, BEFORE INSTITUTING INVESTIGATIONS AND MANAGEMENT.

Table 8.2 Actions to consider given each Vital Sign derangement

Vital	BP	HR	Temp
High	• Recheck manual BP/ different arm • Amlodipine/GTN (glyceryl trinitrate) patch • Give PRN anti-hypertensives • Check for end-organ impact	• ECG • Commence monitoring of other Obs, e.g. BP/ Sats • Bloods • IV Fluids • Rate/rhythm control (with Senior discussion) • +/– Cardiac monitoring if available • Overall very dependent on cause	• Bloods • Blood cultures • Antibiotics (Senior discussion) • Septic screen (CXR, urine MCS, Blood culture) • Paracetamol/anti-pyretic • Encourage oral intake • IV Fluids (+/– bolus) • Other relevant Investigations, e.g. swabs/resp/stool cultures/line cultures
Low	• Encourage oral intake • IV Fluids • Recheck BP manually • Postural BP • Commence monitoring of other Obs, e.g. HR/ Sats • Bloods • Lie/sit down/legs elevated • Withhold anti-hypertensive Medications • Day Team review mane re re-commencing anti-hypertensives • Very cause dependent	• ECG • Monitor BP and other Obs closely, e.g. attach Obs/sats machine • Withhold rate control Medications (Senior discussion first) • +/– Cardiac monitoring if available	• Septic screen as above • Bair Hugger/warm blankets • TFTs (thyroid function tests)

Vital	Sats	RR	BSLs
High	• That's fine • Wean oxygen (if on it)	• Oxygen (if low Saturations) • Monitor Sats and other Obs closely, e.g. attach Obs/sats machine • CXR • Bloods/ABG • ECG • Bronchodilators/Nebulisers	• Give oral anti-hyper-glycaemic agent (OHA) • Insulin (e.g. sliding scale) • Check Ketones/VBG • Endocrine Consult by Day Team
Low	• Oxygen: nasal prongs or Hudson mask • Repeat sats (other hand/fingers) • Sats probe on ear • Bloods/ABG • CXR • ECG	• Re-consider O_2 (if on it) • Review Medications • Opioid reversal • Monitor Sats and other Obs closely, e.g. attach Obs/sats machine	• Withhold insulin • Withhold OHA • Oral glucose (food or drink) • IV dextrose • Glucagon • Endocrine Consult by Day Team

KEY POINTS

- Always seek help if unsure or concerned.
- Seek advice of Seniors, local guidelines, clinical texts.
- Key aim of After Hours is to exclude life-/limb-/organ-threatening Pathology.
- Follow usual principles of Assessment: History, Examination, Differentials, Investigations, Management.
- Consider Review procedure:
  - Call back
  - Fruitful questioning of the caller of Review
  - Note trawling (concurrent)
  - Initiation of basic Ix/Mx
  - +/− Documenting preparation
  - See patient
  - Differentials/Senior advice/further Ix/Mx
  - Chase progress
  - Hand over (if required).
- See Table 8.2 for simple Ix/Mx that can be considered with derangement of each vital sign.

Patient Reviews

Know common types + approach.

These are again extremely variable, from patients having a tingly toe because they kicked it, or a tingly toe because there's a stroke (highly unlikely).

Reassurance lies again in that most people don't have Pathology.

However, as this domain is very clinical and scenario based, you're again directed to real clinical texts/teachers. The principles of action are the same as the above in section 'Clinical Reviews/Yellow Zones', only you usually have more time.

Know the common types of Reviews you'll see and have a systematic approach for each, e.g. History/Examination/Investigation/Management set you'd usually do. These may include:

- Falls
- Aggression
- Delirium/confusion/reduced level of consciousness
- Chest pain (often Clinical Review)
- Abdominal pain
- Limb pain
- Low/high urine output
- Headache
- GI bleeding
- Vague pain of any other body part
- Symptomatic relief
- And many others depending on Institution/Term.

The main thing to remember is *always* to exclude *life-* and *limb-/organ*-threatening causes or other things causing irreversible damage. It's often hard to find the actual cause, but, so long as you exclude the serious ones, it's something that can wait till the morning. If it can't wait or you're not sure, you should notify your Seniors. There also tends to be a higher index of suspicion for new complaints, though you should always remain vigilant.

Do not try to solve minor dilemmas at 3 a.m. You won't solve them and you'll fail to look after your other patients. Keeping people alive is your chief role.

You'll also get many calls/tasks for symptomatic relief. Remember to bring your common armamentarium ready for the legions of complaints, e.g. pain, nausea/vomiting, constipation, etc. However, as you mostly know nothing about the patients, you may need to Review them formally. Use your judgement, especially if symptoms are persisting despite adequate Treatment or unexplained by present Medical condition. Generally only chart stats/PRNs and check if the Team's PRNs have been used. Use these in preference as these are generally more appropriate (the Team should know what's best).

Handover Reviews

You'll be handed over to by various people to review patients for various things. This may be in person, over the phone and/or on 'Multi-Patient Task List'/'Task Manager'.

This is much easier than your own Reviews as they should tell you exactly where/when/what to look for. However, here's a checklist to know exactly what to know and prevent misses/hassles of re-calling.

1. **Precise instructions**: Know exactly what you're doing. You cannot be too meticulous. You're being asked to do something for someone you have no idea of, by someone who should have every idea. All questions are fair. Know at least who, why, when, what to do. If you don't know how to do it, you should decline. As for where, well, usually in the Hospital. You can find the Ward. Get a good clinical context. Also, the requestor should document. Some things you can even decline to do unless there's formal documentation, especially approving major Investigations/Management. You don't want to explain why you've charted all these cytotoxics or mAbs (monoclonal antibodies). To save yourself forgetting, document at least the Plan as they speak. It'll save you fumbling about later and prevent repetition. There are few calls worse than 'Sorry, I forgot the Plan'.

2. **Contingency Plans**: Usually, the Review will depend on a particular Result, which will result in different Investigations/Management instituted. Get each of the contingency plans. Know/ask what scenarios may occur, and then a Plan for each scenario, including if they wish to be notified. Get contacts if yes.

3. **Clarify urgency**: After Hours can be crazy. There are many demands on your time. All Doctors remember and understand. Always clarify when things need to be done by. The one who asks is best able to tell you and it'll save much unnecessary stress. Something for Review in the next shift is very different from Review in the next hour.

4. **Follow instructions**: Once you have the above, enact. Pretty obvious.

5. **Document**: As mentioned. But also note down what the Result was they wanted and consequently the resulting action as approved by them, or the further discussion you've had. Unfortunately, as said, if it isn't documented, it didn't happen.

6. **Handover**: Some Jobs or Reviews span several shifts. Or you were just so smashed you didn't get to it. That's ok. However, *hand over*. Make sure someone will do it eventually.

KEY POINTS

- Precise instructions.
- Contingency Plans for each scenario.
- Clarify urgency.
- Document all above concurrently.
- *Enact.*
- Document progress/Result.
- Hand over as required.

Protocol-based Reviews

Hospitals usually have protocols that automatically trigger Reviews after certain things have been done.

These may include Post-Transfusion Reviews, IVC Reviews (day 3), Post-Procedure Review, nasogastric tube placement.

Usually, the patients needing such Reviews are much more stable, have no idea why you're seeing them and are generally less urgent than all the above Reviews.

Unless otherwise indicated, these Reviews are just like the endless Jobs on 'Task Manager'/JMO Job book and you'll get to them as you come to them.

To get through them:

1. **See the patient**: Review them only for the protocol reason unless there are other complaints. Know how to do a good standard Review.

2. **Auto-text**: The first time you do them, set up the auto-text/Template. You'll do many more. And, soon, the Review will be faster than Documenting for the Review. However, with auto-text, you'll almost never need to type these again for each of the normal Reviews will be nearly exactly the same.

   Besides, your Template always reminds you what to look for, in case, after a 14-hour shift and 18-hour day, your mind isn't quite at peak performance.

   And if the Review is abnormal, well, it becomes a 'Patient Review'.

   We append an auto-text example; however, they're just a guide. Your own will be best.

3. **Document/cross off Jobs List**: It happened, so save the next shift grief.

Example of a Cannula Review (as always, for illustrative purposes only):

[Insert type here] Medical Officer Dr [insert name here]

Asked to review day 3 IVC

Patient consented to review

[insert size] _ G IVC in _ [insert position]
- Nil pain
- Nil erythema
- Nil oedema
- Nil induration or palpable cord along path of cannula
- Patient afebrile
- Nil other complaints
- Visual Infusion Phlebitis Score = _

[obviously adjust above if there were positive signs]

Impression:
- IV site appears _healthy/unhealthy
- Sign of cannula infection/phlebitis: _Yes/No

Plan:
- Keep and observe cannula for further 24 hours/ Please remove IVC and re-site
- Team to review need for cannula mane
- Notify Medical Officer if any concerns

KEY POINTS

- Know what (and what does not) trigger protocol Reviews: review policy if required.
- Perform Review as required.
- Generate auto-text for each type of Review with built-in adjustments for variables, e.g. size/gauge.
- Urgency usually protocol driven/defined and defers to clinical need.

DEATHS

Man is mortal. You certify this is so.

We include deaths in After Hours as this is the time when it happens most by probability (about 16 hours of the time versus about 8 hours) *and*, when happening, there's the least support. Your Team is asleep, there's limited Senior staff (or any staff) and, as to the patient, you probably know nothing about them, and will be seeing them often for the first, and last, time.

Deaths can obviously be a very confronting experience, but we'll address the practicalities of it so you can at least deal with that side. As to the emotional side, well, each in their own way.

Death certification is a two-step process

First examine

Certify the patient is actually dead. Again, save this as a Template as this way it reminds you to check for all things. The exact process of almost all death certifications you'll see is the same. Follow your State's policy. Once you're satisfied, you can proceed to the second stage. Also, depending on the circumstances of the death, try to console the family if you can. If the death was expected, then it's likely they'll be more accepting. However, if it wasn't, discuss with your Seniors or Consultant and see if any further tasks are needed, e.g. reporting to the Coroner.

Then, paperwork

Variable between States. Follow your State's policy. Often, there's a 'death package' that has all paperwork needed, often provided by the Ward staff. Most of it is self-explanatory and you fill in as instructed. Questions involving the History mostly just require some eMR trawling. 'Cause(s) of death' and 'contributing factors' are the main ones that require Senior input, usually Consultant (see section 'Sample death paperwork').

Do only your part (some forms ask for multiple staff to fill). Familiarise yourself early with the forms so you know what to obtain in case no one knows what the 'death package' looks like. If you're also not familiar, ask your Seniors, e.g. Day Team, After Hours NUM/CNC or Med Reg. You can even call your insurance company, as some offer advice 24/7 and you can see if they do.

Sample death paperwork

1. **Cremation certificate**: Pretty straightforward, follow instructions, and the only question that may be hard is the 'radioactive treatments' or if there was a 'battery powered device' attached to the patient. Do some note trawling as needed.
2. **Coronial checklist**: Also pretty standard, usually deaths aren't reportable and, if they are, it's probably above your rank to fill it out anyway (likely ICU/ED Reg/other Seniors). Follow the criteria/instructions it gives you. If reportable, notify Seniors, at least the Med Reg.
3. **Patient death checklist**: As above. Follow instructions.
4. **Death certificate**: The most complex one. In general, it's also follow instructions. However, tricky bits include the following:
   - **Country of birth**: Hard to find. The only place seems to be on the front cover of the patient chart with many of the patient details in boxes.
   - **Cause of death**: If you're the Home Team, then ask your Consultant, who'll tell you what to put in. If you're After Hours, look through the notes to see if it was expected. The Consultant may've documented what they want

written. Otherwise, give the AMO (Attending Medical Officer) a call (each Institution will have its custom of when to call) and they'll tell you what to write. Leave a message if the AMO is uncontactable. In the morning, if possible, notify the Team.

- **Certificate Issued Pursuant to s38 (2)**: Just read the Act on page 1 (turn page over). Usually 'no', as 'yes' means the death is reportable, but you have activated an exception as per the Act (read). However, always check with your Senior or just the Act.
- **AHPRA (Australian Health Practitioner Regulation Agency) number**: Google it.

Remember, always fill in everything as carefully as you can. This is a very serious matter, and if any errors are found, you'll be called to Medical Records to rectify them. So get everything right the first time with multiple checks to save everyone much unnecessary distress.

Documentation

Certifying deaths follows a standard format, which needs to be documented. Consider the following example which you can do *and* write. Of course, always follow your Hospital policy.

XXX[Your Name] (MO [Your role])
Asked to review patient re: no signs of life

Examined patient:
- No response to verbal or painful stimulus
- No carotid pulse
- No breath or heart sounds over 2 minutes
- Pupils non-reactive to light
- No motor (withdrawal) response or facial grimace in response to painful stimulus

Time of death: _

Nursing staff/I have already attempted to contact family/NOK

Cause of death: _

Plan:
1. Cremation certificate completed
2. Coronial checklist completed
3. Death certificate completed
4. Patient death checklist completed
5. Team to complete Discharge Summary [if you're not the Team] or Discharge Summary Completed [if you're the Team]
6. I will update Dr _ (AMO)
7. Will attempt to contact family or Family notified
8. Please leave patient on Ward until family have been given option of visiting patient in room (subject to local policies)

Again, remember, if you're in any difficulties, or anything is out of the ordinary, seek help. Ask your Seniors or After Hours Manager. Someone will know. And, if they don't, they'll know who to call. Don't do anything you're not comfortable with.

KEY POINTS

- Verify death on examination per protocol.
- Save standard death documentation as auto-text and implement (see text for sample).
- Obtain verbal or written advice from AMO regarding cause of death/contributing factors.
- Familiarise yourself early with standard death documentation sets (death packages).
- Seek Senior advice for any unexpected deaths/out-of-ordinary circumstances.

ACKNOWLEDGEMENT

We acknowledge Cerner Corporation as the proprietor of *PowerChart* and *FirstNet* electronic medical record (eMR) programs and related and subsidiary names and terms within those programs. References in this work to eMR predominantly relate to the aforementioned programs. These references and descriptions are made based on the author's experiences, discussions and observations only.

CHAPTER 9

COVID-19

Hopefully, by the time you see this, we will be nearing the end of COVID-19 (or at least nearing the beginning of the end) and are resuming some sort of COVID normal (whatever that is).

Again, in accordance with the spirit of the book, we won't go through the clinical details of COVID management apart from the fact that oxygen, proning, dexamethasone and various biologics/anti-virals are useful. Refer to the constantly evolving local, State and national guidelines.

Depending on your Hospital's rostering structure, COVID Wards can be like your regular Ward job or have an After Hours feel to it with multiple rostered shifts in coverage. The usual advice in the relevant sections still applies: refer to *Chapters 3–6 and 8* as required.

However, there are a few differences from the regular Wards. What with the constant PPE (personal protective equipment), the changing clinical situation, the anxiety, it can make an already stressful work environment even more difficult. Looking after yourself is even more important as you engage in this difficult position.

Below are practical pointers to make it more manageable.

GENERAL HEALTH/PRESSURE AREA CARE

- **Hydration (and nourishment)**: Especially important as it's much harder. You can't simply drink, you have a giant mask and perhaps even a face shield in between. You must make a conscious effort to hydrate regularly and eat. Set up a timer if necessary. Benefits already outlined in *Chapter 3*. However, check with local policy regarding how this can be facilitated re timing of breaks, etc.
- **Mask fitting**: You will all be professionally fitted to a P2/N95 mask, especially if working on COVID wards. If you only fit one mask, well that's that. However, you may successfully fit to multiple masks. Yet not all N95 masks are made the same. Some are more comfortable than others (i.e. cause less pressure

injury), pending your facial geometry. Considering you may be in one for up to 12–14 hours, you may as well get comfortable. You don't want to be fitted to the one that tries to break your nose each time you put it on. Hence, before your fit test, try to suss out which mask (that your Hospital offers) is most comfortable for you. You've probably experienced a few prior to formal fit testing. Then, during the fit test, where possible, try to fit for that mask first. Your nose, mandible and zygomatic arch will all thank you for the attempt.

- **Ear protectors**: Mask lanyard. Mask loops. Mask hooks. Mask extender straps. Ear savers. You get the idea. Your ears are precious, as anyone with ill-fitting glasses knows. Wear a mask that touches your ear in any way for long enough, and you will add pinna pressure injury to the other OH&S (occupational health and safety) hazards of being a doctor. Prevent this from happening. Invest in an ear protector of whatever sort you like. There are some very cheap options online. Alternatively, you can even make your own. A short band of elastic fabric (or other fabric/material) or even a piece of string, it's length customised to your head, and two buttons sown/attached to each end make excellent ear extender straps and your ears will thank you for hearing its pain.

- **Pressure area foam/gel/pads**: The N95s are designed to be very close fitting to keep the virus out, but certainly presses your face in. And your face really doesn't like being pressed in, especially the nasal bridge and cheek bones. Try nasal pads just over the bridge of the nose and over the highest area of the cheek bones to minimise pressure areas. The Hospitals sometimes supply specialised gel or foam to help; alternatively, some dressings are very helpful, ask your friendly nurses for help there.

- **Goggles**: Another great COVID preventer and pressure area inducer, especially around the side of your head or around your usual suspects, the nose and ears. Again, apply the pads as above or wrap the goggle legs in softer material, e.g. fabric, to avoid this. Alternatively, consider a face shield (which unfortunately has its own issues of tension headaches, a band-like headache due to a band around your head).

- **Mental health**: COVID has been extremely stressful. Duh. Especially for HCWs (Healthcare Workers). An already stressful and stretched workplace has just been hit with a once-in-a-generation global pandemic. So there is an even greater need to look after your mental, as well as physical, health. There are many supports both available to the public and dedicated to HCWs pending each facility. All that can be said is be even more aware of your wellbeing, seek out help early if needed and look after each other.

HYGIENE

- **Scrubs**: Wear these where possible as previously stated in *Chapter 2*, but even more so in COVID Wards. It is often Hospital policy that you change to surgical scrubs in COVID Wards to prevent infection spread. They also breathe better than the plastic gowns and you won't feel like you're constantly in a space suit.

- **Shower**: Often offered in various facilities for you after a shift. Worthwhile to take it up. Don't forget your usual toiletries.
- **Comfy shoes**: Essential in any role really, but you have even more excuse to be in them now. Consider a set of shoes for the COVID Ward then cleaning and bagging them after the shift before changing to your regular set. Some clinicians have invested in gum boots also.
- **Loose items**: You have a lot of stuff. Phones. Keys. ID badges. Steths. All can be a route for infection spread. The best way is, of course, frequent cleaning and wiping down all your stuff after each shift. However, things you often use, namely your phone, can be bagged and still work on shift. Try your humble freezer bag +/– new transparent specimen bags. Keeps your stuff clean but functional.

PROTOCOL

With the evolving situation, it can be difficult to keep abreast of the constant developments.

Our best advice is to familiarise yourself with the COVID protocols early and strictly follow the guidelines. Each Hospital usually has its own COVID protocol manual (or district directive). Find, keep, know and refer to this document. If in any doubt, ask. There is usually a COVID Consultant or Senior Medical Officer who has oversight over the COVID response. Refer to this person or their delegate re any queries.

Key areas to familiarise yourself early with include:

- Admission to various COVID pathways, e.g. suspected COVID versus confirmed COVID, and the criteria.
- Routine investigations after COVID diagnosis.
- COVID management: Including the options available and indications.
- COVID isolation/testing pathways, e.g. requirements/duration.
- Escalation of management and its pathways, e.g. ICU admission and inter-Hospital transfers.
- COVID-related deaths: Procedures.
- Release from COVID pathway/release from isolation algorithms.
- Discharge clearance procedures (including isolation at home procedures).
- COVID clinical reviews and emergencies: Procedure and differences from usual medical emergency responses.
- PPE requirements.
- Staffing rules, e.g. surveillance swabbing, isolation requirements.
- Vaccination: Opportunities to vaccinate and patient suitability pending clinical condition.

DOCUMENTING

With the prevalence of COVID, it's now also important to include a COVID Template regardless of whether one works on the COVID ward or not.

Key elements to consider include (pending Team):

- COVID status
  - COVID +ve: Date of symptom onset/first positive swab (if asymptomatic), days post symptom/swab +ve, RAT (rapid antigen test) versus PCR (polymerase chain reaction), location of test, subsequent swab results, key investigations, e.g. serology, Ct values (cycle threshold values), Management already received (days post each type), oxygen requirement, ventilation type.
  - COVID –ve: Date of negative swabs, days of isolation, dates of additional required surveillance swabs, anticipated day of release.
- Past COVID infections? Timing and general clinical course.
- Close contacts?
- Immunosuppression and other risk factors?
- Vaccination: Y/N, number of doses, timing of doses, type of vaccine(s), reactions (if applicable).

The above can similarly be Templated pending which elements your Seniors wish to prioritise.

KEY POINTS

- Be anti-pressure area via use of:
  - o Ear protectors
  - o Pressure area pads
  - o Optimal mask fitting
  - o Goggle pressure area prevention.
- Look after your mental health.
- Extra care with cleaning:
  - o Frequent wiping of equipment/hand hygiene
  - o Use scrubs
  - o Showering post shift
  - o Phone bags.
- Be very familiar with COVID protocols in all situations (see section 'Protocol').
- Use COVID-specific documenting template (see section 'Documenting').

CHAPTER 10

Money matters

Clearly.

Why we talk about money matters is self-explanatory, as money matters.

Sorry, that was irresistible.

But, in all seriousness, it does. For doubtless you have other life goals apart from Medicine, and while money isn't everything, it's a good deal of things, and certainly helps very much in achieving your non-monetary, non-Medicine goals.

And you owe it to yourself, your family and your friends to be prudent and thus to achieve happiness where you can, or, at least, avoid avoidable misery.

Work is a new thing to many JMOs (Junior Medical Officers) and the Admin side is often not much taught. Suddenly, you have income, taxes, super, salary packaging, Contracts, Rosters, etc. It would help to have some string to pull yourself out of the mush.

For many Doctors, work becomes most of your life. And perhaps for many junior Doctors, work is life. What with the Overtime, the nights and the weekends you do, why, you really are a Resident of the Hospital, even before becoming one on your payslip.

You only have limited life. But we imagine most want to have something out of life more than work.

So here are some general pointers on how you can put the piggy bank and general life bank into more tolerable shape, especially when you figure out how this whole work thing, works.

Disclaimer: This includes general advice only. It by no means recommends, or un-recommends, any practice whatever. We disclaim all responsibility whatever. If you go broke, that is not our fault. What you see is what you get. Always seek professional financial/legal/industrial advice to meet your personal circumstances.

NB: IT'S FORTUNATE THAT UNIVERSITY AND JMO TEACHING IS INCREASINGLY TEACHING YOU ABOUT THIS, WHICH IS AN EXCELLENT STEP. DON'T FALL ASLEEP, OR, WORSE, BE ABSENT FROM THESE LECTURES AS THEY'LL BE INSTITUTION SPECIFIC AND OFTEN TELL YOU EXACTLY WHAT YOU NEED TO KNOW. MAKE NOTES AS YOU WOULD FOR A MEDICAL LECTURE. IT'S VERY POSSIBLE YOU'LL REFER TO THEM AGAIN, AND NOT JUST BEFORE EXAMS.

However, as these aren't available to everyone, we think a general section here is needed. This is, as stated, general. There are minutiae that you'll need to figure out by asking your fellow JMOs and/or Hospital Admin, etc. However, the basis here should be sound, for it's largely universal across the Hospitals.

NB: EVERY STATE IS DIFFERENT AND THERE'LL BE SUBTLE (AND SOME NOT SO SUBTLE) DIFFERENCES. WE OFFER BELOW CHIEFLY A CASE STUDY OF NSW. FOR THOSE IN OTHER STATES, THE FOLLOWING WILL ASSIST IN WHAT TO LOOK FOR IN YOUR OWN WORK LIFE, AND THOUGH SOME DETAILS ARE DIFFERENT, THE PRINCIPLES SHOULD LARGELY BE THE SAME. AND IF THERE'S THE REQUEST FOR IT, A SIMILAR COMPILATION, IN COLLABORATION WITH THE FRONT-LINE STAFF, CAN BE MADE. SOME THINGS CAN ONLY BE KNOWN ON THE FRONT LINE.

EMPLOYMENT MATTERS

The Contract: Rules of work – an exhortation to read

> *The contracting parties mutually agree of their own free will to abide in every respect by the Terms set forth in this Agreement.*

The work environment is extremely complex and variable. It's impossible to discuss each scenario, in each Institution with each combination of players. There are many different interests, obligations, responsibilities, entitlements, rights, rules and laws at play. And you, unfortunately, while thrown right into their midst, are likely the one who knows the least about them.

Is there not one rule, manual, guide to show you your way out of all this?

There is.

It's called your Contract.

The Award (generally).

Yes, we're talking about that forty- to eighty-page document that is written in legalese, that many don't know/remember exists and that certainly no one wants to read. Yet it governs most of your job itself.

You have *agreed* to everything in it.

Therefore, it's *binding*.

You should at least *know* what's in it.

You're legally entitled to all that's in your Contract. Anything that you don't get is a breach and you're entitled to recover it (pursuant to the Contract).

Similarly, the responsibilities that you take on are likewise binding. You must do them. You're obliged to do so. If you do not, there'll be consequences, not the least of which is being fired.

However, whatever is *not* in the Contract, you're by no means obliged to perform or obtain. Nobody can make you do it or give you it. And if you do it or get it, in the first, it's a favour you're rendering to others, in the latter, a favour rendered to you. You should not expect one or the other.

Since it tells you what you *should* get, and what you *should* do, *shouldn't* you at least take some time to skim it?

We know, it's rather long and complex, and there's a reason you're in Medicine and not say, Law, not the least of which is the hate of legalese. However, you're working for at least 2 years in the public health system. And, if you continue to train in public Hospitals, you'll be bound by the same Contract as the Award carries forward.

Hence, this is an under one hundred-page document that will govern your entire Hospital working life, i.e. your life, for the next 2–10 years, or more. Perhaps, considering this, it's worth reading. Especially considering how much other, less useful reading we do.

To make this distasteful task slightly less so, Award references are appended in the 'Notes' section and referred to via superscript numerals for areas of general interest. The legalese is copied verbatim, plus a less legalese statement. Section references are also provided if you wish to pursue more in-depth reading.

NB: IT'S STILL BETTER IF YOU READ THE CONTRACT. WHAT'S APPENDED IS MATTERS OF GENERAL INTEREST BUT EVERYONE HAS THEIR NICHE INTEREST THAT WILL BE BEST ANSWERED BY THE ORIGINAL DOCUMENT. IF YOU DO DECIDE TO TAKE THAT BRAVE STEP, NOTE THE AWARD DOESN'T GO BY PAGE NUMBERS BUT BY 'SECTIONS', WHICH KEEP TALKING ABOUT A TOPIC UNTIL DONE. WE SUPPOSE IT LETS THEM ADD TO EACH SECTION AS NEGOTIATIONS CONTINUE. BUT IT DOES MAKE NAVIGATING HARDER. HOWEVER, TO HELP, JUST LOOK FOR BOLD (WHICH ANNOUNCES A NEW SECTION). THERE'S NO NAVIGATION THROUGH THEM SO YOU'LL JUST HAVE TO FLICK THROUGH THE DOCUMENT.

NB: THE AWARD IS LOCATABLE BY GOOGLING '[INSERT STATE] HEALTH AWARD/ENTERPRISE AGREEMENT MEDICAL OFFICERS' OR SIMILAR SUCH SEARCH TERMS.

Documenting

Write, down, everything. Times two.

Just as you should document for all patient affairs in eMR (electronic Medical Records), you should document for all your own affairs. And keep copies of everything. Specifically, consider:

- **Email correspondence everything**: Most effective method. Saves you and the other person time. The only worry is no reply, but that also is kind of a reply. If there's a discussion about anything, you should send a follow-up email promptly, as a memo of what was discussed.
- **Copies of everything**: Photocopy/scan/photo all your official hard copy documents, e.g. Term Assessments, Overtime forms, Leave forms. In other words, file all documents related to your work, or anything else that'll affect your life, especially if it were to go wrong. If you don't save a copy, you shouldn't care if it goes wrong.
- **Save online documents**: As above. Save those that affect you, e.g. Roster changes, Timesheets, Leave documents. Anything can change.
- **Get countersignatures**: You may or may not get these. But if there's an official stamp/signature/docket/reference number of receipt/record of your discussions/documents, you should get these on your documents.

There is often confusion and error. This will save the hassle of all that. People may easily forget or remember incorrectly verbal discussions 3 weeks down the track. Things are sometimes lost to follow-up. Documenting is relatively unforgettable and can always be followed up.

Salaries

> *Money!*

Ah yes, one of the first exciting topics in working life.

So you're working at last. And you're about to receive (for many) your first official pay cheque, ever. And (for almost everyone) the first dollars for saving lives (sort of).

You'd think such an important topic would be in the Award. But apart from a nice note to look elsewhere, there's not much more. Fortunately, we've looked elsewhere, and found for you what you want to know, for years to come.

Essentially, Google 'health professional/medical officer salaries (state) award 20xx' (or similar terms). And this will not only tell you your salary for this year, but for ranks to come, as well as the salary of almost everybody else, for those overly curious. Search for yourself. You're a 'Medical Officer'. Pick your own grade.

Ok, so now you know. Let's see what you need to do to earn it.

Working Hours (s6)

> *Contrary to popular opinion, Residents do NOT live at the Hospital.*

This is generally religious in most occupations, except in Medicine. There is, we suppose, that unpredictable element in it which has so blurred the line between work time and home time, to the point that sometimes it's indistinguishable.

However, there *is* a line, supported by your Award and the government in general. Let it be clear enough to you and hopefully you won't need to waver from it too often, too much.

We'll only discuss Rostered hours here. See section 'Overtime' for anything beyond.

As per your Contract/Award

- Normal (*ordinary*) hours means ≤38 hours/week via 40 hours per 7 days straight or 80 hours per 14 days straight *and* one allocated day off (ADO) per month (s6(i)).[1]
- You should get ≥2 days *off* per week (not including Overtime) or ≥4 days *off* per fortnight from normal hours. Admin will try to make them in runs and in combo with ADOs/other days off (no guarantees) (s6(ii)).[2]
- Your shifts should be in one straight session, not split in any way or <4 hours (s6 (iii),[3] (iv)[4]).

- You should also be working safe hours (Policy Directive 2019_027 s4.1.12 for NSW):[5]
  - You *should* not be Rostered on for >14 hours (inclusive of everything).
  - You *must* have a break of >10 hours between shifts.

> **NB:** YOUR CONTRACT ALSO SUPPORTS ALL THIS, BUT IN LESS EXPLICIT TERMS (S32), AND MAINLY CENTRES AROUND KEEPING SAFE. AS USUAL, IT'S CENTRED AROUND THE MOST FAMOUS LEGAL ENTITY, THE 'REASONABLE'. THIS SEEMS HARD TO DEFINE, ESPECIALLY FOR A DOCTOR. HOWEVER, YOU CAN REFUSE TO DO OVERTIME AS IT'S 'UNREASONABLE', WITH VARIOUS BASES. READ THE SECTION IF YOU'RE CONSIDERING IT.

- Interestingly, you're considered to be 'working' not just when you work, but also when you eat, study, rest, sleep or do anything really, while you wait for something to happen before you do *your* thing (s9 para. 1).[6] So you're allowed to do these things, so long as you have finished as much of *your* job as possible and start the job when you can:
  - This obviously doesn't include official mealtimes in which you actually eat (s9 para. 2),[7] and when you just feel like coming in to work when you're not on or when someone has told you to go home already and you won't (at least you won't be paid for it (s9 para.3)).[8]

In practice

Variable between Institutions, but, officially, your Working Hours are as follows (approximately):

- Medical Terms: approximately 08.30–17.00.
- Surgical Terms: approximately 07.30–16.00.
- Emergency: Three shifts, usually 10 hours:
  - Day shift: approximately 08.00 to approximately 18.00.
  - Evening shift: approximately 14.00–24.00.
  - Night shift: approximately 22.30–08.30 (next day).
- ICU: Two to three shifts (10–12 hours) and similar to Emergency or 1 hour earlier.
- Other Terms, e.g. Paeds, O+G (Obstetrics and Gynaecology), Cardio: Variable, often there's a day and evening shift similar to the ED (Emergency Department), though may be shorter.

Rosters

These are the governors of your life.

Tells you when to work, and when not to.

Get very familiar with these very early to plan life in general. Especially any job where After Hours work is common, e.g. ED. You don't want to come in on a weekend to find you're not on, or not come in when you're on nights.

Usually published on the Intranet and/or emailed to you so know where early.

As JMOs, there's your day job Roster (which is usually the same) and an After Hours Roster detailing all the other shifts you do and On Calls. It's a good idea to save these in your calendar and have it remind you on the day or day before.

These also do change now and then, but you should get notice, as per your Award, i.e. ≥2 weeks' notice for your day job Roster (s6(vii))[9] and hopefully for Overtime too, but Admin can change the latter at any time.

KEY POINTS

- Know your normal working hours per the Award and allowed time off.
- Know your maximum daily hours.
- Know your working hours in each type of Term (regular versus shift work).
- Know your Roster well and plan in advance.

Meal breaks (s10)

Food is not superfluous.

You have these in theory. In practice, well, it's variable.

Unlike Nursing staff, who have quite a systematised breaks system, Doctors aren't quite as religious with their off time. On busy Terms, you may find 'meal breaks', or breaks of any kind for that matter, non-existent. Even that final break called 'home time' may be eaten into.

However, remember, you are granted breaks as per your Award.

There are two circumstances regarding breaks, normal/day shift and After Hours shift.

Day shift (Monday–Friday)

Yes, you may eat. You have a special time dedicated to it, i.e. you're entitled to a ≥½ hour break (s10(ii)),[10] for which you're not actually paid. And if you work them, you should be paid (s10(iii)).[11]

That is why, though you're at work 8.5 hours per day or 85 hours per fortnight, you're only paid for 76 hours per fortnight or 7.6 hours. Approximately 0.4 hours goes to your ADO, 0.5 hours to your meal break, i.e. you're technically 'not working' then.

Try to eat then. It'll do you good (s10(i)),[12] and it even exists in the Award.

After Hours shifts (other than day shifts Monday–Friday)

You may eat then too, but the difference is, *you SHOULD be paid for your 'meal break'* (s10 reference to Circular No. 83/250 of 19 August 1983).[13] We suppose the government recognises that eating 'lunch' at 4 a.m. is not quite the same as at 1 p.m. There isn't exactly anywhere to go at 4 a.m., except perhaps a vending machine.

Note the exact phrase: *Because of the widespread difficulty involved in officers leaving Hospital premises for any purpose (including the taking of meal breaks) during 'Out of hours shifts' ... .*

There. The government, which doesn't exactly work regular night shifts, and has Parliament kitchens open when they do, does know about them, at least some of the practicalities (or lack thereof).

This clause is particularly applicable on ED/ICU shifts, weekend and night shifts, of which the half an hour 'meal break' time should not be deducted from your pay unlike your day job. Similarly, all your Overtime After Hours shifts; evenings, nights, weekends and public holidays all should *not* have meal break times deducted.

Something to be aware of next time you review your payslip or Online Pay Transactions. Though the amount each time is not much, it can easily cumulate to something significant.

KEY POINTS

- You need to eat.
- You're usually not paid to eat during normal hours.
- You're usually paid to eat After Hours (non-normal hours).

After Hours-Penalty Rates (s8)

You're paid in a special way when you work weird hours. Yes, the government also recognises that working 10 hours on a Monday day 8 a.m.–6 p.m. is different from working 10 hours on a Sunday night 10 p.m.–8 a.m.

This is how you should be paid if there are weird hours. You get paid your normal rate, *plus loading*, at the following rates:

(i) Hours worked between 6 p.m. and midnight, Monday–Friday: 12.5%.

(ii) Hours worked between midnight and 7 a.m., midnight Sunday to midnight Friday: 25%.

(iii) Hours worked between midnight Friday and midnight Saturday: 50%.

(iv) Hours worked between midnight Saturday and midnight Sunday: 75%.

Which means ... see Table 10.1.

Table 10.1   Summary of loading schedule

Time	Day		
	Monday to Friday	Saturday	Sunday
12 a.m.–7 a.m.	25%		
7 a.m.–6 p.m.	Normal rate	50%	75%
6 p.m.–12 a.m.	12.5%		

Important: Overtime trumps After Hours. However, only one will be paid. You won't get 75% loading and double time.

> **NB: A NOTE FOR SUNDAYS – GETTING EXTRA ANNUAL LEAVE: YOU CAN ACCRUE EXTRA ANNUAL LEAVE IF YOU WORK MANY SUNDAYS/ PUBLIC HOLIDAYS (S14(II))[14] FOR AT LEAST 8-HOUR BLOCKS AT A RATE OF 38 HOURS OF EXTRA ANNUAL LEAVE PER 35 SUNDAYS/PUBLIC HOLIDAYS WORKED (S14(II)(B)),[15] ROUNDED TO THE NEAREST 1/5 OF AN HOUR (S14(II)(D)).[16]**
>
> **THAT IS, IF YOU WORK 35 SUNDAYS/PUBLIC HOLIDAYS, YOU GET 1 FULL WEEK ANNUAL LEAVE (S14(II)(A)).[17] BUT 35 SEEMS TO BE THE CAPPED MAXIMUM. NOTE THAT IF YOU'RE 'CALLED IN' ON A SUNDAY, THAT IS NOT COUNTED (S14(II)(C)).[18] YOU CAN ALSO HAVE THIS EXTRA ANNUAL LEAVE PAID OUT TO YOU LIKE ANNUAL LEAVE IF YOU DON'T TAKE IT, AS LONG AS YOU HAVE ≥1 WEEK OF THIS EXTRA LEAVE (S14(II)(E)).[19]**

Overtime (s11)

The once inevitable. The future, perhaps dispensable.

As a JMO, this is very likely. It also depends on the Term you're doing. Some hate it, some don't mind it, some take on more of it. Suit yourself.

What will be discussed are your rights and responsibilities with regards to it, so you may know where you stand and what your entitlements are. What you choose to do, lies with you. Just make the choice, yours.

How it's paid
You're paid Overtime when:

- Any work more than normal hours, i.e. *≥38 hours/week or ≥76 hours/fortnight*

  or
- Any hours *≥10 hours in one shift (s6(v)).*[20]

This affects you in a few ways.

- **ED**: If you pick up extra shifts, you'll be paid Overtime, but *not* if you just work weird hours. See section 'After Hours: Penalty rates'.

- **Most other Terms**: If you work more than your 'normal hours', you get Overtime. This means any evening/weekend shifts you pick up.
- **ICU**: If you work 12-hour shifts, you're entitled to Overtime.

The *Overtime payment rates* are as follows (s11(i)):[21]

- Weekdays and Saturday:
  - First *2 hours* of Overtime = 1.5× normal rate.
  - All time beyond *2 hours* = 2× normal rate.
- Sunday: 2× normal rate for all.

> **NB:** YOU SHOULD GET NOTICE OF ALL YOUR SHIFTS AT LEAST ONE SHIFT BEFORE THAT SHIFT. OTHERWISE, YOU SHOULD GET EITHER FOOD OR FOOD MONEY (S11(II))[22] IF YOU'RE WORKING EARLIER THAN 6A.M., AFTER 7P.M., OR AFTER 2P.M. ON WEEKENDS/PUBLIC HOLIDAYS. THAT IS, YOU GET APPROXIMATELY $32 FOR FOOD (PART B, TABLE 1, ITEM 2 AT END OF AWARD).

When it's paid

There are two types: ROT (Rostered Overtime) and UROT (un-Rostered Overtime).

Rostered

These are shifts you *must* go to, unless you swap out/give away. There are people who take and people who give. Your pick. Take note there's not always equal demand and supply, so whichever side you are, get in early and organised to get/ give the adequate amount.

There are also policies to prevent excess of either, i.e. you're not allowed to work too many shifts too close together nor can you give away all your shifts. The first is for your safety, the latter as you need After Hours learning experience. Check with your Hospital for the precise policies.

There's no approval needed for ROT, but still check that you've been paid for it, especially when you've taken extra shifts or if there's been shift swaps. As your pay lags behind your work, keep a pay calendar/notepad and note each Overtime shift you've worked. You can easily lose track and so can Med Admin, especially with the innumerable swaps and gives always going on.

Un-Rostered

The difficult one. It's easy to work it, but less so to get paid.

However, there've been some recent changes that are more understanding of actual circumstances and these are policies you should be familiar with.

Officially, you need UROT to be either (Policy Direction 2019_027 s9 in NSW):

a. Pre-approved

   or

b. One of currently *nine* reasons, as follows.

1. **Medical Emergency**: MET (Medical Emergency Team) calls +/– Clinical Reviews (the government realises that you can't really step out from the middle of an intubation as it's 5 p.m.) (s9.2.1).[23]

2. **Patient transfer**: You won't usually be involved in this, but if a patient needs to be transferred to another facility, there are many logistical issues that may need sorting out. Another time-consuming matter (s9.2.2).[24]

3. **Theatres**: If you're helping in Theatres, you shouldn't really drop the retractor. Overtime will be paid (s9.2.3).[25]

4. **Admitting/Discharging a Patient** (s9.2.4).[26]
   Both of these usually take some time, as you'll know, the first more as a Reg, the second as a JMO. Admitting often requires some Admin/basic Reviews, e.g. reviewing the patient's condition, Charting Meds, Ordering Bloods, effecting Boss (Consultant) Plans, etc. while Discharges similarly have their own set of Admin, e.g. scripts, Discharge Plans, Medical Certificates, Investigation forms. And also one very important piece of paperwork, now paid for, which is … :

5. **Patient transfer/Discharge Summaries**: Yes, you are paid for these! Patients should have them prior to Discharge. Gone are the days (hopefully) of unpaid weekend Discharge parties (coming in on weekends unpaid to do overdue Discharge Summaries and pretending it's a party). You are now paid to party in such a manner (still, do not come in on weekends). If you can't hand over and/or can't finish on time, you get Overtime (s9.1.5).[27]

6. **Late Ward Rounds**: Bosses starting WRs (Ward Rounds) at 5 p.m. is well … Overtime. Yes, they should Round within hours, and if they regularly *don't*, that should be formally Rostered, either into your usual hours or ROT (s9.1.6).[28] However, you *will* definitely, at least, be paid for the 5 p.m. WR (s9.1.6).[29] Even if the WR is in hours, but Ward responsibilities stretch outside it, i.e. Jobs still need doing and it'll be after your shift if you do them, then you can claim Overtime. But hand over if you can (s9.1.6).[30]

7. **Mandatory training**: Should be done when you're Rostered on (i.e. while you're officially at work). If your Boss asks you to do them when you're not, then you get Overtime (s9.1.7).[31]

8. **Clinical Handover**: This should take place in your normal hours, but, if it doesn't, you get Overtime until you finish Handover (s9.1.8).[32]

9. **Outpatient Clinics (in Hospital)**: Any Clinics run by you going out of your hours, you get Overtime until you've finished the Clinic stuff (s9.1.9).[33]

Now, there's not much pre-approval going on usually. So, it'll be one of the Nine. However, if a senior requests your presence, we suppose that usually constitutes approval (pre- or otherwise).

Usually, the approver of Overtime must be accessible, know what you're doing and can re-allocate the UROT work to someone else (s9.2).[34]

You need to submit your claim within 4 weeks of working UROT (to keep Med Admin happy) so submit early. You should get paid the following pay cycle (s9.4).[35]

Follow assiduously their Admin requirements to get paid (see literally s9.3). See the entire Section 9 for very good reading on your rights and responsibilities.

KEY POINTS: NINE REASONS

1. Medical emergency.
2. Patient transfer.
3. Helping in Theatres.
4. Admitting/Discharging a patient.
5. Patient transfer/Discharge Summaries.
6. Late Ward Rounds.
7. Mandatory training.
8. Clinical Handover.
9. Outpatient Clinics (in Hospital).

Getting it paid

This is, of course, a difficult topic and is extremely variable between Hospitals and even between departments, though it should perhaps be universal, unequivocal and standardised.

You'll have to use a lot of your own judgement here. As usual, the best policy is to be well prepared. But exactly how ... think of having the following.

- **Good reasons**: You should be well aware of what grounds UROT is paid (the *Nine*).

- **Good documentation**: Always stash your Overtime forms on yourself or convenient places. Grab the stickers of patients who you had to manage out of hours. Record what you needed to do, why you needed to do it and who asked you to do it. Check it off against the criteria for Overtime.

  The better and more comprehensive your documentation, the better your case for Overtime. Remember that the people approving your Overtime weren't there. But if you bring good documentation, then, naturally, it's far more convincing than if they could only take your word for it. This also links in why documentation is so important, for, by doing so, it shows everyone what you've been doing. So make it a priority after effective patient care.

  You're naturally entitled to pay for work done. Just show that you've done it.

- **Good organisation**: As mentioned, doing Overtime is easy. Getting it paid is ... more involved. So you need to be on the ball. In addition to the above measures, especially when time pressed, create a List for all your patients who you did Overtime for. Thus, so long as you documented at some stage, you can always accurately complete your Overtime forms and you'll no longer need to dredge your brain for who you did that Overtime for last Thursday ... or was it Monday?

Many Hospital networks are also moving towards an online claiming system. Be familiar with that process and, ideally, claim on the day you performed Overtime, right afterwards if possible. It may involve staying back a few extra minutes, but you've definitely locked in the hours you've already spent working and it's more than worth it.

- **Not going over time**: Hand over if possible. The Hospital does have a system for managing patients out of hours. You can and should utilise this system. Alternatively, try to do it tomorrow.

- **Approver**: Find out early who your Term Supervisor is and who approves Overtime. These people are usually senior and difficult to reach, so if you want the forms approved, rather than getting grimy in your locker/folder, you'll need to hunt for these people or make use of any opportunity to reach them.

- **Chat with prior JMO**: Discuss with your previous JMO the Overtime procedure. They probably know how it's paid and the procedure. Some Terms approve Overtime more readily than others.

- **Med Admin/Director of Training**: If you're running into serious difficulties, i.e. working much Overtime but not getting paid it, you may consider discussing this with the Director or Med Admin. It's the Hospital that hires you, the Term is only one of the places you work. If there are issues, you should liaise with Admin to discuss the matter.

KEY POINTS

- Overtime commences per rules, e.g. ≥10 hours in one shift or ≥38 hours/week or ≥76 hours/fortnight.
- Overtime rates at 1.5× for first 2 hours, then 2× any hours after, Sunday always 2×.
- ROT: Scheduled and must attend.
- UROT: Unscheduled. Will be paid if follows criteria; see Key Points: Nine reasons.
- Maximise chance of Overtime being paid by:
  - Good reasons (one of nine).
  - Good documentation (Overtime forms and patient stickers ready).
  - Good organisation (make custom List of Overtime-related patients *and/or* claim directly online).
  - Aim for not going over time (hand over where possible).
  - Process familiarisation (know approver, chat with other JMOs, Med Admin).

Leave

Absence from work exists. Even for Doctors.

See section 'IT matters/Leave' for how to view. This section will deal with how each works.

Leave is important to everyone for stuff happens in life, outside of work. It's also one of your entitlements. Hence, you should know how it works and make use of it to sort out what's left of your non-Hospital existence.

Each common Leave type for JMOs will be discussed. The exact protocol in each Hospital will be different, so you'll need to work those out, but the principles are the same and cannot contradict your Award. For other Leave, you're referred to the Award itself.

The best advice apart from knowing how Leave works is to keep a record, a diary/spreadsheet/other document, of all the days that were not ordinary.

Note down all times you didn't work, i.e. your Leave, e.g. ADOs, sick and other Leave and all times you did too much work, e.g. the Overtime/After Hours/public holiday shifts you've done.

This will help you cross-check things easily and make sure you're receiving the correct pay and leave.

Sick Leave (s16)

You have *76 hours* of sick leave each year paid (s16(i)).[36]

Sick leave *carries forward* over time and between Hospitals (s16(v)).[37]

Admin notes:

- Notify Med Admin and your Team +/– the Consultant you're sick, as early as possible, preferably in <24 hours (s16(i)(c)).[38] ED usually has its Admin or the Admitting Officers you should call.
- Pagers can be rediverted, so don't stress if you've carried the pager home.
- Fill in the Leave form when you return.
- Assiduously follow any paperwork. You don't want to be sick and miss out on your pay.

Provisos:

- You cannot take sick leave if employed for <3 months (s16(i)(b)).[39]
- Max sick leave a day is 8 hours (s16(i)(f)).[40]
- You won't get 'sick leave' for Overtime shifts (s16(i)(e)).[41]
- You may need a Medical Certificate (and no, you can't write it) (s16(i)(a)).[42] See your Institution's policy.
- Worker's compensation affects sick leave (s16(i)(d)).[43]

Annual Leave (s14)

You're entitled to *4 weeks* of Annual Leave each year (s14(i)),[44] during which you're paid your normal rate (s14(viii)).[45] Annual Leave accrues in hours on a pro rata basis, i.e. accumulates as you work, i.e. you have none at the beginning of the year.

- **Admin pointers**:
  - Lodge Leave forms early (by the *deadline*) and chat to Med Admin to get the time you want. Of course, there are no guarantees, but less popular times, e.g. *not* Christmas/New Year, are usually more likely.
  - Watch out that you don't pick up any shifts during Annual Leave else you'll need to come in.
  - You can sometimes combine all your Public Holiday Credits and extra Annual Leave with your normal 4 weeks and hence take more weeks, e.g. 5–6 weeks. Plan well and discuss with Med Admin.

- **Taking it**: You have to take it. We *know*, most people won't complain about that, but just saying. You *must* take it within 12 months of getting it (s14(iv)).[46] That's why it's called Annual Leave, rather than, say, Centennial Leave. Usually, you can't have it paid out (i.e. instead of taking it (s14(vi))).[47]

- **Timing**: Normally, you take Annual Leave in one block. However, if Med Admin agrees, you can take it in two or three blocks (s14(iii)),[48] but usually not less than 1 week, unless you discuss with Med Admin. Know your Leave policies early.

  Some Hospitals mandate you take it in the Relief Term, some don't mind. Whenever it is, you *must* get ≥2 months' notice prior to Annual Leave starting (s14(vii)).[49]

- **Paid out**: If you have *extra* Annual Leave, e.g. due to working many Sundays or public holidays, you can elect to have it paid out whenever you like instead of taking it. See section 'After Hours: Penalty rates' and s15(iv).[50]

- **Annual Leave in advance**: Variable between Institutions but you usually can only take so much Annual Leave as a proportion of time worked unless you have accrued it (i.e. no one as an Intern), e.g. you can't take 4 weeks in Term 1 usually. However, if Med Admin are happy, you *can* take Annual Leave before you're entitled to it. However, you can't really take more Annual Leave until 1 year has passed since this early Annual Leave taken, e.g. if you take it in February, you'll need to wait till next year February before Annual Leave will start accumulating again (s14(v)).[51]

- **Registration**: Bear in mind, as an Intern, you have to do at least one Surgical and one Medical Term (at least one block of 10 weeks each) and at least one ED Term (at least one block of 8 weeks) with a grand total of 47 weeks of full-time Medical experience in order to gain 'General Registration' (otherwise, you remain 'Provisional' until you fulfil the requirements). You'll need to consider this when you apply for Leave (always check Australian Health Practitioner Regulation Agency (AHPRA)/Medical Board policies).

• **End of employment**: If you do quit, you should get all your Annual Leave paid out to you (s14(ix)). However, if you took Annual Leave in advance and you quit before you finish the year, well, you'll only get paid the amount of Annual Leave that you're entitled to, based on how much time you've worked (s14(x)).[52] See s14 (ix),(x) of the Award for more precise details.

KEY POINTS

- Entitled to 4 weeks Annual Leave yearly.
- Plan early: Notify Med Admin.
- Lump all leaves together for longer Leave (conditions apply/variable).
- Accumulates on pro rata basis.
- Must take it yearly.
- Can be taken in blocks/one block.
- Can be paid out if excess.
- Can be taken in advance (conditions apply).
- Beware impact on Registration and satisfying AHPRA requirements re minimum Term times.
- Will be paid out if ending employment.

ADO

Allocated day off. Yes, you get a day off. Legit.

How it works

ADOs are extremely confusing, with the end result being, most people think it's just an extra free day you get for every month of work.

Actually, it's not free. You have earned it. Remember how all your non-Medical friends work 9–5 and you for some reason start at 8.30 a.m.? But you get paid 76 hours, just like them.

What's happened is that you work an extra approximately half hour every working day that is unpaid. Until your ADO. Remember the 0.4–0.5 hours they dock in your 'Employment Pay Transactions'? That's for your ADO.

So, no, the government isn't robbing you. It is paid eventually. In an ADO. A day off where you get paid.

ADOs accrue approximately 0.4–0.5 hours each day you work, approximately 5% of the working hours. When it adds up to a full 8-hour day, you become entitled to a day off. Which is around once every 4 weeks, i.e. 20 working days × 0.4 hours/day.

To keep track of them, see section 'IT matters'.

There are many ways you can use that day. But we hope the following helps you actually take it in some form.

How to take it

The best way to take your ADO is either as per Medical Admin, i.e. a Rostered ADO, or via negotiation with the Team.

- **Principles**: First thing is, you're *entitled* to an ADO. It's granted to you by your Award. You're mandated to take them. As said, it's not a free gift, but something you've earned, your right and right of way. So you will take them, the question only being when. And if you do decide to give up your right, it's because you choose, and not others on your behalf.

  NSW Health supports and mandates you take your ADO as per Policy Document 2019_027 s4.1.9.[53] Also, as per the same section, if there are any untaken ADOs at the end of a District's rotation, they must be taken or paid out, the first three ADOs at normal rates, any after at Overtime rates as ADOs don't transfer between Districts (s4.1.9).[54]

- **Med Admin/Rostered**: This is a great way to take an ADO as it's third-party mandated so there are no awkward conversations. Several Hospitals already do this. If yours doesn't, you can discuss with your Med Admin. If you don't like the allocated day, unless Med Admin has organised formal cover for you on that day, they're usually amenable to adjusting it with the Team's concurrence.

- **Team negotiated**: Very Team dependent. Crazy Terms can't do without their JMOs. Chill Terms won't mind if you take a few extra. The main thing is to get a compromise. Choose a day of least inconvenience to your Team. No, least inconvenience doesn't mean not taking it (though that may be least inconvenient). But avoid days where your Team is Post take/On Call, where the patient load is much higher than usual, and when there are going to be many Discharges. Remember, so long as you and the Team agree, it's usually a settled matter.

- **Pre-ADO**: So the Team doesn't miss you too much, however close you all may be, try to pre-empt as many of the Jobs as you can before the ADO. Prep the Discharges, write scripts/Outpatient forms, order Bloods like it's a weekend, order the Jobs and give Handover if there's cover. Optimally, there's a covering JMO, but there isn't always. In short, do as much of tomorrow's Jobs as you can anticipate. You have around 10 weeks per Term. You may have up to three ADOs in that Term. If the first ADO wasn't a disaster, the second ADO will come much easier.

- **Post-ADO**: Not much to say except you may see a List explosion. Just remember to pick up the Jobs accrued from the day before and carry on with life.

- **As Annual Leave**: Sometimes, ADOs can be appended onto Annual Leave and you can take a longer holiday. Check with your Institution and always let Med Admin know your plans early.

- **Not taking**: For those who wish, you can opt not to take ADOs and have them paid out. This will be at Med Admin's discretion so discuss with them. Of course, with the reduced amount of leave, always beware exhaustion and burnout. Most of you are already working much more than the usual working population. You may well need that Leave.

- **Nights**: Note you are *not* to be Rostered an ADO the day a night shift finishes (PD 2019_27 s4.1.9).[55]

KEY POINTS

- Approximately 1 day off per month as you work an extra approximately 30 minutes every day.
- It is your entitlement.
- Take it via Rostered (via Admin) or Team negotiation.
- Do as many Jobs in advance as possible to assist Team so your ADO day goes smoothly.
- Aim to take on a relatively chill day.

Public holidays (s15)

Ideally, you'll have your public holidays off. That doesn't always happen. Luckily, however, those days, unlike your weekends, don't just disappear. You'll get them back, at some point. All you need to do is keep track of them, and perhaps the thought of working all through Christmas and New Year won't be so devastating when you think about the 5 weeks of Annual Leave you'll get instead.

Essentially, *whenever you should get a public holiday and you don't, you'll get more Annual Leave*, e.g.

- If you're working on a public holiday, you get an extra day of Annual Leave (s15(ii)).[56]

- If you're officially Rostered off on a public holiday, you get an extra day off (s15(iii)).[57] This is inclusive of public holidays falling on a weekend, an ADO, ED days off or pre-/post-nights days off.

- If you're on Annual Leave and there's a public holiday (especially consider Christmas/New Year period), you get an extra day Annual Leave for each one (s14(i)).[58]

Rate: You're paid 1.5× if working on public holidays (s15(ii)).[59]

Keep track and keep organised: Make a record of what public holidays you've worked to ensure you get your entitlements. Rosters are usually published only directly prior to the Term, so, once you know, that longer holiday may well be possible. Just keep organised and aware. Notify Med Admin early if you plan to thus use your public holiday credit.

Study Leave

Very needed as you begin to sit your numerous College exams. Hence, consider the following.

- Interns don't get Study Leave (s25 (i)).[60]

- You get *4 hours per week, for ≤27 weeks/year OR ½ hour study time for every hour of compulsory Lectures/Tutes.*

- The day job needs to be sorted before you study (obviously) (s25(iv)).[61]

- You can accumulate Study Leave *up to 7 days* for study before an exam (let Admin know at the beginning of the year) (s25(vi)).[62]
- Max Study Leave you can accumulate is *14 days* (s25 (vii)).[63]
- Courses eligible are essentially anything that will help you get into one of the Colleges, e.g. Uni degrees, diplomas, FRACP, FRACS, FRACGP (see definition of 'higher medical qualifications' in s1) (as per s25(ii)).[64] Ask with Med Admin. Most probably will be approved.
- As per Med Admin, but you may need to provide a timetable and evidence of you studying for said course (s25(iii)).[65]
- Please don't use Study Leave to get Overtime (s25(v)).[66]

Maternity/Adoption/Parental Leave (s17)

Another important topic, where we trace the Award as follows (see the original Award for precise details):

A. Maternity Leave.

(i) Eligibility: You need to have worked *40 weeks* first before giving birth.
     You don't need to work 40 weeks again for another eligibility *unless* you've stopped then started work again *or* have had LWOP (Leave Without Pay) (excluding Sick, Maternity, Worker's Compensation) for >40 weeks.

(ii) Portability: If you've worked in the government before, that time counts to the 40 weeks (conditions apply). You do need to start working with the Hospital though within 2 months of changing from the previous government job.

(iii) Entitlements: You get *14 weeks PAID leave*, starting *up to* 14 weeks before birth. You can get it paid as a *lump sum* or *normally* or as ½ pay for 28 weeks (and combine it with Annual Leave/Long Service Leave to get full pay). You don't have to take it, but, if you don't, you still need to be able to do your normal work.

(iv) Unpaid Leave: You get an *additional 1 year maximum* of *unpaid* leave after the baby's date of birth whether eligible for paid maternity leave or not.

(v) Applying: You need to let the Hospital know (*written*) *at least* 8 weeks prior (preferably ASAP). Bring a Medical Certificate indicating expected date of birth.

(vi) Changing Leave: As much as you like if the Hospital agrees after it starts. You get to change it *once* without agreement *but* with 2 weeks' notice.

(vii) Your Relief: Should know that they're only filling in, and you can come back when you like.

(viii) Leave accrual: Leave accrues as per: if you were on *full pay* Leave, then *normal* Leave accrual, if *half pay* gets *half* accrual. LWOP doesn't accumulate Leave.

(ix) Illnesses related to pregnancy: If this happens, you can use *any* type of Leave to be off work *or* Sick LWOP. At 9 weeks prior to birth, that other type of Leave stops and Maternity Leave begins.

(x) Changing jobs: If due to pregnancy-related illness/risks, you can't do your current job, your boss *must* find you another job (within possibility) as close to your current job as possible in pay and position.

(xi) Miscarriage: Sick Leave covers for this.

(xii) Stillbirth: Sick Leave (with Medical Certificate) or Maternity Leave can cover this. You can start work again when you like as long as you get another Medical Certificate saying you're ok.

(xiii) Premmie: Leave starts on the day you go to have the baby. If you come back to work early, Maternity Leave ceases.

(xiv) Right to return: You have a *right* to resume your old job. If that job doesn't exist, they must find you a job as close as possible in position and pay, and that you can do.

(xv) Pregnant again: If you become pregnant while on Maternity Leave (paid or not), you get another block of Maternity Leave. If you start it before you've finished your first lot, then the leftover from the first lot disappears.

B. Adoption Leave: Very similar to Maternity Leave, date of birth being now date of taking custody of the child. See s17B (pretty self-explanatory). Main difference is less notice time as rather unforeseeable when custody is granted.

C. Parental Leave: This is if your spouse/partner is pregnant/adopting. You get *up to* 52 weeks of Leave, 1 week paid at full or half rate (for 2 weeks). Eligibility conditions are essentially the same. You should give at least 4 weeks' notice. The 52 weeks is mainly if you're the *main* one looking after the child and hence usually can't be while your spouse/partner is taking Maternity/Adoption Leave. Again, you need Medical Certificates/Adoption papers.

D. Requests: You can request various other things, e.g. ≤8 weeks of simultaneous Maternity, Parental and Adoption Leave, extend unpaid Leave by another ≤1 year, come back to work as part-time till the child is school age. Then, you and the employer will just have to negotiate.

E. Communication: While you're off work, your boss should let you know about major changes, and you should let the boss know if there are any major changes with you.

Other Leave

These are not as often used. We have appended Award references as usual but it's best to discuss with your Med Admin regarding these.

FACS (Family and Community Services Leave) (s18A)

There are many circumstances for this, almost every 'life' stuff that happens, e.g. looking after sick/old relatives, parent–teacher interviews, funerals, community service, representing Australia/the State in sport competitions, dangerous weather conditions. See the Award s18A(i)(b) for details.

People who you often take FACS for include (s18A(i)(a)):[67]

- Relative = Person related by blood, marriage or 'affinity'.
- Affinity = Any of the in-law's family.
- Household = Family group living under the same roof,

You can get the greater of (s18A(iv)(a)):[68]

- **3 days FACS leave per year** on average (after first year, you can get 6 days in 2 years) (i.e. 24 hours per year for most of us).
- **1 day cumulative every year**, after working 2 years, minus FACS already taken since 1995.

NB: YOUR FACS IS BASED ON HOW LONG YOUR WORKING DAY IS, I.E. MOSTLY 8 HOURS PER DAY. THE RATE FACS IS PAID IS BASED ON THE RATE OF THE ROSTERED SHIFT, I.E. THE RATE OF THE ACTUAL HOURS YOU WERE AWAY (S18A(IV)(B)).[69]

You use FACS based on how many hours you were absent (s18A(iv)(b)).[69]

Deaths: You may also get an extra ≤2 days of FACS if all your FACS is used up for bereavement, e.g. due to death of a relative/household member (s18A(v)).[70]

If Admin agrees, you can also use this other Leave for FACS purposes (s18A(vi)).[71]

Personal Carer's Leave (s18B)

You can also use sick leave for this (s18B(ii),[72] (c)),[73] again likely needing a Medical Certificate/Statutory Declaration (you choose which) (s18B(ii)(e),[74] (f)).[75] See s18B(i) for who are the exact qualifying family members. Sometimes, Admin can approve extra Sick Leave from earlier than 3 years (s18B(ii)(d)).[76] You don't have to disclose what the illness is (s18B(ii)(g)).[77] Again, you need to tell Admin early (s18B(ii)(h)).[78]

You can also use *other Leave including Annual Leave (≤10 days), Long Service Leave and LWOP (see s18B(iii)).*

You can also use *Overtime* (performed within 1 year of so asking) to get extra Leave instead of being paid (if Admin agrees), i.e. you can get the same number of hours Leave as Overtime worked, one to one (see s18B(iv)(a),[79] (b)).[80] If you end up not taking it, you'll get paid as usual (see s18B(iv)(c),[81] (d)).[82]

You can also use *'make up' time,* i.e. work some other time and get time now off. Discuss with your Admin. The shift loading rates of those times off can still apply (see s18B(v)).[83]

Leave Without Pay

Sort of Leave, but since you don't get paid … . Main thing is to look out for it in your payslip. Per PD 2019_027 s4.1.11,[84] you're not supposed to have any LWOP *unless* you applied for it and had it approved. So watch that it doesn't appear unless you wanted it.

On Call (s12)

Get ready to go to work. But don't go. Yet.

Yes, we know the anxious feeling on a weekend at approximately 7–10 a.m. then at around 7–9 p.m. when you wonder if you'll be called in. And also the constant enquiries regarding the health of your colleagues who are on that week, with more than a little personal interest.

On Calls.

A period when you're literally waiting for the phone to ring, or, rather, for it not to ring. Well, it usually isn't so bad, and often more a matter for Regs and Consultants who may be called at any time to make decisions and/or to do something. As a JMO, it's mostly to cover another JMO who's sick. Mostly you shouldn't be called in. However, you should know the processes if you do.

- **Each On-Call period** (for pay) is 24 hours max (s12(ii)).[85]
- **Not called in**: For being On Call, you get approximately $16 if you were Rostered on (i.e. are working anyway that day) or approximately $33 if you were Rostered off. It's capped at approximately $116 per week (s12(iii),[86] Table 1 near the end of Award).
- **Called in**: You get the On-Call amount *plus* the relevant Overtime rate for a minimum of *4 hours* (s12(iv)).[87]
  - If you do whatever you need to do after being called in, and the Hospital/Seniors *formally* tell you to go home, you can go home, if it's 4 hours yet or not (s12(v)).[88] And if you unfortunately get called in again, that counts as another 4-hour period for you (s12(viii)).[89] However, make sure they have *formally* let you go, else if you're called in again, you won't be paid any extra until the 4 hours are up (s12(vii)).[90]
- **Phone/remote advice**: If you *don't* get called in, *but* give phone/remote advice/reports, you'll be paid *like* you were called in, for a minimum of *1 hour* (s12(ix)). You need to do a whole phone/email History, Exam, Investigations, Diagnosis, Management or provide a report on images (mainly for Radiologists) to be eligible (s12(xi) – *read yourself,* it's *long*). Main hinge point is *if* you didn't do the above, you would *have to* have come in (s12(xii)).[91] You also only get paid while you work, i.e. while you're remotely appraising the patient (s12(xii)).

IT MATTERS

Know this as well as eMR and you'll sort yourself out as well as the patients.

You need to know how to see your stuff. Which is not always shown you in detail, nor is there consistently much education on it. Hence, *you* need to figure it out, through asking, through friends, through Admin, through Google searches or never.

Do this early. You're working the whole time. It's useful to know you're getting paid for it. As the barest minimum, work out your Roster, payslips, HR stuff, email and mandatory education.

Email

Email is quite important for State Health blocks everything, even the Clinical Information Portals and MIMS sometimes (such sites can be used for potentially non-work-related purposes … ?), so if you need to send/receive anything, especially various forms, this is a very useful medium, especially if you're not carrying around a laptop and you need to interface with Hospital computers.

Plus, some people need to receive certain reports; surprisingly, not by fax, as in the Hospital world, but actually via email. So use this instead of stressing about life without Dropbox/Drive and normal email.

How to use (often, variable between States)

- Use State Health website – it has link to email.
- Your own email is generally [your full name]@[standard state health portal suffix]. Identify early in your State.
- The login is often the same across all the Systems. Call your State-wide Help Desk for issues.

Pay

We know you're all busy, but it's probably a good idea to check these fortnightly. Since you've taken the trouble to work (not that you had much choice), it's worth taking far less trouble to ensure you're paid right. It's true you have a choice here, but if you don't check, then that choice lies with chance and the IT gods.

Now, though the IT system is usually quite good, what with all the random Overtimes, ADOs and After Hours, etc. that you do, it's quite easy for things to get missed so do check yourself.

First rule of Medicine: Trust no one. Including about your pay.

Check early as, however great your memory, you won't remember all that has passed in the last 2 weeks. Sometimes not even what happened yesterday. Even ADOs fade into the ether, and you wonder if you took them or if you were at work… And as for the infinite number of After Hours shifts you did, well, they were all yesterday, right?

Moral of the story: keep a record.

How to use

- Google StaffLink or your HR/pay system.
- Login, i.e. common login.
- Go to Navigation Bar (top left ≡ sign).
- Find 'Payslip'
- It may also be emailed to you.

Pay is usually delayed a cycle, which is usually 2 weeks, i.e. you work and get paid approximately 2 weeks later.

Payslip

If you've never received a payslip before, it can be an exceedingly annoying document to read. There are many numbers, and the ones you care about seem invisible. Find a brief de-annoying agent below.

Summary of earnings this pay

- Weekly Base Rate = How much you're paid assuming smooth sailing, i.e. nil Overtime or days off.
- Total Gross Earnings = What you wish you had (grand total of income).
- Deductions Before Tax = Things you requested to be deducted off your pay. Pre-tax deductions include salary packaging, job-related expenses e.g. union fees.
- Taxable Income = Total gross earnings – deductions before tax.
- Deductions After Tax = Like deductions before tax, only after tax. Includes most other things that aren't tax deductible.
- Tax = Bane of existence.
- Nett = What appears in the account (= taxable income – deductions after tax – tax).
- HELP (Higher Education Loan Program) = HECS Higher Education Contribution Scheme) (will be 'Y' till you're 60).
- YTD = Year to date, a cumulative balance of whatever it's attached to, based on the financial year, i.e. July to next year's June; for example, gross income, taxable, tax, nett, super.
- Super = To keep you alive when old.
- Super This Pay = Super contribution this pay.
- Leave balances = Shows how much of each main type of Leave you have left, especially Annual Leave and Sick Leave.

Earnings and allowances

This you'll need to check: shows your Overtime, etc. Comes in table format. Headings include:

- Factor = Number of times your money is being multiplied by.
- Units = Usually hours, sometimes the number of units, e.g. number of On Calls.
- Rate = Your hourly pay rate usually, sometimes unit rate, e.g. rate per On Call.
- Amount = Rate × units × factor = Dollar amount for each item.

Hence, count the numbers of each item type. There'll be a separate item row for each type of work you do, including normal hours, Overtime (time and a half *and* double time), various penalty rates (e.g. After Hours, weekends and public holidays, *and* each grade of penalty, i.e. 12.5%, 25%, 50%, 75%), On Calls and Leave taken/accrued, e.g. ADOs/Sick Leave, etc. Also included here are any adjustments made to your pay if there were errors and their details.

Other payments

Self-explanatory if applicable.

Pre-tax and post-tax deductions

Details of the above. They'll tell you what's included, e.g. Admin fees and Employer Share of your salary packaging.

Disbursements

Where/which account they paid your money to and how much.

Leave/absences processed this pay

Shows what Leave you've taken during this period and when.

Online pay transactions

As the payslip shows grand totals of everything, and that sometimes may not tally with your totals, you need to find the details. These can be found at 'Online Pay Transactions' (under 'Payslip').

This, unfortunately, is much longer than the payslip itself. But you need to read it.

Why?

Disparities, disparities. There'll always be disparities. You need to keep a particular eye on disparities in Overtime (especially un-Rostered, which usually gets paid one or two pay cycles later), After Hours loading, Leave calculations, meal breaks, ADOs, etc. Pretty much everything out of 'normal hours' (which are sometimes so rare they're the abnormality).

Most of the time, the disparities exist because you're just bad at reading the payslip. So, this way, you can explain it to yourself. Or wait 2 hours for the HR helpdesk to explain it, who may end by asking you to chat to Med Admin.

However, sometimes there is an error, and that's some cool hundreds to thousands of dollars you may miss out on.

As our Union tells us, there are millions of dollars waiting to be recovered. Some of those millions may be yours. Well, you can wait for your money to get lost first and get the Union to recover it for you. Or you can just have those millions paid to you before they need recovering. That is, get the right pay, now.

The longer you wait, the more columns of numbers you'll need to look over till you give up through exhaustion. And that's your money given up also. So, to avoid, do it now to avoid future headaches and get money STAT. You've earned it. So get paid it.

How to read

Bad news. It's long (mentioned).

Good news. You don't need to read all of it.

Besides, the whole thing only looks super-confusing, but is only repetitive.

The columns include:

- **Description**: Type of transaction e.g. normal hours, Overtime, penalty rates, various Leave.
- **Date**: Chief guide. Go on day-by-day basis.
- **Time in/time out**: Start and finish Rostered times.
- **Factor**: Multiplication rate.
- **Rate**: Your pay rate per hours.
- **Units**: Number of hours or units, e.g. On Calls.
- **Amount**: Dollar value.

The two main things to follow are Date and Units:

1. **Dates**: Look at only the transactions in one day, make sure it's right, then move to the next day. Only 10 business days in a fortnight + Overtime days worked (max 14).
2. **Units**: Make sure the correct number of units under each item is entered. You should know, just correlate.

FAQs

- **What is the −0.4?**
  - The extra 0.4 hours you work to generate your ADO. You're not paid it until you take the ADO.
- **Why is it 8 hours? We work 8.5 hours?**
  - 0.5 hours taken off for meal break. Shouldn't be taken if non-ordinary hours.
- **How are penalty rates calculated?**
  - As a separate percentage, e.g. 12.5% of ... normal hours are already included directly above. An additional item and amount is simply added for the penalty rates.

- **What does the 'Adj' mean?**
  - There's been some change since lodging your original timesheet. Usually due to UROT or some error. Check if it's right. The date is often the event's date and is a good guide.
- **Why is UROT not paid?**
  - Check back one or two pay cycles later. It'll usually appear at the top of the pay transactions for the cycle it's paid, as it'll be back dated to the date you worked it. Just look at the date you worked it and add everything up. If it adds up, it's right. You don't have to worry about all the numbers.
- **Why is there a '+8 units' then '–8 units' when there are adjustments (and general complexity)?**
  - Not really relevant to you. The extra columns are merely an Admin thing where they need to recreate you working on that day to create the transaction, then delete it, as they've paid you already for that day (the normal hours). It's for self-cancelling purposes. But if they don't create it, they can't add on Overtime transactions. For you, ignore the numerous recreated +8, –8, +0.4, –0.4 hours and just check the Overtime is right. Also, make sure there are the same number of +/–8 or 0.4 to prevent over-/underpayment. There may be a stack of these at the bottom of your pay transactions just cancelling each other out.
- **My ROT is not paid right.**
  - Not likely unless you've made some swaps/takes. If so, notify Admin. Usually, you'll see it paid in the 1.5× and 2× tranches. Add up the units and it should make up your total Overtime performed. There'll usually be the 2 units of 1.5× (first 2 hours at 1.5×) and the remaining as 2×. This time, there won't be a separate entry for 'normal hours' as in penalty rates, but all as one as it's not 'normal hours'.

Everything else is quite self-explanatory, e.g. Leave and ADOs. Just check the amounts are correct, i.e. units mainly.

After all this, tally the total hours/units and these should add up to the number of units of each type of Overtime or other non-normal hours you've worked in your main payslip. If the units are right, then the dollar amount generally will be.

This sounds long. Trust me, it's shorter to do than explain.

Issues

If there's an issue, do the following:

- **Contact State-wide Helpdesk/Payroll:** They can clarify any questions you have. It may just be an Admin matter or an incorrect entry or an explanation you need. They can view all that's been lodged and explain it to you. However, if there's an error, often they can't change it, unless it's at their end.

- **Contact your Med Admin/JMO manager**: They can amend any errors or explain disparities. Remember to bring any supporting documentation, e.g. relevant payslips, Rosters, correspondence with State-wide Help Desk, Overtime forms.
- **Document**: Email them as you discuss the matter, confirming what has happened/been done, especially once you have a resolution confirming the details and, that way, you'll make sure everything is properly documented to prevent confusion. It's not just patient notes that need documenting.

KEY POINTS

- Important to confirm you're getting the right pay – errors have and do occur – costing you thousands.
- Know how to read your payslip: See component key terms in section 'Payslip'.
- Know how the payslip is compiled, i.e. via the summation of pay transactions, and how to read each transaction.
- Amount = pay rate × units (e.g. hours) × factor (multiplication rate).
- Contact State-wide Payroll or Med Admin if issues and document process/solutions.

Leave

Another important part of your Admin is Leave accruals. Here you can see all your cumulated ADOs and other leave balances. Make sure you're receiving the correct entitlement.

The names are self-explanatory. Go to StaffLink→Navigation Bar ≡→Leave Accruals. They're in hours or days so, when you've used them, check the right amount was deducted, e.g. a Sick Leave on a normal day will be 8 hours deducted.

Remember to check each Leave type, especially when you've accrued or used them, probably a cycle or two after the event. Especially useful if you're adding public holiday credit or extra leave due to working Sundays to your Annual Leave.

Mandatory training

Get the perfect green pie.

You're going into the workplace and there's obviously a stack of new rules. Rather than tell you face to face, online modules are often used to convey this needed though not-exactly-thrilling information. There's often good education within them so pay attention.

Find these early and know which ones are mandatory. Login usually via Google search/Intranet search of your learning portal, e.g. 'My Health Learning' in NSW Health.

Just slug through them else your Med Admin/Director of Training will be onto you. Something legit to do on chill Terms. Some places may even allocate times for you to do them, e.g. half a day off. Check with your Institution.

There's also practical training, e.g. CPR or fire safety, so make sure you find time to attend these, particularly during non-crazy rotations.

FINANCIAL MATTERS

You'll manage money based on your own habits and goals and we won't dictate. But, in addition to the salary you get, there are also a few extra financial matters you should be aware of, specific to the workplace.

Salary packaging (s31)

To package or not to package? Package. Generally.

We leave this to the packaging experts but usually this is a good idea.

Take note, we aren't offering financial advice in any way. Please refer to your financial advisor for personalised advice. Usually your parents/finance-savvy friend/fiancé/spouse/family or no one.

Policy

Please refer to the salary packaging policy document regarding this. It's long, but the PDF is searchable and clickable, just go to the section you want. Also, most of it is examples (many not relevant to you). Use on PRN basis.

The Contents is *very good* and is very fine in splitting the expenses. Just check what's relevant to you.

The chief benefit (s2.2 PD2018_044) is allowing you to spend approximately $9000 pre-tax generally and an additional approximately $2600 on meals and entertainment. See below for details.

Catches

- **Fees**: Variable and may be hefty. Each packager is different. Some packagers charge just one fee for the year, some charge that and extra fees for every packaging contribution you make. You'll need to figure out if it's worth your while.

- **Tax savings split**: You don't get all the tax savings. Rather, it'll be split with the Hospital. An incentive we guess for the Hospital to support the programme. Hence, in the example above, your expected tax saving of $300 is split so you may get approximately $150. Check with your Hospital how much they take.

- **Direct deduction**: You don't see your tax-savings directly. What you'll see is Payroll taking the amount directly. You may package $1000, and your Payslip will show a deduction of $1200. The $200 is the Hospital's share. Hence, as the Hospital's share is directly deducted from your pay or gross income, you can't really claim it back with tax deductions like you can tax.

- **Tax deductions**: Don't package otherwise tax-deductible expenses, e.g. Registration fees. You can only deduct *once* and it's better against tax than in salary packaging (the tax benefit is not split). Besides, you're not allowed (PD 2018_044 s4.1).

- **FBT (fringe benefits tax)**: Though packaging appears to reduce your taxable income, it counts as a fringe benefit, i.e. full salary packaging attracts a fringe benefit of approximately $17 000 (subject to yearly change). This can have implications for anything involving FBT, e.g. if you're getting other fringe benefits *or* HECS repayment rate *or* Medicare Levy Surcharge (MLS). The last two take into account both taxable income *and* fringe benefits when calculating how much to charge so be aware where your income (with the addition of the fringe benefit of salary packaging) sits relative to the MLS/HECS payment tiers/grades.

Thus, very generally, how worthwhile salary packaging is depends on your total taxable income, i.e. gross income less deductions:

- **At taxable income > approximately $29 000 = Generally worthwhile** as the tax-free income is approximately $20 000 (including low-income tax offset, check your own eligibility/when the scheme ends) and the approximately $9000 is the full tax benefit of salary packaging. You can add approximately $2500 to this if you intend to use the 'meal and entertainment' benefit that year.

- **At approximately $20 000 < taxable income < approximately $29 000 = Possibly worthwhile**. You'll need to do the maths, e.g. fees versus tax benefits.

- **At taxable income < approximately $20 000 = Unlikely worthwhile**. Since you won't be paying any tax anyway, not much point to split 'tax benefits' with the Hospital (which you may or may not be able to get back) and paying fees to minimise no tax.

> **NB**: ABOVE OF COURSE IS GENERAL ADVICE. FIGURE OUT THE DETAILS FOR YOUR OWN CIRCUMSTANCES.

However, considering the Medical Officer starting income, unless you have vast tax deductions, it's likely worthwhile.

NB FOR INTERNS: FOR EVERYONE BEYOND, YOU'LL BE PAID MORE AND MORE, SO YOU'LL ALMOST CERTAINLY HAVE INCOME >$29 000 (UNLESS YOU'VE TAKEN SOME TIME OFF WORK OR ARE VERY PART TIME). HOWEVER, FOR STARTING INTERNS, THIS IS MORE A CONSIDERATION. YOU'RE MORE LIKELY TO FALL INTO THE ZONE OF UNCLEAR BENEFIT IN THE FIRST SALARY PACKAGING YEAR, I.E. THE YEAR YOU ENTER INTERNSHIP UP TO 31 MARCH MAY OR MAY NOT BE WORTHWHILE. NOTE YOU'LL NEED TO CALCULATE ALL YOUR TAXES IN THE YEAR PRIOR, I.E. 31 JULY OF THE YEAR BEFORE WORKING. SOME OF YOU ARE WORKING IN MED SCHOOL AND INCOME THEN IS APPLICABLE. ALSO, SEVERAL GOVERNMENT BENEFITS ARE ALSO TAXABLE. SO DO SOME SERIOUS CALCULATIONS OR GET FORMAL TAX ADVICE TO SEE IF THE PACKAGING IS WORTHWHILE.

History

This whole thing was created when it appears the government wanted to give HCWs (Healthcare Workers) a pay rise but didn't want to give them actual money. So, instead, they gave them a tax break, and allowed them to pay less tax, by paying their own private expenses as pre-tax dollars, effectively extending a pseudo-deduction, with various provisos.

How it works

1. **Set up**: With your salary packaging representatives who'll go through the Admin stuff with you and how to lodge claims, etc.

2. **Mechanisms of benefitting**:

   a. **Paying expenses direct**: You decide what expenses you want to pay, e.g. rent, and direct your packaging people to pay it directly to your people, from your salary. There'll be Admin, but follow their instructions to set up. You've paid them hence with pre-tax money.

   b. **Package credit**: You decide how much salary you want to package. This amount will then be taken *out* of your pay. For example, if it was $2000 before gross, and you package $500, then you'll only have $1500, which will then be taxed, instead of $2000. $500 (less the Hospital's share) will now sit with the packaging people, ready to give you dollar for dollar when you lodge expenses. It's pre-tax money ready to spend.

   c. **Credit card**: Some packaging people offer a 'credit card' that you can put money into. It works like a debit card +/– with credit card options. You can now spend your money as if it were a debit card, but all pre-tax. The 'meal and entertainment card' works similarly, only they may restrict the retailers you can use it to outlets that provide meals and entertainment.

3. **Lodge expenses**: If you have package credit, you now submit your expenses, e.g. utilities, credit card, to the salary packaging people. They'll look at it, and if it's a valid expense (99% will be), they'll give you your money by direct bank transfer or other method you choose. For example, if you have a $900 credit card bill, and you have paid it, they'll give you $900 in hand *or* if you don't have that much salary packaged, say only $500, they give you $500.

4. **Keep lodging expenses and packaging**: When you have lodged more expenses than you have packaged, the extra will just sit there. For example, from above, the $400 of extra expenses will sit there until you package more salary. Once you package more salary, they'll pay out as much of the expenses as possible. Similarly, if you have packaged too much and there are no expenses, then your packaged money will sit there until you lodge expenses. Then they'll pay you however many expenses you lodge, till you have no package credit left.

5. **Aim expenses >> package credit**: Generally a good idea as, that way, the *full* amount you package, will always be paid directly to you, and not sit with the package people. It's your salary after all. Note that we aren't advocating reckless spending. Spend responsibly. Not to make up your packaging credit.

6. **Tax savings achieved**: You have now paid your expenses with pre-tax dollars, instead of post-tax dollars as either you've directly paid them (the salary packaging people doing it for you) or paid it yourself with after-tax dollars, then received back pre-tax dollars.

Packages

Three main packaging packages you can benefit from:

1. **Salary packaging**: Approximately $9000 or so to spend pre-tax, which is effectively spent on almost anything you like. See the salary packaging policy document for exactly what but includes almost everything, such as rent, utilities, credit card expenses.

2. **Meal and entertainment**: Approximately $2500 you can spend on 'sit down/ social gathering' meals/entertainment and especially functions like weddings. See the salary packaging policy document for details.

3. **Novated leasing for your car**: Beyond the scope of this work. The idea is similar, but there are much more complex fee structures (you need to pay interest), and different benefits (you can package petrol, but you could also if you paid on your credit card). As it's much more complex and everyone's circumstances are different, we'll leave it to the experts. Read the policy document.

Carrying forward: A very handy thing when you have many expenses that you can't exhaust in 1 year. As the expenses keep rolling forward, they can be used against next year's salary packaging cap. That is, if your wedding costs $25 000, you can collect the salary packaging benefit of $2500 for 10 years to come, even if you never eat out ever again. And, if you do, you just keep adding to your expenses.

Hence, unlike tax expenses, which mostly expire in that year, salary packaging expenses keep carrying forward indefinitely, though, for the precise time, please check with the packagers.

Actual dollar benefits

Difficult to calculate generally. The tax savings will roughly be your marginal tax rate for the extent you package up to approximately $9000. In other words, you pay around 50% less tax on the final or highest $9000 of your income (the other 50% going to the Hospital). If this final $9000 straddles tax brackets, then each tax rate is applied. Hence, if your marginal tax rate (or the highest tax bracket or tax rate applicable to you) is 32.5%, and you package $9000, total tax savings is approximately $2900, and you get approximately $1400.

If your marginal tax rate is higher, then your savings will be greater. However, consider fees, etc.

Admin details

- **Enquire**: You'll probably only have one packager so call them and have them run through things with you. Of course, they are salespeople too so you'll need to do your own calculations to make sure it's worthwhile.

- **JMOs**: If you intend to package, start early, e.g. during Orientation or as soon as you have your employee number. Main reason is you're least busy then. Also, you can thus get the salary packaging benefits for the first FBT year, i.e. up to 31 March of the year you start Internship. For example, if you start Internship 2020, by packaging early, e.g. in January 2020, you can potentially enjoy the FBT tax savings for the FBT year 2019/2020 and then 2020/2021 (notify the packagers early). Of course, confirm with them how much they let you package (potentially the full $9000) and check how much you'll be earning before 31 March (may well be >$9000, especially if you do Overtime).

- **Website**: Most of the daily things are done online/via an app, e.g. lodging expenses. Be familiar with it, their websites are usually quite accessible, and you can just scan and upload your expenses or have them paid automatically for you. Just follow their instructions. If you have trouble, call them and let the rep guide you through. You should be checking your packaging credit balances and expenses you've uploaded.

- **Receipts**: Keep all of them. Easier if you pay all by credit card as this hence captures most of your payments. As for other things you want to package, but don't want to direct debit, you'll need to file these and submit online. A useful practice is to have a file/folder/box for each year and put all tax-related receipts into it. You can throw them out after approximately 7 years (check tax laws). That way, you'll be resistant to auditing.

- **The Award**: Mentions some things about packaging but not too many details except you get FBT exempt for $17000 grossed up. Also, you don't have to package, only if you want to. Best to read the salary packaging policy document/tax laws/financial experts.

KEY POINTS

- Main idea is to pay your usual expenses directly with pre-tax, rather than after-tax, dollars, i.e. some tax goes to paying your personal expenses = tax savings.
- Main catches:
  - o FBT impacts (especially on MLS and HECS repayments).
  - o Fees charged by packagers.
  - o Hospital also takes portion of savings.
- Types:
  - o Salary packaging (approximately $9000 available to package).
  - o Meals and entertainment (approximately $2500 available).
  - o Novated car leasing (complex).
- Mechanism:
  - o Pay expenses, e.g. rent directly via packager.
  - o Get reimbursed in money by packager for expenses paid.
  - o Use packager's credit card function and spend pre-tax dollars like a debit/credit card.
- Keep lodging expenses aiming for expenses >> packaged amount so all savings are crystallised.
- Many items can be packaged: See policy document or discuss with packager.
- Package early (if intending to), keep receipts and speak to your packaging expert regarding your circumstances.

Taxes

Immensely complex subject. That's why there are whole degrees on them. Also, everyone's circumstances again are different so consider this very general.

However, for those who haven't had to fill out a tax return (not, at least, one with much in it) and wish to do so without the tax agent, consider the following basic pointers:

- **The ATO website**: Has very good (and the most legit) information and hyperlinks to anything you don't quite understand. Many tax returns are done entirely online. Just follow guidelines.

- **Income**: Quite straightforward usually (see corresponding thinness of legislation compared with deductions). Money = Income. Just check it's correct against your payslips.

- **Deductions**: Where most of the work will be. Subject to the tax laws/guidelines, really many things work related are considered a deduction so you can use it to reduce your income and hence pay less tax. See the tax deductions section on ATO for precise details but many of your new expenses are tax deductible. Consider AHPRA fees, union fees, application fees, courses you do, scrubs, steths, registration checks, telco expenses (if you use your phone/data to work) etc. The best way is simply collect the receipts of all your expenses you think are work related and then cross-match them against the various categories. Try to be familiar with those categories beforehand.

> NB: MANY ORGANISATIONS THAT WANT YOU TO SPEND MONEY WILL DECLARE THE TAX DEDUCTIBLE-NESS OF THEIR STUFF. THIS IS GOOD AND REMINDS YOU. HOWEVER, TAX DEDUCTIBILITY DOESN'T MEAN FREE. YOU'RE SIMPLY GETTING A 'DISCOUNT' ON WHATEVER YOU'RE BUYING. THAT IS, IF YOU WERE GOING TO SPEND ON SAID THING IRRESPECTIVE IF TAX DEDUCTIBLE OR NOT, THEN BEING TAX DEDUCTIBLE IS ALWAYS A GOOD DEAL. *BUT* IF SPENDING OR NOT DEPENDS ON TAX DEDUCTIBILITY, WELL, CONSIDER THE AFTER-TAX DEDUCTED PRICE. IF YOU WOULDN'T SPEND EVEN THE AFTER-TAX AMOUNT, THEN NO. FOR EXAMPLE, IF A COURSE IS $100 AND THE MARGINAL TAX RATE IS 30%, AFTER TAX THE COURSE IS STILL $70. IF YOU WOULDN'T PAY $70 FOR IT, DON'T GO. THE $30 DOLLAR SAVING IS ONE, ONLY IF YOU WOULD'VE GONE EVEN IF IT WAS $100.

- **Beyond**: Tax goes far beyond the above. The main idea is to keep records and know what deduction categories there are. However, more complex matters are beyond the scope of this work.

If you have complex tax matters, you're either versed yourself or have someone to do them for you. If neither, consider getting a good tax agent. There are sometimes good tax people specifically for Doctors so use them PRN.

KEY POINTS

- Use ATO website for the most reliable information.
- Income = Money coming in from all sources.
- Deduction = Money spent to earn money, e.g. all those new expenses for being a Doctor.
- Tax deductible is only worthwhile if the after-tax deducted price is still acceptable to you *or* you would've spent the money thus anyway.
- Get a tax consultant if you have complex matters or don't want to manage all this tax stuff.

Superannuation

Look after it now. It'll look after you when you're old.

There are usually two options. You either have your own fund or the Hospital gives you one. You can also self-manage, but those people don't need to read this.

Also a very personal matter, subject to everyone's circumstances.

However, you should at least know it exists and seek your own financial advice for your financial goals.

If you're happy with your super fund, there's no reason to use another one. Why pay two sets of fees?

If you don't have one, you can give the Hospital one a go. Give them a call early to make sure all your details are correct and make sure the super's investment setting is what you'd like.

Read the statements when they come. Read especially the returns and the fees. See if you're happy. Shop around. You may not care now. But the >70-year-old you will care very much. Sort these things out early. Your future self will thank you infinitely.

And if you're too confused about it all, get a financial planner/adviser/person (fees may apply).

OTHER AREAS OF INTEREST

It is slightly possible that, after reading the above, you have become inspired to read more of the Award yourself. Though that is probably wishful thinking, we still append below some other areas of interest, to some, at some point. They're quite self-explanatory, so have a look if you're affected.

The best way to use the Award is as a reference guide. When certain areas affect you, look it up. If it doesn't, well, it isn't the most thrilling read.

- **S3 – Payment of salaries**: How you're paid. Mainly fortnightly and there's a specific process if you're under- or overpaid. Refer to this if you're having issues. Generally, underpayment will be fixed in 3 working days, Overpayment will be recovered as a one-off lump sum next pay or at 10% of gross pay if a lump sum deduction would cause hardships/difficulties.
- **S4 – Qualification allowance**: If you get a qualification meeting the 'higher medical qualification' definition, you'll get this (approximately $60/week).
- **S5 – In charge allowance**: Probably not while you're junior, but, higher up, you get this if you're 'in charge' during After Hours for every period ≤12 hours, i.e. approximately $20.
- **S7 – Part-time employees**: Your main section is Section 7. Most of it's the same as everyone else, only proportionally less depending on how part time you work.

– **Casual employees**: Has own set of rules governing Leave, e.g. Maternity set and s18C. Refer as needed or just search the doc for 'casual'. There aren't that many hits.

- **S13 – Higher duties allowance**, i.e. informal promotions: More applicable the more senior you become. Sometimes, when your Reg is on leave, you may 'become' the Reg. If you truly do so for >5 days straight, do a good job and assume the Reg responsibilities, you're entitled to the Reg-level pay (s13).[92]

- **S17A – Lactation breaks**: Self-explanatory. You're entitled to these if relevant.

- **S18A – Family violence Leave**: There are provisions here for these circumstances if you're unfortunately affected by them.

- **S19 – Long service Leave**: Not applicable until after 7–10 years' service, by which time you'll be experts in everything already. But read early if you wish.

- **S20 – Board and accommodation**: Applicable if you live/are given meals at the Hospital and how your pay will be deducted. Mainly you'll pay according to standards if you live/eat at the Hospital.

- **S21 – Uniform and laundry allowance**: If you have to wear a uniform. Mainly you should either be given one or get around $2.50 a week to buy one.

- **S22 – Getting fired**: Mainly that you should get 4 weeks' notice or pay if less notice. But not if you stuffed up.

- **S23 – Dispute settlement**: If you and State Health don't agree. Tells you how to escalate. Mainly speak with Med Admin first, then it goes way up, e.g. CEOs and union secretaries. Hope it doesn't come to that but it's there if you need it.

- **S24 – Anti-discrimination**: Pretty obvious. But if you feel you've experienced it, there are provisions here to protect your rights.

- **S26 – Travelling allowance**: If you're seconded to another Hospital or have to go somewhere other than your normal Hospital, e.g. for Clinics, other Hospitals ('official business'), you should get money back for the extra travel, whether petrol costs or public transport costs. Doesn't include call-backs. It does refer to other legislation about the exact amount but makes precise references so Google it. Or ask Med Admin.

- **S27 – Mobility, excess fares and travelling**: If you have to travel away from your usual place of work to work. There are reimbursements or you can travel during the actual work hours, especially the extra time needed to get there, greater than your usual time. The excess will be paid for or used as working hours. If they decide you must work somewhere else now, they should let you know and discuss with you. However, a Reliever is not reimbursed unless it's more than $5 extra.

- **S28 – Secondment**: If you're seconded to a rural Hospital (listed in Table C at the end of the Award), you're entitled to more pay (not if you're an Intern) and travel allowance (you get an economy class return trip every 7 weeks).

- **S29 – Relocation**: If you're relocating, you get some of your expenses back.

- **S33 – Salary sacrifice to superannuation**: Option available. You can sacrifice 100% if you like. If you're considering this, it's imagined you're already quite financially savvy and don't need our advice. The Award has some useful clauses so peruse according to your circumstances.

Policy Directive 2019_027 'Employment Arrangements for Medical Officers in the NSW Public Health Service' (or its more updated versions) also has some useful other information and back-up for what's in your Award.

Read its Contents to pick what you're interested in. This may include:

- **S5 – Overseas MOs.**
- **S6 – Rotations to Country Locations.**
- **S7 – Rotations outside NSW Health.**

Again, very variable considering everyone's individual circumstances but these are guides to begin with.

ACKNOWLEDGEMENT

We acknowledge NSW Health as the author of any references to and/or quotations of the NSW Health Award: PUBLIC HOSPITAL MEDICAL OFFICERS (STATE) AWARD 2021 and Policy Directive 2019_027 'Employment Arrangements for Medical Officers in the NSW Public Health Service' © State of New South Wales NSW Ministry of Health.

NOTES

1. The ordinary hours of work shall not exceed an average of 38 hours per week. This shall be achieved by rostering officers for duty over either forty hours in any period of seven consecutive days or eighty hours in any period of fourteen consecutive days and, in addition, then granting officers roster leave additional to that prescribed in subclause (ii) of this clause to the extent of one additional day per calendar month.

2. Officers shall be free from ordinary hours of duty for not less than two days in each week or, where this is not practicable, four days in each fortnight. Where practicable, days off shall be consecutive and where possible additional rostered days off shall be combined with other rostered time off.

3. No shift shall be less than four hours in length.

4. No broken or split shifts shall be worked.

5. Maximum rostered hours.
   Employees must not be rostered for shift periods totalling more than 14 consecutive hours (inclusive of meal breaks and handover).
   Break after rostered shift periods.
   Rosters must be arranged so that there's a break after rostered shift periods of at least 10 hours.

6. Time worked means the time during which an officer is required by the employer to be in attendance at a Hospital for the purpose of carrying out such functions as the employer may call on him to perform, and it shall include times when the officer, in waiting to carry out some active function, is studying or resting or sleeping or engaged in any other activity.

7. Provided that time worked doesn't include breaks allowed and actually taken for meals.

8. Provided further that where an officer attends of his/her own volition outside of hours rostered on duty, or where an officer remains in attendance when formally released from the obligation to perform professional duties, the employer shall not be liable to make any payment for such attendance.

9. Officers shall be given at least two weeks' notice of rosters to be worked in relation to ordinary hours of work and also, where practicable, in relation to additional (overtime) rostered hours of work, provided that the employer may change the rosters without notice to meet any emergent situation.

10. There shall be a uniform meal break of 30 minutes except where locally agreed arrangements for a longer period are made (which shall not exceed one hour).

11. If officers are required to work during their meal break they shall be paid for the time worked.

12. In the interests of patient care and the health and welfare of medical staff, officers must have a break from duty for the purpose of taking a meal.

13. As per s2.2(ii) Page 2: Shifts Other Than Day Shifts Monday to Friday:
   Because of the widespread difficulty involved in officers leaving Hospital premises for any purpose (including the taking of meal breaks) during 'Out of hours shifts', it has been decided that except where agreement is reached between a Hospital and the Association in respect to arrangements for the taking of meals breaks (in which case the time involved shall not count as time worked), henceforth in all shifts other than Monday to Friday days shifts, all time an officer is required to be in attendance shall be regarded as working time and paid for accordingly. Payment for the whole of the elapsed time between the starting and finishing times of the shifts will be made irrespective of whether the work is overtime or forms part of the officer's ordinary hours.

14. Officers who are required to work on Sundays and/or public holidays during a qualifying period of employment for annual leave purposes shall be entitled to receive additional annual leave in respect of each complete period of eight hours so worked as follows:

15. [I]f less than 35 such periods on such days have been worked – leave proportionately calculated on the basis of 38 hours leave for 35 such periods worked[.]

16. The calculations referred to in paragraphs (a) and (b) of this subclause shall be made to the nearest one-fifth of the ordinary hours worked, half or more than half of one-fifth being regarded as one-fifth and less than half being disregarded.

17. [I]f 35 or more such periods on such days have been worked – one week[.]

18. [W]ork performed by reason of call backs pursuant to clause 12, On Call and Call Back, of this Award shall be disregarded when assessing an officer's entitlement under the subclause.

19. An officer with accrued additional annual leave pursuant to this subclause can elect at any time to be paid an amount equivalent to the value of accrued additional annual leave in lieu of taking additional leave, provided that the amount is a minimum of one week's accrued additional leave and that the salary for the period of additional leave paid out will be calculated as if the period of leave was actually taken.

[20] All time worked in excess of ten hours in any one shift shall be paid as overtime.

[21] All time worked by officers in excess of the ordinary hours specified in clause 6, Hours of Work, of this Award, shall be paid at the rate of time and one-half for the first two hours, and double time thereafter provided that all overtime performed on a Sunday, shall be at double time.

[22] An officer who works authorised overtime and was not notified on or prior to his/her previous shift of the requirement to work such overtime shall be paid in addition to payment for such overtime:
(a) as set out in Item 2 of Table 1, Allowances, for breakfast when commencing such overtime work at or before 6.00 a.m.;
(b) as set out in Item 2 of Table 1, Allowances, for an evening meal when such overtime is worked for at least one hour immediately following his/her normal ceasing time, exclusive of any meal break and extends beyond or is worked wholly after 7.00 p.m.;
(c) as set out in Item 2 of Table 1, Allowances, for luncheon when such overtime extends beyond 2.00 p.m. on Saturdays, Sundays or holidays;
or shall be provided with adequate meals in lieu of such payments.

[23] In the event that a medical officer is treating a critically ill patient or a patient's condition has changed dramatically at the completion of a shift, they may undertake unrostered overtime until adequate medical attention can be arranged.

[24] In the event that a medical officer is treating a patient who requires transfer, they may undertake unrostered overtime until the transfer process is complete.

[25] In the event that a medical officer is already working in theatre and the procedure continues past the scheduled end of shift, they may undertake Unrostered overtime until their responsibilities conclude.

[26] In the event that a medical officer is responsible for the admission and/or Discharge of a patient at the completion of a shift, they may undertake Unrostered overtime until their responsibilities conclude.

[27] Patient transfer/discharge summaries should be provided to the patient on transfer/discharge. In the event that a medical officer is unable to complete this documentation during their normal rostered hours, or the task is unable to be handed over to another medical officer to finish, they may undertake unrostered overtime until this work is complete.

[28] Visiting Medical Officers/Staff Specialists are expected to undertake ward rounds within the medical officer's normal working hours. Where ward rounds are regularly held before or after the medical officer's rostered shifts or at weekends (i.e. it is known in advance that a medical officer will be required to attend those times), then the roster must be updated to allocate these hours as normal hours or rostered overtime.

[29] In the event that a medical officer is requested by a superior to attend a late ward round outside of their rostered shift, they may undertake unrostered overtime until their ward round responsibilities conclude. Or where it is feasible for this work to be handed over to another medical officer to complete.

[30] In the event that a ward round occurs during a medical officer's rostered shift but they have ongoing ward round responsibilities that extend beyond the length of their rostered shift, they may undertake unrostered overtime until their ward round responsibilities conclude or where it is feasible for this work to be handed over to another medical officer to complete.

[31] Mandatory training should be completed in rostered hours. In circumstances where a medical officer is required and directed by their employer to complete mandatory training outside of their rostered hours, they may undertake unrostered overtime.

[32] Clinical handover should occur during the medical officer's normal rostered hours. Where designated clinical handover cannot be undertaken within rostered hours, a medical officer is permitted to undertake unrostered overtime until clinical handover is complete.

[33] When a medical officer is assigned to work in a hospital-based outpatient clinic and the clinic extends beyond their rostered hours, the medical officer may undertake unrostered overtime until they have completed their clinic duties.

[34] • The approver must be accessible to the medical officer when the request to work unrostered overtime is made.
• The approver should have a knowledge of the work undertaken by the medical officer so as to be able to determine the unrostered overtime requirement.
• The approver should be in a position to reallocate.

[35] The NSW Health Agency should process, where practicable, unrostered overtime claims in the next pay cycle after the medical officer submitted the claim.

[36] An officer shall be allowed sick leave on full pay calculated by allowing 76 'ordinary' hours per year for each year of continuous service less any sick leave on full pay already taken (conditions apply).

[37] Sick leave as defined, shall accrue and be transferable between Hospitals, at the rate of 76 hours per year of continuous service, minus hours taken.

[38] [E]ach officer shall take all reasonably practicable steps to inform the employer of his or her inability to attend for duty and as far as possible state the estimated duration of the absence. Where practicable such notice shall be given within twenty-four hours of the commencement of such absence[.]

[39] [A]n officer shall not be entitled to sick leave until the expiration of three months' continuous service[.]

[40] [A]n officer is not entitled to more than 8 hours' sick leave in respect of any one day.

[41] [A]n officer is not eligible for sick leave during periods when he would have normally been rostered on overtime shifts[.]

[42] [T]he employer may require the sickness to be certified to by the medical superintendent or by a legally qualified medical practitioner approved by the employer, or may require other satisfactory evidence thereof[.]

[43] [A]n officer shall not be entitled to sick leave on full pay for any period in respect of which such officer is entitled to accident pay or workers' compensation; provided, however, that where an officer is not in receipt of accident pay an employer shall pay to an officer who has sick leave entitlements under this clause, the difference between the amount received as workers' compensation and full pay. The officer's sick leave entitlements under this clause shall, for each week during which such difference is paid, be reduced by that proportion of hours which the difference paid bears to full pay. On the expiration of available sick leave, weekly compensation payments only shall be payable[.]

[44] All officers shall be allowed four calendar weeks leave of absence on full pay in respect of each twelve months' service plus one day on full pay in respect of each public holiday occurring within the period of such leave.

[45] The employer shall pay each officer before entering upon annual leave his or her ordinary rate of salary for the period of leave. For the purposes of this subclause 'ordinary rate of salary' means the Award rate of salary and qualification allowance if applicable.

[46] Annual leave shall be given and shall be taken within a period of six months after the date when the right to annual leave accrued; provided that the giving and taking of the whole or any separate period of such annual leave may, by mutual agreement between the employer and the officer, be postponed for a further period not exceeding six months.

[47] Except as provided by this clause, payment shall not be made by the employer to an officer in lieu of any annual leave or part thereof nor shall any such payment be accepted by the officer.

[48] Annual leave shall be given and shall be taken in one consecutive period, or, if the officer and the employer so agree, in either two or three separate periods, but not otherwise.

[49] The employer shall give the officer at least two months' notice of the date from which his or her annual leave is to be taken.

[50] Provided that an employee who has accrued additional annual leave referred to in subclauses (ii) and (iii) of this clause can elect at any time to be paid an amount equivalent to the value of the accrued additional annual leave in lieu of taking additional leave, provided that the amount is a minimum of one week's accrued additional leave and that the salary for the period of additional leave paid out will be calculated as if the period of leave as actually taken.

[51] If the officer and the employer so agree, the annual leave or any such separate periods, may be taken wholly or partly in advance before the officer has become entitled to that leave, but where leave is taken in such circumstances a further period of annual leave shall not commence to accrue until the expiration of the twelve months in respect of which the annual leave or part thereof has been so taken.

[52] (x) Where the annual leave under this clause or any part thereof has been taken in advance by an officer pursuant to subclause (v), of this clause; and

(a) the employment of the officer is terminated before he/she has completed the year of employment in respect of which such annual leave or part was taken; and

(b) the sum paid by the employer to the officer as ordinary pay for the annual leave or part so taken in advance exceeds the sum which the employer is required to pay to the officer under subclause (ix) of this clause;

(c) the employer shall not be liable to make any payment to the officer under the said subclause (ix) and shall be entitled to deduct the amount of such excess from any remuneration payable to the officer upon the termination of the employment.

[53] Allocated days off (ADOs) for eligible medical officers are an Award entitlement and rosters must make provision for them to be taken. Medical officers are to be directed to take all rostered ADOs. The medical officer's supervisor must ensure that the medical officer is able to take his or her ADO entitlement.

[54] Where at the end of a rotation to a District by a medical officer there are any untaken ADOs, those ADOs must either be provided to the medical officer or paid out – at ordinary time rates for the first three untaken ADOs and at appropriate overtime rates for any additional ADOs after the first three. ADOs may only be taken in whole days.

Where a medical officer starts a new rotation with a new District, the District from which the medical officer has rotated must either provide or pay out any accrued or untaken ADOs for that medical officer before the medical officer commences the new rotation. There is no transfer of untaken ADOs between Districts.

[55] ADOs must not be rostered on the same calendar day that a night shift finishes.

[56] Where an officer is required to, and does work on any of the public holidays set out in this clause, the officer shall be paid for the hours worked at the rate of time and one-half. In addition, the officer shall have one day added to annual leave for each public holiday so worked unless time off in respect of time worked on such public holiday has been granted.

[57] Where a public holiday falls on a rostered day off, the officer shall have one day added to annual leave.

[58] All officers shall be allowed four calendar weeks leave of absence on full pay in respect of each twelve months' service plus one day on full pay in respect of each public holiday occurring within the period of such leave.

[59] Where an officer is required to, and does work on any of the public holidays set out in this clause, the officer shall be paid for the hours worked at the rate of time and one-half. In addition, the officer shall have one day added to annual leave for each public holiday so worked unless time off in respect of time worked on such public holiday has been granted.

[60] Subject to the terms of this clause the employer may grant to officers other than interns, study leave without loss of pay as follows:

Face-to-face courses: Half hour study time for every hour of compulsory lecture and/or tutorial attendance, up to a maximum of four hours study time per week. Where no face-to-face course is provided: A maximum of four hours study time per week for a maximum of 27 weeks per year.

[61] The grant of study leave is subject to the convenience of the employer and should not interfere with the maintenance of essential services or with patient care.

[62] Study leave granted subject to the terms of this clause, may be accrued to a maximum of seven working days for the purpose of enabling the officer to study prior to a written, oral or clinical examination. An option to accumulate study leave in terms of this subclause shall be exercised at the commencement of each academic year and the officer shall notify the employer accordingly[.]

[63] Officers who have given continuous service of more than one year shall be allowed to accrue study leave not taken up to a maximum of fourteen calendar days.

[64] (ii) Study leave shall only be granted in respect of a course:

(a) leading to higher medical qualifications as defined in clause 1, Definitions, of this Award; and

(b) in respect of a qualification which when obtained would be relevant to the needs of the Hospital.

[65] The officer shall submit to the employer a timetable of the proposed course of study and evidence of the officer's enrolment in the course.

[66] Periods of study leave granted shall not be taken into account for the purposes of calculating overtime payments.

[67] '[R]elative' means a person related by blood, marriage or affinity;

'[A]ffinity' means a relationship that one spouse because of marriage has to blood relatives of the other; and

'[H]ousehold' means a family group living in the same domestic dwelling.

[68] (a) The maximum amount of FACS leave on full pay that may be granted to an employee is:

(1) 3 working days during the first year of service, commencing on and from 1 January 1995, and thereafter 6 working days in any period of 2 years; or

(2) 1 working day, on a cumulative basis effective from 1 January 1995, for each year of service after 2 years' continuous service, minus any period of FACS leave already taken by the employee since 1 January 1995,

whichever method provides the greater entitlement.

[69] For the purposes of calculating entitlements under (vi)(a)(1) and (2) above, a working day for employees working 38 hours per week shall be deemed to consist of 8 hours, and a working day for employees working 35 hours per week shall be deemed to consist of 7 hours. The rate at which FACS leave is paid out and utilised shall be on actual hours absent from a rostered shift.

[70] (v) Additional FACS leave for bereavement purposes:

Where FACS leave has been exhausted, additional FACS leave of up to 2 days for bereavement may be granted on a discrete, 'per occasion' basis to an employee on the death of a relative or member of a household as defined in subclause (i)(a) of Part A of this clause.

[71] Use of other leave entitlements:

The employer may grant an employee other leave entitlements for reasons related to family responsibilities or community service, by the employee.

An employee may elect, with the consent of the employer, to take annual leave; long service leave; or leave without pay.

[72] Use of sick leave to care for the person concerned – entitlement:

(a) The entitlement to use sick leave in accordance with this subclause is subject to:

(1) the employee being responsible for the care and support of the person concerned; and

(2) the person concerned being as defined in subclause (i) of Part B of this clause.

[73] Sick leave accumulates from year to year. In addition to the current year's grant of sick leave available under (b) above, sick leave untaken from the previous 3 years may also be accessed by an employee with responsibilities in relation to a person who needs their care and support.

[74] The employee shall, if required, establish either by production of a medical certificate or statutory declaration that the illness of the person concerned is such as to require care by another person.

[75] The employee has the right to choose the method by which the ground for leave is established, that is, by production of either a medical certificate or statutory declaration.

[76] The employer may, in special circumstances, make a grant of additional sick leave. This grant can only be taken from sick leave untaken prior to the period referred to in subclause (c) above.

[77] The employee is not required to state the exact nature of the relevant illness on either a medical certificate or statutory declaration.

[78] The employee shall, wherever practicable, give the employer notice prior to the absence of the intention to take leave, the name of the person requiring care and that person's relationship to the employee, the reasons for taking such leave and the estimated length of absence. If it's not practicable for the employee to give prior notice of absence, the employee shall notify the employer by telephone of such absence at the first opportunity on the day of absence.

[79] An employee may elect, with the consent of the employer, to take time off in lieu of payment of overtime at a time or times agreed with the employer within 12 months of the said election.

[80] [O]ne hour off for each hour of overtime worked.

[81] If, having elected to take time as leave in accordance with (iv)(a) above and the leave is not taken for whatever reason, payment for time accrued at overtime rates shall be made at the expiry of the twelve month period from the date the overtime was worked, or earlier by agreement, or on termination.

[82] Where no election is made in accordance with paragraph (iv)(a) above, the employee shall be paid overtime rates in accordance with the provisions of clause 11, Overtime.

[83] (v) Use of make-up time:

(a) An employee may elect, with the consent of the employer, to work 'make-up time'. 'Make-up time' is worked when the employee takes time off during ordinary hours for family or community service responsibilities, and works those hours at another time, during the spread of ordinary hours provided for in clause 6 of this Award, at the ordinary rate of pay.

(b) An employee on shift work may elect, with the consent of the employer, to work 'make-up time' (under which the employee takes time off during ordinary hours and works those hours at another time) at the applicable shift work rate which would have been applicable to the hours taken off.

[84] Leave without pay can only be entered into a roster where a medical officer has formally applied for leave without pay, and this application has been approved.

[85] For the purposes of calculation of payment of on-call allowances and for call-back duty, an on-call period shall not exceed 24 hours.

[86] An officer shall be paid for each on-call period which coincides with a day rostered on duty an allowance as set out in Item 3 of Table 1, Allowances, and for each on-call period coinciding with a rostered day off an allowance as set in the said Item 3 with a maximum payment as set out in the said Item 3 per week.

[87] Subject to subclauses (v)–(ix) below, officers who are recalled for duty, whether notified before or after leaving the employer's premises, shall be paid for all time worked at the appropriate overtime rate, with a minimum of four hours at such rates.

[88] Officers may be required to perform other work that arises during the recall period. Officers shall not be required to work the full four hour minimum payment period if they complete the work they were recalled to perform and any additional work they're required to undertake, within a shorter period.

[89] Officers who are advised they won't be required to perform any additional work and are formally released and who are subsequently recalled again during the four hour minimum payment period, shall be entitled to another four hour minimum payment.

[90] Officers who are not formally released and who are recalled again during the four hour minimum payment period are not entitled to any additional payment until the expiration of the four hour period.

[91] A clinical appraisal provided remotely pursuant to subclause (xi)(a) above shall attract a minimum payment of one hour at the appropriate overtime rate only in circumstances where, if it had not been provided remotely, the on-call resident medical officer or registrar would have otherwise needed to have returned to the workplace. Any additional requirement to provide further clinical appraisal falling within the hour from which the initial clinical appraisal commenced shall not attract an additional payment. Any time worked beyond the expiration of one hour shall be paid at overtime rates. Time where work is not being performed won't be counted as time for the purposes of overtime payment.

[92] An employee who is called upon to relieve an employee in a higher classification continuously for five working days or more and who satisfactorily performs the whole of the duties and assumes the whole of the responsibilities of the higher classification, shall be entitled to receive, for the period of relief, the minimum pay of such higher classification.

CHAPTER 11

To conclude

The reason we listen so little is people talk too much.

So this completes our little guide or rant or whatever else it might've been for you. We hope it has been helpful, informative and eased the transition into your working life from a Student to a real Doctor. And if you're working already, we hope it has made working in Medicine a little clearer.

Now, just go ahead and be the Doctor you really want to be.

We all know why we entered. But the real world isn't like that. Can we not have both? Most say no. Some try to strain into both and are often broken as a result. But with a little thought, a little care, a little help and a little luck, you may run over the hard ruts of Medicine and life, and yet be cushioned in your vision within.

Index